L SCIENCE, MATERIALS AND TECHNOLOGY

RENDS IN PERIODONTICS
IPLANT DENTISTRY

DENTAL SCIENCE, MATERIALS AND TECHNOLOGY

Additional books in this series can be found on Nova's website under the Series tab.

Additional e-books in this series can be found on Nova's website under the e-book tab.

DENTAL SCIENCE, MATERIALS AND TECHNOLOGY

CURRENT TRENDS IN PERIODONTICS AND IMPLANT DENTISTRY

VISHAL ANAND
AND
MINKLE GULATI
EDITORS

NOVA BIOMEDICAL

New York

For permission to use material from this book please contact us:
Telephone 631-231-7269; Fax 631-231-8175
Web Site: http://www.novapublishers.com

Library of Congress Cataloging-in-Publication Data

ISBN: 978-1-62618-819-8

Library of Congress Control Number: 2013938556

Published by Nova Science Publishers, Inc. † New York

Contents

Preface

Periodontal diseases are multifactorial infectious diseases wherein the presence of periodontopathogenic species seems to play a key role in the etiopathogenesis and results in a progressive loss of the hard and soft tissue around the teeth, and if left untreated, ultimately leads to the loosening and subsequent loss of teeth. Similarly diseases affecting peri-implant tissues, if not managed and treated properly results in an implant failure. However, the nature and severity of the periodontal and peri-implant diseases depend on the patient's oral hygiene, interaction between the bacterial agent, the environment and the host defense mechanisms, and the presence of various risk elements for periodontal/peri-implant diseases like genetic factors, diabetes, smoking etc. Periodontal diseases itself can also act as a potential risk factor for several systemic conditions and may significantly enhance the probability for certain systemic diseases or alter their natural course. Fortunately, periodontal and peri-implant diseases are largely preventable and treatable conditions; and their successful long-term management and treatment requires a treatment strategy that integrates non-surgical, surgical and supportive periodontal/peri-implant therapy along with patient motivation and reinforcement of excellent oral hygiene measures.

Impressive research advances in the epidemiology of periodontal/peri-implant diseases; their specific bacterial etiology and the immunoinflammatory mediators involved in periodontal/peri-implant tissue destruction have greatly altered the way clinicians detect and classify periodontal/peri-implant diseases. This has also led to the development of potential novel therapeutics to prevent, slow or arrest periodontal/peri-implant disease progression. Hence, in this volume the current trends in periodontics and implant dentistry have been explored; reviewing the literature that highlights recent trends in classification of periodontal diseases, periodontal-systemic interrelationship, periodontal diseases in children and adolescents, major breakthroughs in the understanding of essential mechanisms that mediate and resolve periodontal/peri-implant tissue destruction, peri-implant complications and their management, host modulation, as well as advances in nonsurgical and surgical treatment strategies. The volume also includes original researches exploring the role of human cariogenic bacteria, oral spirochetes and herpes virus in the pathogenesis of periodontal diseases, as well as the effect of bisphosphonate adjunctive therapy in postmenopausal women with chronic periodontitis and osteoporosis. Thus, this book all in all offers up-to-date information on the current state of periodontology and implantology.

Chapter I - Periodontal disease is not a single disease entity but a set of inflammatory diseases affecting the periodontium, i.e. the tissues that surround and support the teeth. It can present in different forms and typically progresses from simple inflammatory condition of gingiva to severe destruction of periodontium. Hence, several classification systems have been developed over the years to reflect the variety of forms of gingivitis and periodontitis. The development of various periodontal classification systems has largely been influenced by the paradigms that reflected the understanding of periodontal diseases at that given historical period. Though such systems have provided clinicians a way to organize the health care needs of their patients, yet because of the multifactorial nature of the periodontal diseases, any endeavor to categorize this vast group of diseases in an orderly and extensively accepted manner is often fraught with difficulty and considerable controversy. Inconsistencies and inaccuracies in the classification system that is current at that time are revealed as the knowledge of periodontal disease grows and subsequently leads to the modification or evolution of a new classification system. This chapter presents a comprehensive review of the various forms of periodontal diseases and their classification systems that have evolved over time, the drawbacks and rationale for the emergence of new classification systems and scope for the future revisions needed in the current classification system.

Chapter II - The modern hypothesis of periodontitis pathogenesis suggests that periodontitis is a complex disease, which means it is likely associated with the effects of multiple genes in combination with lifestyles and environment factors, i.e. it is a multifactorial disorder. Other human complex diseases include autoimmune diseases, diabetes, heart diseases, hypertension, mood disorder such as depression, obesity and so on. Interestingly many of these systemic complex diseases are associated with periodontal disease such as diabetes, heart diseases, autoimmune diseases and mood disorder. The reason could be these diseases share some common pathogenic pathway or common risk factors. In addition, it is well-known that many other systemic diseases or conditions can affect periodontitis onset, severity of the symptoms, progression and treatment responses. This chapter will mainly focus on the effects of systemic complex diseases and other systemic diseases and conditions on periodontal disease. The discussion will be about periodontal manifestations of different systemic diseases, the effects of systemic conditions on periodontitis diagnosis, treatment and prognosis. Hopefully it can help medical and dental clinicians to understand more about periodontitis and other systemic diseases, and provide a general guidance for them when facing a periodontitis patient with systemic diseases or systemic disease patients seeking periodontal therapy.

Chapter III - Substantial evidence indicates that susceptibility to periodontal disease varies among patients and is modulated by both acquired and intrinsic risk factors. Genetic, systemic, medication induced, behavioral, and tooth-related local factors have been reported in various scientific investigations to be related to periodontitis. The central intent of this chapter is to discuss the genetic and behavioral risk factors associated with periodontitis. Polymorphism of genes that affect the expression of the inflammatory mediators might be associated with severity of periodontal diseases. It appears that there is at least a weak association between polymorphisms in the interleukin-1 genes and chronic periodontitis. As is the case for the association of smoking and periodontitis, cross-sectional and longitudinal studies provide strong epidemiologic evidence of a positive association between the two (2-8-fold increased risk for periodontal attachment loss and/or bone loss). Certain micronutrients such as antioxidants might be beneficial in periodontitis by downregulating proinflammatory cascades. Antioxidants such as vitamin C, E, GSH, folic acid, catechin (green tea), and melatonin have been associated with periodontal health. Stress might be associated with more severe periodontal disease and a poorer healing response to periodontal therapy. Furthermore, low levels of physical activity might be associated with an elevated prevalence of periodontitis. However, up till now no evidence documents that improved physical activity could influence the periodontal condition.

Chapter IV - Gingiva forms an important part of oral mucosa as well as periodontium. The prevalence of gingivitis in children is as high as 99% but periodontal diseases are not common. The control of gingivitis in young children by its early detection, treatment and prevention may be a realistic approach to the reduction of the prevalence and severity of periodontal disease in adulthood. Components of periodontium are same in childhood, adolescence and adulthood. Clinical and radiographic images differ owing to the significant changes that take place during growth and development. "The periodontium during childhood and adolescence is in a constant state eruption of teeth. This makes a general description of the normal periodontium difficult because it varies with the age of the patient". The chapter would cover detailed description about periodontium stating the differences in adulthood and childhood and also various gingival and periodontal diseases in children.

Chapter V - There is accumulating evidence that periodontal infections could influence overall health and the course of some systemic diseases. Periodontal disease is characterized by inflammation and bacterial infection of the gums surrounding the teeth. The bacteria that are associated with periodontal disease can travel into the bloodstream and consequently to other parts of the body, and that puts health at risk. People think of gum disease in terms of their teeth, but they don't think about the fact that gum disease is a serious infection that can release bacteria into the bloodstream resulting in additional health risks in people whose health is already affected by other diseases or leading to serious complications like heart disease. Periodontal medicine is a term used for different purposes in different parts of the world. In certain countries, it relates to the study of the dynamic relationship between periodontitis and systemic conditions, such as cardiovascular and cerebrovascular disease, pre-term labour and low-birth-weight babies, diabetes mellitus, osteoporosis and disorders of respiratory tract. Such studies investigate the peripheral impacts of periodontal inflammation on systemic health and also the influence of systemic diseases on the progression of chronic periodontitis such as type II diabetes mellitus, where evidence exists for a bi-directional relationship with periodontitis. In the other countries, "periodontal medicine" is a term used to describe the periodontal (and gingival) manifestations of medical conditions. This includes their investigation, diagnosis and therapeutic management and how management of the oral conditions integrates with the patient's medical management as a part of a holistic approach within defined care pathways. The text is a comprehensive analysis of research on periodontitis and its link to systemic conditions. It supports what many scientists have suspected for years-oral infections such as periodontal disease can adversely affect conditions outside the mouth. The basis of periodontal medicine is treating periodontitis to preserve the structure, function and esthetics of the dentition, which will further prevent any untoward affects on a patient's over all health. Periodontology brought awareness and education to the public of the fact that infections in the mouth can cause health problems in other parts of the body as well. Periodontal diseases have been linked to diabetes, heart disease, osteoporosis, preterm births, stroke, respiratory disease and renal disease. Periodontal medicine is the emergence of a new branch of periodontology. The goal of the campaign will be to educate patients about periodontal infection and its associated general health risks. Oral health is often a good indicator of what is happening in the rest of the body. Therefore, a visit to a periodontics may benefit more than an older person's gums. It is important for patients to have regular oral check-ups to not only maintain oral health, but to identify possible risks for serious medical conditions.

Chapter VI - Though bacteria are the primary etiologic factor of periodontal diseases, yet the extent and severity of tissue destruction seen in periodontal diseases is determined by the host immuno-inflammatory response to these bacteria. This increasing awareness and knowledge of the host-microbial interaction in periodontal pathogenesis has presented the opportunity for exploiting new therapeutic strategies for periodontitis by means of targeting host response via host modulating agents. Host modulation means supplementing the natural inherent defense mechanisms of the host by modifying or modulating destructive or damaging aspects of the inflammatory host response that develops in the periodontal tissues as a result of the chronic challenge presented by the subgingival bacterial. This chapter discusses the host-modulating role of various systemically delivered (Tetracycline analogues, NSAIDs, lipoxins, resolvins, protectins, maresin, anti-cytokines, bisphosphonates, probiotics, periodontal vaccine and certain nutrients) and locally delivered agents (Enamel matrix proteins, bone morphogenetic protein, platelet derived growth factor, hypochlorous acid and taurine-N-monochloramine and cimetidine). These host-modulating agents are potentially non-invasive, have fewer side effects, do not require complicated application method and tip the balance between periodontal health and disease progression in the direction of a healing response, when combined with conventional treatments aimed at reducing the bacterial burden.

Chapter VII - The benefits of periodontal maintenance therapy (PMT) in maintaining the homeostasis of periodontal tissues obtained after active periodontal therapy, which includes surgical and non-surgical procedures, has been extensively documented in numerous studies. A classic problem in PMT programs is difficulty in maintaining the patient's cooperation and in scheduling regular maintenance visits. However, without establishing a regular program of clinical re-evaluation, adequate biofilm control, and reinforcement of oral hygiene instructions, the benefits of PMT cannot be maintained. Several indicators or risk factors and biological, behavioral, and social conditions can influence the periodontal status of individuals undergoing PMT. Moreover, neglecting a regular PMT program has been associated with a higher risk of recurrence and with the progression of periodontitis. In this chapter, smoking, diabetes, and poor oral hygiene were strongly associated with recurrence, progression of periodontitis and tooth loss in individuals under PMT. The efficiency of surgical and non-surgical periodontal procedures in the context of periodontal therapy has been widely reported. Review studies on surgical or nonsurgical periodontal therapy have concluded that: (a) the comparison of the efficacy of surgical and nonsurgical procedures revealed that scaling and root planing alone or in combination with flap procedures are effective methods for the treatment of chronic periodontitis; (b) the consistent message is that in treating deep pockets, open-flap debridement results in greater probing pocket depth reduction and clinical attachment gain than nonsurgical modalities; (c) Nonsurgical modalities in shallower pockets consistently involve less post-therapy recession and are clearly recognized as being more conservative. Additionally, recurrence of periodontitis and tooth loss has been reported in studies in the absence of periodontal treatment, as well as in many PMT retrospective and prospective studies. However, these results have been very controversial, primarily related to the type of surgical or non-surgical procedures performed during PMT. In this sense, several issues related to the recurrence, progression of periodontitis and tooth loss during periodontal maintenance therapy require clarification. The aim of this chapter is to review the periodontal literature and summarize the main findings of different study designs, in attempt to a greater understanding of the influence of risk factors associated with surgical or non-surgical procedures performed during periodontal maintenance therapy on the occurrence of these adverse outcomes.

Chapter VIII - Chronic periodontitis is an infection disease caused by an opportunistic microflora. The infection triggers host inflammatory responses resulting in the destruction of the tooth supporting tissues. Periodontal maintenance measures implicate the elimination of plaque and calculus, and an assessment geared toward categorizing aspects that may impede with oral health. Scientific exploration has established that with meticulous day-to-day plaque removal and periodontal maintenance procedures, the reappearance and progression of periodontal disease can be minimized.

Chapter IX - With the introduction of endosseous dental implants for rehabilitating partial and completely edentulous patients, dental treatment has been revolutionized. The high survival rates of osseointegrated dental implants have validated these implant supported restorations as a predictable method for oral rehabilitation. It is becoming increasingly clear that successfully integrated implants are susceptible to disease conditions and complications that may eventually lead to the loss of the implant. Therefore, careful treatment planning based on accurate preoperative anatomic assessments and an understanding of all potential implant related complications is very important for the successful placement and functioning of an implant. It is also necessary to know the various types of biological, technical, surgical and esthetic failures and the management of these failures.

Chapter X - *Streptococcus mutans* and *S. sobrinus* have been implicated as the most important etiologic agents of human dental caries. The mechanism of caries induction by these bacteria has been well characterized; however, little is known about the relationship between periodontal inflammation and these bacteria, although it has been shown that bacterial lipoproteins trigger an innate immune response mediated via the Toll-like receptor 2 (TLR2) displayed on the host cell. In this chapter,the induction of inflammation triggered by *S. mutans* and *S. sobrinus* is characteraized. Lipoproteins were extracted from cells of *S. mutans* 109c and *S. sobrinus* NIDR6715 by treatment with Triton X-114. Interleukin 8 (IL-8) production by THP-1 cells stimulated with either bacterial cells or extracted lipoproteins was measured by ELISA (Enzyme-linked immunosorbent assay). Nuclear factor-kappa B (NF-κB) activation in Human embryonic kidney (HEK) 293 cells transiently producing TLR2 was determined by relative luciferase reporter assay. Results of these experiments revealed that cells of both streptococcal species induced IL-8 production and NF-κB activation via TLR2. Lipoproteins extracted from *S. mutans* and *S. sobrinus* also induced IL-8 production and NF-κB activation via TLR2. This TLR2-mediated activation was abolished by pre-treatment of the lipoprotein fraction with a lipoprotein lipase. These results strongly suggest that lipoproteins of human cariogenic bacteria *S. mutans* and *S. sobrinus* induce inflammatory responses through TLR2.

Chapter XI - Periodontal disease, as typified by periodontitis, has a varied and highly complex polymicrobial etiology. Oral spirochete bacteria, all of whose members belong to the genus *Treponema*, constitute one bacterial group that has been consistently associated with the occurrence and severity of periodontal infections. However, disease associations may be complex, as diverse communities of oral spirochete bacteria have been shown to be present within the human oral cavity. This chapter primarily discusses the positive association of oral spirochetes with periodontal diseases; their diversity within periodontal environments; as well as putative virulence factors that may play important roles contributing to the initiation and progression of periodontal diseases.

Chapter XII - The human chronic periodontitis is a disease that leads to tooth loss in the patients and naturally implicates in a decrease of self esteem and many other healthy problems related to this disease. Some species of bacteria are implicated in the pathogenesis of the periodontitis, however, the presence of these bacteria does not merely explain the inflammatory processes completely. Some authors have suggested that association between bacteria and viruses, especially herpes viruses, could play a role in the pathogenesis of periodontitis affecting the immune response against microbes. In this chapter the association between herpes virus, specifically cytomegalovirus, and human chronic periodontitis has been investigated. Twenty chronic periodontitis affected patients and 12 healthy subjects were biopsied during surgical treatment and tissue fragment analyzed by polymerase chain reaction and imunohistochemistry to detect cytomegalovirus DNA and antigen, respectively. None of the samples collected from healthy subjects presented positive results to cytomegalovirus either by polymerase chain reaction or immunohistochemistry. Yet, samples from 30% of the periodontitis affected patients were positive to cytomegalovirus DNA, though none of them showed a positive result for cytomegalovirus antigen. The results suggested that cytomegalovirus could play a role in the pathogenesis of periodontitis; however, patients probably presented latent infection instead of active infection. Due to this contrast, additional studies are necessary for better investigation of the association between herpersviruses and chronic periodontitis.

Chapter XIII - The objective of this chapter was to present the effect of mechanical periodontal treatment on clinical, microbiological and radiological parameters in chronic periodontitis patients with postmenopausal osteoporosis using oral alendronate. A total of 20 female patients were included. All of the patients were diagnosed as postmenopausal osteoporosis with a T score ≤ -2.5 and defined to be in need of alendronate treatment by their gynecologists. The test group (n=10) consisted of patients who confirmed to undergo oral alendronate treatment whereas the control group (n=10) was made up with patients refusing any type of medication. Both of the groups received mechanical periodontal therapy. At baseline and 6 months after periodontal treatment, periodontal condition was assessed, subgingival microbial samples were evaluated by culturing, bone mineral density (BMD) of lumbar spine, femur and mandible was analysed by dual energy xray absorptiometry and mandibular cortical width (MCW) was measured by dental panoramic radiographs. Clinical evaluation revealed statistically significant periodontal improvements within both groups ($p<0.01$). Intergroup comparisons revealed a statistically significant difference for sulcus bleeding index only ($p<0.05$). The proportion of obligate anaerobes decreased significantly in both groups ($p<0.05$), however, no significant difference was found between the groups. While BMDs were decreased in the control group, significant increases were observed in the test group ($p<0.01$). Similarly, the MCW increased in the test group but decreased in the control group. Furthermore, a significant positive relationship was detected between the mandibular BMD and MCW ($p<0.05$). The results presented in this chapter suggest that oral alendronate therapy may have an adjunctive effect to mechanical periodontal treatment in terms of resolution of gingival inflammation in postmenopausal women with chronic periodontitis and osteoporosis. In addition, no side effect of orally administered alendronate was observed during this period.

In: Current Trends in Periodontics and Implant Dentistry
Editors: Vishal Anand and Minkle Gulati
ISBN: 978-1-62618-819-8

Chapter I

Periodontal Diseases and Their Classification

Vishal Anand[1,*] and Minkle Gulati[2]
[1]Department of Periodontics, Faculty of Dental Sciences,
KGMU, Uttar Pradesh, India
[2]Department of Periodontics, BBDCODS,
Uttar Pradesh, India

Abstract

Periodontal disease is not a single disease entity but a set of inflammatory diseases affecting the periodontium, i.e. the tissues that surround and support the teeth. It can present in different forms and typically progresses from simple inflammatory condition of gingiva to severe destruction of periodontium. Hence, several classification systems have been developed over the years to reflect the variety of forms of gingivitis and periodontitis. The development of various periodontal classification systems has largely been influenced by the paradigms that reflected the understanding of periodontal diseases at that given historical period. Though such systems have provided clinicians a way to organize the health care needs of their patients, yet because of the multifactorial nature of the periodontal diseases, any endeavor to categorize this vast group of diseases in an orderly and extensively accepted manner is often fraught with difficulty and considerable controversy. Inconsistencies and inaccuracies in the classification system that is current at that time are revealed as the knowledge of periodontal disease grows and subsequently leads to the modification or evolution of a new classification system. This chapter presents a comprehensive review of the various forms of periodontal diseases and their classification systems that have evolved over time, the drawbacks and rationale for the emergence of new classification systems and scope for the future revisions needed in the current classification system.

---

[*] Correspondence: 1/288, Viram Khand, Gomti Nagar, Lucknow, Uttar Pradesh, India, Zip Code: 226010, Contact No: +91-9621280850, Email: drvishalanand@yahoo.co.in.

Introduction

Our understanding of the etiology and pathogenesis of periodontal diseases is continually changing with increasing scientific knowledge. [1] Any attempt to group the entire constellation of periodontal diseases into an orderly and widely accepted classification system is fraught with difficulty and considerable controversy. [2]

- *Classification* is defined as the act or method of distribution into groups
- *Diagnosis* is defined as the act of identifying a disease from its signs and symptoms

The Need for a Periodontal Classification System

Direct research aimed at learning more about the diseases concerned: [3]

- Help determine the evidence base for better-targeted therapy.
- Guide practitioners towards the best method for treating a disease.
- Enable the international community to communicate in a common language.
- Guide public health planning and targeting of therapy.
- Help practitioners plan treatment protocols to maximize benefit to all their patients.
- The ideal way to classify any disease is to use the name of the etiological agent.
- Periodontal diseases are poly-microbial and poly-immuno-inflammatory in nature.

A Historical Perspective of Periodontal Classification

The first classification system for periodontal disease was recorded in 1806 when Joseph Fox attempted to classify "gum-disease". In 1823, Alphonse Toirac, called it "Pyorrhea Alveolaris". [4] The development and evolution of the periodontal classification system was largely influenced by paradigms that reflect the understanding of periodontal diseases at the given historical period. [3, 5, 6]

1. The Clinical characteristics paradigm (1870-1920)
2. Classical pathology paradigm (1920-1970)
3. Infection / Host response paradigm (1970-the present)

Classification systems should be viewed as dynamic works-in progresses that need to be periodically modified based on current thinking and new knowledge.

1. Clinical Characteristics Paradigm (1870-1920)

Very little was known about the etiology and pathogenesis of periodontal diseases during this period and most of the diseases were classified almost entirely based on their clinical characteristics and also on unsubstantiated theories about their cause.

Many authors considered these diseases to be caused by local factors. [7] Some believed that systemic disturbances played a dominant etiological role. [8, 9, 10, 11] John M. Riggs called periodontitis as Riggs disease.

- First: Margins of the gums showed inflammatory action and bleeding at slightest touch of the brush.
- Second: Inflammation extends over the thinner alveolar border causing absorption of bone and gum tissue, forming small pockets filled with pus.
- Third: Thicker portions of the process are involved absorbing it most rapidly.
- Fourth: The disease has swept away all of the alveoli and much of the gum.

A classic example was the paper published by C.G. Davis (1879) who believed that there were 3 distinct forms of destructive periodontal disease. [12]

1. Gingival recession with minimal or no inflammation
2. Periodontal destruction secondary to "Lime deposits"
3. "Riggs disease" the hallmark of which was 'loss of alveolus without the loss of gum'

Similarly G.V. Black (1886) classified periodontal disease into 5 categories [13]

1. Constitutional gingivitis
2. A painful form of gingivitis
3. Simple gingivitis
4. Calcic inflammation of the peridental membrane
5. Phagedenic pericementitis (phagedenic - spreading ulcer or necrosis). In a later publication, the term 'phagedenic pericementitis' replaced with 'chronic suppurative pericementitis (1915). [14]

By 1929 Becks H. estimated that there were over 350 theories of pyorrhea and much more confusing terminologies such as [15]

- Pyorrhea alveolaris
- Calcic inflammation of the peridental membrane
- Phagedenic pericementitis
- Chronic suppurative periodontitis

2. Classical Pathology Paradigm (1920-1970)

According to this concept there were at least two forms of destructive periodontal disease-inflammatory and non-inflammatory (degenerative or dystrophic). Gottlieb in particular postulated that certain forms of destructive periodontal disease were due to degenerative changes in the periodontium. [16, 17, 18] In 1923 he described the disease and called it "the diffuse atrophy of the alveolar bone".

Gottlieb classified periodontal disease into four types:

1. Schmutz - pyorrhoe
2. Alveolar atrophy or diffuse atrophy
3. Paradental - pyorrhea
4. Occlusal trauma

McCall and Box (1925) introduced the term 'Periodontitis' to those inflammatory diseases in which all components of periodontium are involved. [19] Wannenmacher (1938) given the term Paradontosis marginalis progressive. [20] In 1940, Thoma and Goldman called the disease as Paradontosis. [21] Orban and Weinmann (1942) coined the term Periodontosis. [22, 23]

Classification systems were dominated by the Orbans principles during this time.

1. Periodontal disease follows the same pattern as do diseases of other organs.
2. The basic pathologic tissue changes however are the same as those of other organs.
3. Environmental factors however dictate the inclusion of a third and different category of pathologic reaction in periodontology i.e., 'pathologic reactions' produced by occlusal trauma.

Orban's Classification (1942)

This was the first classification scheme to be accepted by AAP. He grouped them according to the "Pathologic" categories of inflammation.

- Inflammation
  Gingivitis: Local / Systemic
  Periodontitis: Simplex / Complex
- Degeneration
  Periodontosis: Systemic disturbances / Hereditary / Idiopathic
- Atrophy
  Periodontal atrophy: Local trauma / Senile / Disuse / Idiopathic
- Hypertrophy
  Gingival hypertrophy: Chronic irritation / Drug action / Idiopathic
- Traumatism

In 1966 world workshop questions were raised about the existence of 'Periodontosis' as a distinct disease entity. [24] The term 'Juvenile Periodontitis' was introduced by Chaput and colleagues in 1967 and by Butler (1969).

In 1971 Baer defined it as "a disease of the periodontium occurring in an otherwise healthy adolescent who is characterized by a rapid loss of alveolar bone about more than one tooth of the permanent dentition. The amount of destruction manifested is not commensurate with the amounts of local irritants."

3. Infection/Host Response Paradigm (1970 to Present)

W.D. Miller (1890), in particular, was an early proponent of the infectious nature of periodontal diseases. [25] His work had very little impact on convincing his contemporaries that periodontal diseases were infections. He was however, an early advocate of the 'Infection/Host Response Paradigm'. The classical 'experimental gingivitis' studies published by Harald Loe and his colleagues from 1965 to 1968 that the Infection/Host Response Paradigm began to move in the direction of becoming the dominant paradigm. [26, 27, 28, 29]

The next major discovery in periodontal microbiology was the preliminary demonstration in 1976 - 1977 of microbial specificity at sites with periodontosis. [30, 31] This finding, coupled with the demonstration in 1977 - 1979 that neutrophils from patients with juvenile periodontitis (periodontosis) had defective chemotactic and phagocytic activities, marked the beginning of the dominance of the Infection/Host Response paradigm. [32, 33]

In 1977, convincing arguments were provided that there was no scientific basis for retaining the concept that there were non-inflammatory or degenerative forms of periodontal disease. [34] It was concluded that 'Periodontosis' was an infection and 'Juvenile Periodontitis' should become the preferred term.

The 1977 World Workshop Classification

1. Juvenile periodontitis
2. Chronic Marginal Periodontitis

Page and Schroeder (1982) suggested four different forms of periodontitis. [35]

1. Prepubertal periodontitis: Localized / Generalized
2. Juvenile Periodontitis
3. Rapidly progressive periodontitis
4. Adult periodontitis

Prepubertal Periodontitis

Patients under 11 years of age, Sex ratio approximately equal, localized or generalized lesions, minimal tooth associated material, Caries rate low, depressed neutrophil chemotaxis AMLR has not known Genetic implications and possible medical implications.

Juvenile Periodontitis

Patients between 12 - 26 years of age, females affected more than males, first molar and incisor involvement, lack of clinical inflammation with presence of deep pockets, minimal tooth associated material, depressed neutrophil chemotaxis, AMLR slightly increased, genetic implications, and possible medical implications.

Rapidly Progressive Periodontitis

Age of onset is between puberty and 35 years, lesions are generalized, affecting most of the teeth, without any consistent pattern of distribution, some but not all patients may have had juvenile periodontitis. Severe and rapid bone destruction, after which the destruction process may cease spontaneously or greatly slow. During active phase acutely inflamed gingiva and arrested phase the tissues appear free of inflammation. Microbial deposits highly variable, functional defects in neutrophils or monocytes, systemic manifestations, weight loss, mental depression and general malaise.

Adult Periodontitis

Patients over 35 years of age, approximately equal sex distribution, variable lesions, plaque and calculus present, host-response apparently normal, genetic implications unknown.

In 1986, AAP Adopted the Following Classification [5]

I. Juvenile periodontitis
   - a Prepubertal periodontitis
   - b Localized juvenile periodontitis
   - c Generalized juvenile periodontitis

II. Adult periodontitis

III. Necrotizing ulcerative gingivo-periodontitis

IV. Refractory periodontitis.

Grant, Stern and Listgarten Classification (1968) [36]

- Bacterially induced diseases
  1. Gingivitis
  2. Periodontitis: Adult type / Post-juvenile / Early onset periodontitis
  3. ANUG
  4. Acute abscess
  5. Pericoronitis

6. Functionally induced diseases: Traumatic occlusion / Disuse atrophy
7. Trauma: Habits

Suzuki Classification (1988) [37]

1. Adult periodontitis
2. Rapidly progressive periodontitis: Type A / Type B
3. Juvenile periodontitis
4. Post juvenile periodontitis
5. Prepubertal periodontitis

Rapidly Progressive Periodontitis: Type A

Patients usually between 14 and 26 years of age, females affected more than males (2:1 to 3:1), generalized lesions, minimal tooth associated materials, caries rate variable, depressed neutrophil chemotaxis, depressed AMLR, genetic implications, possible medical considerations.

Rapidly Progressive Periodontitis: Type B

Patients generally over 26 years of age, sex distribution not established, generalized lesions, plaque and calculus present, caries rate variable, neutrophil chemotaxis normal or depressed, AMLR within normal limits, genetic implications not known, possible medical considerations

Post Juvenile Periodontitis

Patients generally between 26 and35 years of age, females affected more than males (3:1), first molar and incisor lesions, plaque and calculus present, caries rate variable, neutrophil function not determined, AMLR slightly increased, genetic implications not known, possible medical considerations.

Classification of Periodontitis Recommended by the 1989 Workshop in Clinical Periodontics

I. Adult periodontitis
II. Early-onset periodontitis
    a. Prepubertal periodontitis
        1. Generalized
        2. Localized
    b. Juvenile periodontitis
        1. Generalized
        2. Localized
    c. Rapidly progressive periodontitis
III. Periodontitis associated with systemic disease
IV. Necrotizing ulcerative periodontitis

V. Refractory periodontitis

This classification, although soundly based in the Infection/Host response Paradigm, depended heavily on the age of the patients and the rates of progression.

Problems with the 1989 Classification

The uncertainty about the proposed "Rapidly progressive Periodontitis" as a single entity and secondly the questionable criteria used to determine its presence they were:

1. That the clinician had to actually document that rapid progression had occurred prior to giving the patient the diagnosis.
2. The term rapid was not defined in terms of progression and time period.
3. The disease had to be assumed from a single examination in an adolescent or young adult with massive attachment loss.
4. The concept that the rate of progression might be a useful criterion may itself be flawed.

Shortcomings of the 1989 Classification

1. Lack of a category for gingival diseases.
2. Overlap between the disease categories.
3. Difficulty in fitting the patients into any one of the existing categories.
4. Similarity of microbiological and host response features in different categories.
5. An emphasis on age of onset that became a problem as patients aged into a new category.
6. Unclear classification criteria.

As a consequence the 1989 classification was criticized and a new system of classification was proposed by Ranney in 1993. He eliminated the Refractory periodontitis category since it was a heterogeneous group and it was impossible to standardize treatment. He also recommended the elimination of the "Periodontitis associated with systemic disorders category since the expression of all forms of periodontitis is affected by systemic diseases.

I. Gingivitis
   A. Plaque bacterial, not systemically aggravated
   B. Plaque bacterial, systemically aggravated
      1. Sex hormone related
      2. Drug related
      3. Systemic disease related
   C. Not plaque bacterial
      1. Dermatologic disease associated
      2. Allergic
      3. Infective

- D. Necrotizing ulcerative
  - 1. Systemic determinants unknown
  - 2. HIV related
- II. Periodontitis
  - D. *Adult Periodontitis*
    - Not systemically aggravated
    - Systemically aggravated
      1. Diabetes mellitus
      2. Neutropenias
      3. Leukemias
      4. Acquired immunodeficiency syndrome
      5. Crohn's Disease
      6. Addison's Disease
      7. Lazy leukocyte syndrome
  - E. *Early Onset Periodontitis*
    - 1. Localized (Juvenile)
      - a. Neutrophil functional abnormality
      - b. Systemic deficiency uncertain
    - 2. Generalized (Rapidly Progressive)
      - a. Neutrophil functional abnormality
      - b. Immunodeficient
      - c. Systemic deficiency uncertain
    - 3. Systemic disease related
  - F. *Necrotizing ulcerative*
    - 1. Systemic determinants unknown
    - 2. HIV-related
    - 3. Nutritionally related
  - G. *Periodontal Abscess*

The Consensus Reached By the First European Workshop on Periodontology in 1993 was that Existing Disease Classifications were Unsatisfactory Due to: [6]

- ✓ Extensive overlap
- ✓ The necessity to assume what the previous disease progression had been (progressive periodontitis)
- ✓ The lack of detailed information on the quality of treatment previously provided and the patient's compliance and tissue response (refractory)
- ✓ The lack of a consistent basis for classification

The European Workshop in Periodontics (1993)

The recommendation was that classification should be based on causative factors and host response factors, and a simple classification was proposed that omits the forms ''periodontitis associated with systemic disease'' and ''refractory periodontitis''.

1. Early-onset periodontitis
2. Adult periodontitis
3. Necrotizing ulcerative periodontitis

Problems, inconsistencies and deficiencies associated with the 1989 classification led to many clinicians and investigators to call for a revision in the classification system. What emerged was a classification that was more firmly based on the Infection /host response paradigm. In reality, the changes were a "course correction" or "fine tuning" of the 1989 classification.

Changes in the Periodontal Classification System

1. Addition of a gingival disease component.
2. Replacement of "Adult Periodontitis'' with "Chronic Periodontitis".
3. Elimination of "Refractory Periodontitis" as a separate entity.
4. Replacement of "Early-onset periodontitis" with "Aggressive periodontitis".
5. Sub classification of "Periodontitis as a manifestation of systemic diseases.
6. Replacement of "Acute Necrotizing Ulcerative Gingivitis" and "Acute Necrotizing Ulcerative Periodontitis" with "Necrotizing periodontal diseases".
7. Addition of a category for "Periodontal abscesses and "Periodontic and Endodontic Lesion".
8. Addition of a new category for "Acquired deformities and conditions".

Addition of a Gingival Diseases Category

Gingivitis represents a spectrum of diseases whose onset is commonly attributed to the presence of bacteria. Gingival diseases were classified as:

1. Dental plaque induced gingival diseases
2. Non-plaque associated gingival disease

The AAP International Workshop for Classification of Periodontal Diseases (1999)

Gingival Diseases

1. Dental plaque-induced gingival disease
   I. *Gingivitis associated with dental plaque only*
      A. Without local contributing factors
      B. With local contributing factors
   II. *Gingival disease modified by systemic factors*
      A. Associated with the endocrine system
      B. Associated with blood dyscrasias
   III. *Gingival diseases modified by medications*
      A. Drug-influenced gingival diseases
         1. Drug influenced gingival enlargements
         2. Drug influenced gingivitis
   IV. *Gingival diseases modified by malnutrition*
2. Non-plaque induced gingival lesions
   I. *Gingival diseases of specific bacterial origin*
   II. *Gingival diseases of viral origin*
   III. *Gingival diseases of fungal origin*
   IV. *Gingival lesions of genetic origin*
   V. *Gingival manifestations of systemic conditions*
      A. Mucocutaneous lesions
      B. Allergic reactions
   VI. *Traumatic lesions*
      A. Chemical injury
      B. Physical injury
      C. Thermal injury
   VII. *Foreign body reactions*
   VIII. *Not otherwise specified*

Replacement of "Adult Periodontitis with "Chronic Periodontitis"

Adult periodontitis was defined as a disease characterized by an age of onset of 35 years or older, the presence of microbial deposits commensurate with the amount of periodontal destruction, generalized or localized bone loss seen, but of a pattern different from that of juvenile periodontitis, and no evidence of rapid progression, no predisposing systemic diseases and no blood leukocyte abnormalities. Chronic periodontitis was defined as an infectious disease resulting in inflammation within the supporting tissues of the teeth, progressive attachment loss, and bone loss. It is characterized by pocket formation and or gingival recession.

Clinical Features and Characteristics of Chronic Periodontitis [3]

1. Most prevalent in adults but can also occurs in children and adolescents
2. Amount of destruction is consistent with the local factors
3. Sub gingival calculus is a frequent finding
4. Slow to moderate rate of progression but my have periods of rapid progression
5. Can be associated with local predisposing factors (Tooth related, Iatrogenic factors)
6. Associated with variable microbial pattern
7. May be modified by and or associated with systemic diseases
8. Can be modified by factors other that systemic diseases such as cigarette smoking and emotional stress
9. Can further be classified on the basis of extent and severity

Extent	:	Localized or Generalized
Severity	:	
Slight	:	1 - 2 mm Clinical Attachment Level
Moderate	:	3 - 4 mm Clinical Attachment Level
Severe	:	>5 mm Clinical Attachment Level

Elimination of "Refractory Periodontitis" Category

Refractory periodontitis refers to continued attachment loss in spite of adequate treatment. The term recurrent periodontitis is now used to refer to the return of periodontitis and not as a separate disease. Potentially any patients with a past history of periodontitis can develop recurrent periodontitis if adequate oral hygiene is not maintained.

I. Chronic Periodontitis
   A. Localized
   B. Generalized
II. Aggressive Periodontitis
   A. Localized
   B. Generalized
III. Periodontitis as a Manifestation of Systemic Diseases
   A. Hematological disorders
   B. Genetic disorders
IV. Necrotizing Periodontal diseases
V. Abscesses of the periodontium
VI. Periodontitis associated with endodontic lesions

Replacement of "Early onset Periodontitis with "Aggressive Periodontitis"

In the 1989 classification patients were placed into this category based on the age in so the term was replaced. In 1999 "Aggressive Periodontitis" was defined as a disease in patients who were systemically healthy but had rapid loss of attachment and alveolar bone loss and a high incidence of familial link.

Features Common to Both Localized and Generalized Aggressive Periodontitis [39]

I. Primary features
   1. Except for periodontitis patients are usually healthy
   2. Rapid attachment loss and bone destruction
   3. Familial aggregation

II. Secondary features
   1. Amounts of microbial deposits are inconsistent with the severity of periodontal tissue destruction
   2. Elevated proportions of Aggregatibacter actinomycetemcomitans and in some populations Porphyromonas gingivalis may be elevated
   3. Phagocyte abnormalities
   4. Hyper responsive macrophage phenotype including elevated levels of PGE_2 and IL ß
   5. Progression of attachment loss and bone loss may be self arresting

Localized Aggressive Periodontitis

- Circumpubertal onset
- Robust serum antibody to infecting agents
- Localized first molar/incisor presentation

Generalized Aggressive Periodontitis

- Usually affecting persons under 30 years of age
- Poor serum antibody response
- Pronounced episodic nature of destruction
- Generalized interproximal attachment loss affecting at least three permanent teeth other than first molars and incisors

Periodontitis as a Manifestation of Systemic Diseases

The term "periodontitis as a manifestation of systemic diseases is a misnomer as the conditions listed are strictly systemic diseases that affect the periodontal tissues and are present within them rather than periodontal diseases arising de novo. Diabetes mellitus has not been included in this category as it can modify all forms of periodontal diseases.

Introduction of the Term "Necrotizing Periodontal Diseases"

The workshop participants acknowledged that Necrotizing Ulcerative Gingivitis (NUG) and Necrotizing Ulcerative Periodontitis (NUP) are clinically identifiable conditions although they were unsure if both were two different diseases or part of the same disease.

Diagnostic criteria for NUG:

1. Lesions are painful
2. Lesions are gingival ulcers, punched out crater like and involve the interdental papilla
3. The ulcers bleed spontaneously or readily

Diagnostic criteria for NUP:

1. Deep interdental craters with denudation of interdental alveolar bone
2. Sequestration of interdental and possibly buccal and /or lingual alveolar bone

Addition of a Category for "Periodontal Abscesses" and "Periodontic-Endodontic Lesion"

Periodontal abscess present diagnosis and treatment challenges they deserve to be classified apart from periodontal diseases. Only one category of Periodontic-Endodontic lesions i.e. 'Combined lesion' was added.

Addition of a Category for "Developmental or Acquired Deformities and Conditions"

This category is difficult to interpret and it seems inappropriate to include it in the classification of periodontal diseases as the conditions within this group are modifying factors which alter susceptibility to diseases rather than being discrete diseases entities.

Developmental or Acquired Deformities and Conditions

A. Localized tooth related factors that predispose to plaque induced gingival diseases or periodontitis
B. Mucogingival deformities and conditions around teeth
C. Mucogingival deformities and conditions on edentulous ridges
D. Occlusal trauma

Shortcomings of the 1999 Classification

1. The classification is very long and extensive.

2. Removal of the term "Localized Juvenile periodontitis" is most unfortunate because it is the most clearly defined of all periodontal diseases.
3. There is no provision for the category of "Historical" or "previous disease" for a patient who has suffered periodontal disease in the past and is no longer currently active.
4. The developmental and acquired conditions/deformities are not strictly periodontal conditions.
5. NUG and NUP together called as necrotising periodontal diseases, they should remain as separate terms.
6. The term 'Necrotising Stomatitis' does not appear in the Necrotising periodontal diseases list.

For Administrative and Third-Party Insurance Reporting Purposes, the American Academy of Periodontology Classifies Gingivitis and Periodontitis into Five Broad Case Types (1997)

- Plaque-associated gingivitis is designated as Case Type I
- Case Type II (Early Periodontitis) is characterized by progression of inflammation into the deeper periodontal structures with slight bone and attachment loss
- Case Type III (Moderate Periodontitis) is classified as a more advanced state with increased destruction of the periodontal structures and noticeable loss of bone support, possibly accompanied by increased tooth mobility and furcation involvement on multirooted teeth
- Case Type IV (Advanced Periodontitis) is characterized by further progression of periodontitis with major loss of alveolar bone support that is usually accompanied by an increase in tooth mobility. Furcation involvement is a common finding
- Case Type V (Refractory Periodontitis) includes those patients that continue to demonstrate attachment loss after good conventional therapy

Classification based on the Extent of the Disease [40]

	Permanent/Mixed dentition No. of Teeth Present		Primary dentition
	$n \geq 14$	$n \leq 14$	
Incidental	1 tooth	1 tooth	1 tooth
Localized	2-7 teeth	2-7 teeth	2-4 teeth
Semi-Generalized	8-12 teeth	-	5-9 teeth
Generalized	≥ 14 teeth	8-14 teeth	≥ 10 teeth

Based on the Severity of Disease per Tooth [40]

Minor	Bone loss ≤ 1/3 of the root length or attachment loss ≤ 3 mm
Moderate	Bone loss > 1/3 and ≤ 1/2 of the root length or attachment loss 4-5 mm
Severe	Bone loss > 1/2 of the root length or attachment loss ≥ 6 mm

Based on the Age [40]

Early onset periodontitis	
Prepubertal periodontitis	≤ 12 years
Juvenile Periodontitis	13 - 20 years
Postadolescent periodontitis	21 - 35 years
Adult periodontitis	≥ 36 years

Based on the Clinical Characteristics [40]

Necrotizing periodontitis	Interdental gingival necrosis, bleeding and pain
Rapidly progressive periodontitis	Documented rapid breakdown (at any age), i.e. rapidly progressive periodontitis patients showing a progression of ≥ 1 mm interproximal attachment/bone loss per year at affected sites
Refractory periodontitis	Documented, no or minimal pocket depth reduction at single rooted teeth after proper initial therapy and/or further attachment loss despite the proper execution of various treatment modalities

Conclusion

It is very likely that "Chronic periodontitis" is a constellation of diseases i.e. it is not a single entity, one of the main problems with any attempt to classify this or any other forms of periodontitis is that these infections are polymicrobial and polygenic, in addition the clinical expression of these diseases is altered by important environmental and host-modifying conditions. The facility to study gene expression and the genetic factors underlying the differences in host response to periodontal pathogens between patients may help inform the classification systems of *2010-2020*. Future systems are likely to be controversial, stimulate much debate and require further modification.

References

[1] Carranza's Clinical Periodontology 11th ed- E-Book. Google Books Result.

[2] American Academy of Periodontology. Committee Report and Discussion. The Etiology of Periodontal Disease. World Workshop in Periodontics (Proceedings). Chicago: American Academy of Periodontology, 1966:167-177.

[3] Armitage GC. Development of a classification system for periodontal diseases and conditions. *Ann. Periodontol.* 1999;4:1-6.

[4] Carranza FA, Camargo PM: In: Newman MG, Takei HH, Carranza FA, ed. Carranza's clinical periodontology, ed 10. Philadelphia: Saunders; 2006.

[5] American Academy of Periodontology. Consensus report. Discussion section I. Eds: Nevins M, BeckerW, Kornman K. Proceedings of the World Workshop in Clinical Periodontics. Chicago: American Academy of Periodontology. 1989:I23-I32.

[6] Attström R, van der Velden U. Consensus report (epidemiology). In: Lang NP, Karring T, editors. Proceedings of 1st European Workshop on Periodontics. London: Quintessence Publishing Co., 1994:120-126.

[7] Black GV. Diseases of the peridental membrane and the uric acid diathesis. *Dent. Rev.* 1894; 8:449-472.

[8] Dunbar LL. Oral manifestations in arthritic and gouty conditions. American Medical Association - Section on oral and dental surgery (Proceedings). *Dent. Cosmos.* 1894; 36:724-726.

[9] Mills GA. What I know about Riggs's disease (so-called). How does it happen that this title has come into existence? *Dent. Cosmos.* 1877;19:70-73.

[10] Mills GA. Some of the phases of Riggs's disease (so-called). *Dent. Cosmos.* 1877; 19:185-187.

[11] Mills GA. Some phases of Riggs's disease (so-called). *Dent. Cosmos.* 1877;19:254-256.

[12] Davis CG. Gum and alveolar diseases. *Dental Cosmos.* 1879:21:192-201.

[13] Black GV. Diseases of the peridental membrane having their beginning at the margin of the gum. In: Litch WF editor. American System of Dentistry, Vol. I. Philadelphia: Lea Brothers, 1886:953-979.

[14] Black GV. Chronic Suppurative Pericementitis. A Work on Special Dental Pathology, 1st edn. Chicago: Medico-Dental Publishing Co. 1915:158-184.

[15] Becks H. General aspects of pyorrhea research. *Pac. Dent. Gaz.* 1929;37:259-282.

[16] Gottlieb B. Die diffuse Atrophie des Alveoarknochens. Weitere Beiträge zur Kenntnis des Alevolarschwundes und dessen Wiedergutmachung durch Zementwachstum. *Z. Stomatol.* 1923;21:195-201.

[17] Gottlieb B. The formation of the pocket: Diffuse atrophy of alveolar bone. *J. Am. Dent. Assoc.* 1928;15:462-476.

[18] Gottlieb B. The new concept of periodontoclasia. *J. Periodontol.* 1946;17:7-23.

[19] McCall JO, Box HK. The pathology and diagnosis of the basic lesions of chronic periodontitis. *J. Am. Dent. Assoc.* 1925;12:1300-1309.

[20] Wannenmacher E. Umschau auf dem Gebiete der Paradentose Dtsch Zahnartzl Mund Kieferheilk. 1938;3:81-96.

[21] Thoma KH, Goldman HM. Wandering and elongation of the teeth and pocket formation in parodontosis. *J. Am. Dent. Assoc.* 1940;27:335-341.

[22] Orban B, Weinmann JP. Diffuse atrophy of the alveolar bone (periodontosis). *J. Periodontol.* 1942;13:31-45.

[23] Orban B. Classification and nomenclature of periodontal diseases. (Based on pathology, etiology, and clinical picture). *J. Periodontol.* 1942;13:88-91.

[24] American Academy of Periodontology. Committee Report and Discussion. The Etiology of Periodontal Disease. World Workshop in Periodontics (Proceedings). Chicago: American Academy of Periodontology. 1966:167-177.

[25] Miller WD. Original Investigations Concerning Pyorrhea Alveolaris. The Micro-Organisms of the Human Mouth. Philadelphia: The S.S. White Dental Mfg. Co. 1890:328-334.

[26] Jensen SB, Löe H, Schiött CR, Theilade E. Experimental gingivitis in man. IV. Vancomycin induced changes in bacterial plaque composition as related to the development of gingival inflammation. *J. Periodontal Res.* 1968;3:284-293.

[27] Loe H, Theilade E, Jensen SB. Experimental gingivitis in man. *J. Periodontol.* 1965; 36:177-187.

[28] Loe H, Theilade E, Jensen SB, Schiott CR. Experimental gingivitis in man. III. The influence of antibiotics on gingival plaque development. *J. Periodontal Res.* 1967; 2:282–289.

[29] Theilade E, Wright WH, Jensen SB, Loe H. Experimental gingivitis in man. II. Longitudinal clinical and bacteriological investigation. *J. Periodontal Res.* 1966;1:1-13.

[30] Newman MG, Socransky SS, Savitt ED, Propas DA, Crawford A. Studies on the microbiology of periodontosis. *J. Periodontol.* 1976;47:373-379.

[31] Newman MG, Socransky SS. Predominant cultivable microbiota in periodontosis. *J. Periodontal Res.* 1977;12:120-128.

[32] Cianciola JL, Genco RJ, Patters MR, McKenna J, van Oss CJ. Defective poymorphonuclear leukocyte function in a human periodontal disease. *Nature.* 1977; 265:445-447.

[33] Lavine WS, Maderazo EG, Stolman J, Ward PA, Cogen RB, Greenblatt I, Robertson PB. Impaired neutrophil chemotaxis in patients with juvenile and rapidly progressing periodontitis. *J. Periodontal Res.* 1979;14:10-19.

[34] Ranney RR. Position report and review of the literature. Pathogenesis of periodontal disease. In: *International Conference on Research in the Biology of Periodontal Disease.* Chicago: American Academy of Periodontology. 1977:223-300.

[35] Page RC, Schroeder HE. Discussion. *Periodontitis in Man and Other Animals. A Comparative Review.* Basel: S Karger. 1982:222-239.

[36] Grant DA, Stern IB, Everett FG. Classification of periodontal diseases. Orban's Periodontics, 3rd edn. St Louis: C.V. Mosby Co. 1968:119-120.

[37] Suzuki JB. Diagnosis and classification of the periodontal diseases. *Dent. Clin. North Am.* 1988;32(2):195-216.

[38] Flemmig TF. Periodontitis. *Ann. Periodontol.* 1999;4:32-37.

[39] Lang N, Bartold PM, Cullinan M, Jeffcoat M, Mombelli A, Murakami S, Page R, Papapanou P, Tonetti M, Van Dyke T. Consensus report: Aggressive periodontitis. *Ann. Periodontol.* 1999;4:53.

[40] Van Der Velden U. Purpose and problems of periodontal disease classification. *Periodontol.* 2000. 2005;39:13-21.

In: Current Trends in Periodontics and Implant Dentistry ISBN: 978-1-62618-819-8
Editors: Vishal Anand and Minkle Gulati

Chapter II

Influences of Systemic Diseases on Periodontal Health

***Lei Chai*[1] *and W. Keung Leung*[2]**
[1]School of Dentistry, University of Queensland, Australia
[2]Faculty of Dentistry, The University of Hong Kong,
Hong Kong SAR, China

Abstract

The modern hypothesis of periodontitis pathogenesis suggests that periodontitis is a complex disease, which means it is likely associated with the effects of multiple genes in combination with lifestyles and environment factors, i.e. it is a multifactorial disorder. Other human complex diseases include autoimmune diseases, diabetes, heart diseases, hypertension, mood disorder such as depression, obesity and so on. Interestingly many of these systemic complex diseases are associated with periodontal disease such as diabetes, heart diseases, autoimmune diseases and mood disorder. The reason could be these diseases share some common pathogenic pathway or common risk factors. In addition, it is well-known that many other systemic diseases or conditions can affect periodontitis onset, severity of the symptoms, progression and treatment responses. This chapter will mainly focus on the effects of systemic complex diseases and other systemic diseases and conditions on periodontal disease. The discussion will be about periodontal manifestations of different systemic diseases, the effects of systemic conditions on periodontitis diagnosis, treatment and prognosis. Hopefully it can help medical and dental clinicians to understand more about periodontitis and other systemic diseases, and provide a general guidance for them when facing a periodontitis patient with systemic diseases or systemic disease patients seeking periodontal therapy.

Keywords: Chronic disease, periodontitis

Introduction

Human periodontitis is a chronic infectious disease that is characterized by plaque induced destruction of periodontal soft tissue and alveolar bone. The etiology of the disease is unclear but is commonly believed to be a bacterial infection interacting with host defense which is modified by a multitude of agents, such as genetic, behavioral, and environmental factors. [1] Based on this hypothesis, periodontitis is believed to be one of the complex chronic diseases like diabetes and cardiovascular diseases. Evidence has shown that systemic complex diseases can affect periodontal status, which will be discussed in the chapter later. Moreover, as an infectious disease, any systemic disease or condition that can modulate immune and inflammatory responses can theoretically affect periodontal status. The third category that can affect periodontal status is medication effects. It has been shown that a number of medication can induce distinguish periodontal changes. In the following chapter, the current understanding of influences of systemic diseases on periodontitis categorised as systemic complex diseases which may share pathogenesis with periodontitis; systemic diseases and conditions which modulate immune and inflammatory responses; and medication effects will be discussed.

Influences of Systemic Complex Diseases on Periodontitis

Diabetes and Metabolic Syndrome

The association between diabetes and chronic periodontitis has been extensively studied for more than 50 years. The complications of diabetes are related to long-term elevation of blood glucose concentrations (hyperglycaemia) that results in the formation of advanced glycation end-products (AGEs). These products are associated to: peripheral neuropathy, retinal degeneration, renal insufficiency, atherosclerosis including coronary- and micro-angiopathy. [2] The accumulation of AGEs increases the intensity of the immune inflammatory response to different pathogens, because inflammatory cells such as monocytes and macrophages have receptors for AGEs with consequent increased production of IL-1β and TNF-α. [2] The AGEs-enriched gingival tissue has higher risk for greater vascular permeability, greater breakdown of collagen fibers and accelerated destruction of both non-mineralized connective tissue and bone occurs. Diabetes can also affect neutrophil adhesion, chemotaxis and phagocytosis, making patients more susceptible to periodontal destruction. The effects of the hyperglycemic state include the inhibition of osteoblastic proliferation and collagen production.

Several studies indicate that diabetes is associated with an increased prevalence, extent and severity of chronic periodontitis. For example a study in Hong Kong has investigated more than 200 type 2 diabetes patients and shown that 80.3% of the diabetes patients suffer with periodontitis (at least one site with probing pocket depth $\geq$ 5mm) and 93.8% patients show moderate to severe clinical attachment loss, [3] which is higher than seen in the healthy population. For this reason this disease has been defined as the sixth complication of diabetes; thus, prevention and control of chronic periodontitis must be considered an integral part of diabetes control strategy. [4, 5] Periodontal treatment, leading to a reduction of gingival tissue inflammation may contribute in obtaining reduction of systemic inflammation, thereby improving glycaemic control. [5] A recent systematic review has shown that poorly controlled diabetes increases the odds for periodontitis severity. [6] In addition, periodontitis is associated with poor glycaemic control and diabetes-related complications. However, it is inconclusive that periodontal therapy with or without the use of adjunctive antibiotics results in improvements of glycaemic control and of markers of systemic inflammation. Evidence is also lacking that implant therapy in subjects with diabetes yields long-term outcomes comparable with those without diabetes. [6]

Metabolic syndrome is a group of conditions including obesity, hypertension, impaired glucose tolerance, hyperinsulinemia, and dyslipidemia that leads to an increased risk for heart disease and diabetes. [7] Because both chronic periodontitis and metabolic syndrome are associated with systemic inflammation and insulin resistance, these two diseases may be linked through a common pathophysiological pathway (increased serum levels of products derived from oxidative damage) and a bidirectional association has been hypothesized. [8, 9] Patients with metabolic syndrome have also been associated with poor periodontal health. [10, 11] Although further studies are needed to confirm such association, people affected by metabolic syndrome should be encouraged to undergo a regular periodontal check up and intensive periodontal therapy.

Cardiovascular Diseases

Cardiovascular diseases (CVDs) are a group of diseases affecting the heart and blood vessels. According to the definition of the International Classification of Diseases, 9th Revision, CVDs include: 1) ischemic heart disease, 2) cerebrovascular diseases, and 3) diseases of arteries, arterioles and capillaries. [12] Although it is a chronic process, it can cause acute clinical events such as acute coronary syndromes (ACS), myocardial infarction and stroke. [13] Atherosclerosis is the main cause of all cardiovascular diseases. [13] Inflammation has been considered as a direct, causative factor in atherogenesis and in all stages of cardiovascular diseases. There are enormous studies about periodontitis affecting CVDs and it has been proved by meta-analysis and systemic reivews that periodontitis is a risk factor to CVDs. [14] However the number of studies investigating effects of CVDs on periodontitis appears much fewer.

Studies have been carried out to evaluate the periodontal status in ACS patients. ACS is a severe form of CVD characterized by progressive or unstable angina and non-ST segment elevation myocardial infarction, all of which are associated with localized coronary atherothrombotic events leading to ischemia. In one small study involving 43 ACS patients in Chile, 100% of ACS subjects aged 41–83 years have shown chronic periodontitis, with 58% having severe periodontitis, and 42% with mild disease. [15] A study in Poland also reported chronic periodontitis in all ACS cohorts. [16] Consistent with these studies, a group in Israel studied about 201 ACS patients and reported that 100% patients exhibited clinical signs of chronic periodontitis. [17] These findings indicate a higher prevalence of periodontitis in patients with ACS compared to healthy controls.

An observation study about periodontal status in atherosclerosis has also found that patients with atheroma plaque had the highest percentage of severe periodontitis when compared to atheroma plaque free control group. [18]

Although the mechanism of CVDs affecting periodontal status is unclear yet, there are hypotheses about the biological links between CVDs and periodontitis: 1) periodontal pathogens seems able to influence CVD onset, progression and prognosis; 2) subjects with monocytic hyper-inflammatory phenotype are at increased risk for both CVDs and periodontitis indicating the two diseases may share some common aetio-pathogenetic pathway; and the fact that 3) molecular mimicry- cross-reactivity was observable between periodontal pathogens and host antherosclerosis related auto-antigens indicating certain common immune responses are in operation for both the diseases. [19] Such links could possibly explain the reasons for the higher periodontitis prevalence in subjects with CVDs. Further studies demonstrating influence of CVDs on periodontitis are required.

Autoimmune Diseases

Rheumatoid arthritis is an autoimmune inflammatory disease that affects several organs and systems. It is characterized by persistent synovitis with the destruction of joint connective tissue (cartilage) and bone, resulting in structural damage, decreased mobility and loss of articular function. [20] The aetiology of rheumatoid arthritis remains unclear, but infectious agents may play a role in the loss of self-tolerance and consequent development of an autoimmune disease. [21]

Clinical studies have indicated a plausible association between periodontitis/tooth loss and rheumatoid arthritis, [22, 23] hypothesizing the possibility of a common genetic trait predisposing to both conditions, that are associated to the destruction of bone mediated by inflammatory cytokines; so, periodontitis may be a causal factor in the pathogenesis of rheumatoid arthritis and vice versa. Immune genetic studies of patients with rheumatoid arthritis have established an association with specific human leukocyte antigens (HLA), in particular in the HLA-DR4 locus. The same genetic locus has been associated with development of severe and rapidly progressive periodontitis. [24] In periodontal lesions and rheumatoid synovium, local immune responses are amplified with the recruitment of inflammatory cells from the systemic circulation into the target tissue (gingival mucosa or synovial membrane).

In addition, rheumatoid arthritis may influence the pathogenesis of chronic periodontitis through its motor and emotional damage; in fact, impaired mobility and disability in the upper extremities of the body reduced manual dexterity, making oral hygiene more difficult with consequent increased risk of caries, chronic periodontitis and tooth loss. [23] The salivary flow reduction, due to medication or secondary Sjögren's syndrome, may increase supragingival plaque formation in these subjects. Therefore it is common to detect high plaque accumulation and severe gingivitis and periodontitis in patients with rheumatoid arthritis as well as low salivary flow. The patients may suffer from other dry mouth symptoms due to low salivary flow. Diagnosis of periodontitis in rheumatoid arthritis patients should not only focus on the severity of periodontitis and oral hygiene status, but also salivary flow rate as well as patients' disability level since the latter affects patients' own oral hygiene home care. Accordingly, treatment of periodontitis in patients with rheumatoid arthritis should also take consideration in managing all adverse factors such as medications to relief dry mouth, oral hygiene maintenance and oral health instruction considering patients' disability levels.

Scleroderma is symptom of a group of diseases that involve abnormal growth of connective tissue, which supports the skin and internal organs. [25] It has two broad categories i.e. localized scleroderma and systemic sclerosis (SSc). [26] Compared to localized scleroderma, SSc represents a more extensive skin involvement coinciding with severe internal organ manifestations. It is a clinically heterogeneous, systemic disorder, which affects the connective tissue of the skin, internal organs, and blood vessel walls. Diagnosis of SSc is largely dependent on medical history and physical examination. The signs include changed skin appearance and texture, calcium deposits developing under the skin and changes in the tiny blood vessels at the base of the fingernails. [25] Patients suffering from SSc usually exhibit CREST syndrome, i.e. calcinosis-calcium deposition in soft tissue, Raynaud's phenomenon-color change in fingers and toes, esophageal dysfunction-decreased mobility of esophagus, sclerodactyly-deformity of extremities, and telangiectasia-dilation of terminal vessels. CREST syndrome also presents with various degree of connective tissue fibrosis. [25]

The oral manifestations of SSc include constriction of the oral orifice, [27] periodontal disease, widening of periodontal ligament space, loss of tongue mobility, oral mucosal telangiectasia, and salivary hypofunction. [28-35] Periodontally a study in Hong Kong has shown that all the SSc patients are suffering from gingivitis. 97% SSc patients in the study had calculus and 76% patients had periodontally involved teeth, which was significantly higher than the control SSc free group (55%). [36] However this study did not find the correlations between presence of periodontal pocket and salivary flow rate or extent of mouth opening. [36] The same group reported that SSc patients exhibit higher levels of periodontal inflammation and wider radiographic periodontal ligament spaces compared to age and sex matched controls. [37] Such findings indicate that the higher prevalence of gingivitis and periodontitis in SSc patients may associate more with patient's impaired oral hygiene and limited mobility. Thus, dental practitioners should pay more attention on how to improve and maintain SSc patient's oral hygiene when managing such patients.

Sjögren's syndrome (SS) is a slowly progressing immune-mediated disorder of exocrine glands, which is characterized by intense lymphocytic infiltration. Involvement of the salivary and lacrimal glands leads to the development of xerostomia and keratoconjunctivitis sicca, respectively. SS may be primary, which is not associated with another underlying autoimmune disorder, and secondary, when it is associated with a connective tissue disorder such as rheumatoid arthritis, systemic lupus erythematosus, scleroderma, polymyositis and primary biliary cirrhosis. [38]

Whether SS can directly influence patients' periodontal status in addition to xerostomia is still controversial. A study in Greece compared the periodontal status of SS patients, patients with any other autoimmune disease and subjects who experienced dry mouth but without any underlying disease, and found no difference among three groups. [39] Several other studies also reported no difference in gingival and periodontal disease between SS patients and age-, sex-matched controls. [40-42] However some later studies have reported higher gingival inflammation levels and detected higher proportion of *Candida albicans* in individuals with SS indicating SS may be associated with gingivitis and *Candida* infection in oral cavity. [43, 44] Further investigations on influence of SS on periodontal status are required.

Osteoporosis

Osteoporosis is a systemic skeletal disease characterized by low bone mass and micro-architectural deterioration of bone tissue, with a consequent increase in fragility and susceptibility to fracture of bones. [45] It is considered nowadays as a heterogeneous chronic systemic condition, which can occur at any age, and its aetiology is attributed to various endocrine, metabolic and individual factors. Furthermore, osteoporosis has recently received increasing attention in relation to the susceptibility to chronic periodontitis in postmenopausal women. [46, 47] The production of estrogen drops drastically at menopause leading to osteoporosis in skeletal bones (loss of bone mass and reduction of bone density) with a consequent increase in bone fragility and susceptibility to fracture. Total skeletal mass reduction in postmenopausal women may include jawbones, particularly the mandible. [48]

A number of studies have shown that bone changes in osteoporosis are associated with a loss of periodontal attachment, loss of teeth, and reduction of the height of the residual ridge. [49, 50] Based on these findings, it has been hypothesized that osteoporosis could be a risk factor for the progression of chronic periodontitis. [51] Both osteoporosis and chronic periodontitis, in fact, are bone resorptive diseases sharing common aetiologic agents/risk factors (e.g. gender, cigarette smoking, alcohol consumption, systemic diseases, and heredity) that may either affect or modulate the course of both diseases. [46] Regarding the treatment of osteoporosis-related periodontitis, randomized, controlled trials have shown the potential of bisphosphonate to reduce the progression of periodontal bone loss in patients with osteoporosis. [52, 53] Furthermore, Lane et al. have shown that bisphosphonate therapy improves the outcome of scaling and root planing in a 12-month randomized, placebo-controlled trial. [54] The effects of bisphosphonate in periodontitis will be discussed in detail in the later section. Therefore for managing osteoporosis-related periodontitis, collaboration between both dental and medical practitioners is recommended.

Chronic Kidney Disease

Chronic kidney disease is defined as a progressive decline in renal function associated with a reduced glomerular filtration rate (as measured clinically by the creatinine clearance). [55] The incidence of chronic kidney disease continues to rise worldwide and the effects of the disease on oral tissues, especially in children, including xerostomia, delayed tooth eruption, calcifications leading to obliteration of pulp chamber and canals, enamel hypoplasia, decreased caries rates and altered salivary pH levels are well documented. [56] Moreover, patients with chronic kidney disease receiving haemodialysis may exhibit a characteristic malodour or bad breath and experience metallic taste which are due to the high urea content in saliva and its subsequent breakdown to ammonia. [57] In addition to renal replacement therapy which is discussed later in the immunosupressant section, studies report increased levels of plaque, calculus and gingival inflammation and possible increased prevalence and severity of periodontitis in chronic kidney disease patients on dialysis maintenance therapy. [58]

Dental management of chronic kidney disease patients is complicated by some systemic consequences (e.g. anaemia, crisis of bleeding and cardiovascular or endocrine diseases). Moreover, untreated dental infection in immune-suppressed individuals can potentially contribute to morbidity and transplant rejection. [59] For these reasons, to improve the health status of these patients, a collaborative plan between dental and renal professionals must be established. So many transplant centres plan a dental check in their pre-transplant protocol. Specific effects of chronic kidney disease and renal replacement therapy on periodontal tissues include gingival enlargement and increased gingival inflammation. [60] Interventional studies are also needed to assess the effect of periodontal treatment on systemic inflammation and chronic kidney disease patients experiencing such complications.

Psychological Stress and Depression

Epidemiological studies have suggested a possible association between emotional stress, depression and periodontitis. [61] The association between occupational stress and progressive periodontitis has been further investigated by a number of studies. [62-64] These studies indicate that life events related stress might exert an unfavourable effect on the progression of periodontitis.

In contrast, some earlier studies showed negative results. [65, 66] However more recent systematic reviews appear to agree, despite the methodological variaties or even flaws in many studies, that stress and depression are important risk factors related to periodontitis progression and severity. [67, 68] The hypotheses of the mechanisms include stress-induced immunosuppression resulting in activation of the central nervous system and autonomic nervous system leading to periodontitis, stress-induced behavioral changes and stress-induced impaired wound healing. [68] Based on sufficient evidence, psychosocial stress and depression should be considered when managing periodontitis. Proper diagnosis and treatment should be administered for patients with such problems.

Alzheimer's Disease

Alzheimer's disease is a progressive neurodegenerative disorder that affects older people, characterized by irreversible cognitive and physical deterioration. It has a multifactorial aetiology including infectious agents and other vascular risk factors. [69] Inflammation has been suggested to play a role in the pathophysiology of Alzheimer's disease, [70] and certain pathogens may speed up the inflammatory response and increase oxidation, causing inflammatory reactions and oxidative damage with consequent vascular injuries. [71]

Some cross-sectional [72, 73] and longitudinal studies [74, 75] have investigated the oral health status of dementia or Alzheimer's disease patients, reporting poor oral conditions in those affected. However, it must be noted that the progression of dementia is accompanied by a gradual inability to perform self-care, including adequate oral hygiene, due to self-neglect and loss of cognitive and motor skills. For this reason, patients with Alzheimer's disease are expected to exhibit more plaque, gingival bleeding, and calculus compared to age and gender matched healthy adults.

Systemic Diseases and Conditions Modulating Immune and Inflammatory Responses

Hormones

Hormones, especially sex hormones, have potent effects on the major determinants influencing development and integrity of human skeleton and oral cavity, thus can have an enormous impact upon periodontal status. During different life stages such as pregnancy, menstruation and puberty, the dramatic changes in hormone level influence the human body including periodontal status. The mechanisms that drive these changes are alteration of cytokine secretion, modified immune cells functions, adjusted osteoblasts and fibroblasts physiology in periodontium in response to hormones and local stimulators. [76]

It is well established that pregnancy causes a modification in the host's response to dental plaque but this is largely confined to the soft tissues and manifests as an increase in the severity of gingival inflammation or pregnancy epilus. [77] Several cross-sectional studies have shown the incidence and severity of gingival redness, swelling, bleeding, and exudation increase from the third month of gestation to the eighth month and then decrease. [77-80] It is evident that with more gingival enlargement false pocketing will become prevelant and thus the quantity and anaerobicity of the subgingival microflora will increase but there are no published studies, which might implicate periodontal attachment loss as sequela to hormone-modified plaque-induced chronic gingival inflammation. [81, 82]

Other clinical indications of a hormonal effect include the effects of oral contraceptives on the gingivae and fluctuations in the level of plaque-induced gingivitis with phases of the menstrual cycle. [83] Furthermore, puberty is often accompanied by increased gingival inflammation and this heightened response to plaque has been attributed to the concentration of circulating sex hormones. [84] An alternative explanation for increased gingivitis during puberty is that it is a period of mixed dentition where erupting and exfoliating teeth present in many patients favour plaque retention. The fact that gingivitis decreases after puberty may reflect the general improvement seen in children as they improve their dexterity and become more aware of oral hygiene. Evidence suggests that hormone levels may alter the inflammatory response to plaque and, although this predominantly results in gingivitis alone, an increased risk of periodontitis in these patients cannot be ignored.

Smoking

Tobacco smoking is the most important risk factor associated with periodontitis. Many studies have been carried out on this topic over decades.

Smoking is probably one of the most harmful human habits affecting periodontium. The harmful effects manifest themselves by interfering with vascular and immunologic reactions, as well as by undermining the supportive functions of the periodontal tissues. [85] A prospective study over 20 years offers convincing evidence that smokers exhibit greater bone loss and attachment loss, as well as more pronounced frequencies of periodontal pockets, than non-smokers do. In addition, tooth loss is more extensive in smokers. [86] Smoking, thus, considerably increases the risk for periodontitis. Depending on the definition of disease and the exposure to smoking, the risk is reported to be at least 2-fold elevated for a smoker compared to a never-smoker. [87, 88]

Chemical products and toxins in tobacco smoke may delay wound healing by impairing the biologic progression of healing and by inhibiting the basic cellular functions responsible for its initiation. [89] Smokers have a decreased response to periodontal therapy compared to non-smokers. [90, 91] Smoking has a strong negative influence on regenerative therapy, which includes osseous grafting, guided tissue regeneration or a combination of these treatments. [92] It has been seen that the hemorrhagic response of periodontium upon probing is decreased in smokers compared to nonsmokers, [93] which could be due to chronic tobacco-induced angiogenic suppression. [94]

On the whole, smoking related periodontal diseases consist of an increased and accelerated destruction of the supporting tissues of the teeth, with clinical signs and symptoms of bone loss, pocket formation, and finally tooth loss. The decreased inflammatory responses of periodontium may conceal the severity of periodontitis. The outcome of periodontal treatment is less favorable or even unfavorable in smokers. Because of the notorious treatment responses in smokers with periodontitis, the dental practitioner shall always consider discusssion with patients to arrange smoking cessation as an integral initial therapy for periodontitis if they want to achieve acceptable predictable treatment outcome.

Aging

The mechanisim of aging affecting periodontal tissues possibly are: 1) alterations in differentiation and proliferation of osteoblasts and osteoclasts; 2) an increase in periodontal cell response to the oral microbiota and mechanical stress leading to the secretion of cytokines involved in osseous reabsorption; and 3) systemic endocrine alterations in elderly persons. [95] However there is conflicting evidence for the role of aging on periodontitis progression. Some longitudinal studies indicate age to be a risk indicator for alveolar bone loss or clinical attachment loss, [96-98] while others show no association. [99, 100] It seems aging alone may not cause a significant loss of periodontal attachment. [95] While increasing age has been found to be associated with the prevalence, extent and severity of periodontitis, this relationship is considered to be a reflection of individual cumulative periodontal breakdown over time rather than because of factors related to the aging process itself. [101-103]

When considering identification of individual's susceptibility to disease progression, age is an important factor. The amount of tissue destruction in relation to a patient's age is a good predictor of future disease progression. A young patient with aggressive disease and advanced attachment loss is considered at higher risk for further disease progression than an older individual with the same level of attachment loss. [104]

Down Syndrome

Down syndrome (DS) is characterized by central growth deficiency with delayed mental and physical development. All individuals with DS are mentally impaired to some degree, ranging from mild to severe. DS itself is not a disease; however affected individuals have a greater risk of acquiring many systemic conditions. Persons with DS are susceptible to upper respiratory tract and chest infections. Approximately 50% have some forms of heart defect, usually ventricular septal defect; some may require antibiotic cover for invasive dental treatment. Alzheimer disease is a problem in later life of DS individuals. [105] The oral manifestations of Down Syndrome include large and fissured tongue, cracked lips, shelf-like or 'stair-palate', malocclusions, microdontia of permanent dentition, altered crown morphology and shape, short root, enamel hypoplasia and hypocalcification, thinner enamel and dentine in the permanent dentition, taurodontism, hypodontia and supernumerary teeth, asymmetry and delayed eruption. [105-107]

In terms of periodontal status, DS individuals usually present with poor oral hygiene manifested as marginal gingival inflammation, acute and subacute necrotizing gingivitis, advanced chronic periodontitis, loss of attachment in form of gingival recession and increased probing pocket depth, alveolar bone loss, suppuration or periodontal abscesses, furcation involvement in the molars, increased tooth mobility, and even loss of teeth. [105, 108] DS individuals had a prevalence of 60 to 90% periodontitis and increased severity of periodontal disease compared with normal age-matched controls and subjects with other mental disabilities of similar age. [105] Studies suggested that majority of DS children had poor oral hygiene, but at the same time, there was only moderate relationship between dental plaque and periodontal disease severity in DS individuals. [109, 110] Thus, it seems the rapid and severe periodontal destruction in DS individuals cannot be explained by poor oral hygiene alone.

Regarding periodontal treatment, it is apparent that DS individuals have higher treatment needs from dental practitioner's perspective. However one must pay attention to the challenges in periodontal treatment to DS individuals. Cichon et al. have reported that there is no improvement in clinical and microbiological parameters after a single session of scaling and root planing and oral hygiene instructions. [111] The conventional standard periodontal therapy could neither eliminate periodontal pathogens nor even had any remarkable effect on subgingival microbiota. The authors attributed these unsatisfactory clinical outcomes to poor plaque control and impaired host defense mechanisms. [111] However, later studies have shown more frequent recalls and more active intervention such as adjunctive use of chlorhexdine gel and mouthrinse can overcome the adverse factors in periodontal management of DS individuals. [112-114] Although there is currently no gold standard available indicating how periodontal disease in DS individuals can be best managed, appropriate modification of periodontal therapy involves non-surgical periodontal therapy adjuncted with regular use of chemical plaque control agents, and frequent recall schedule in DS individuals appears to be a promising way forward.

Blood Disorders

Common and rare blood disorders may influence periodontal status by the mechanisms such as direct infiltration by abnormal hematologic cells, deposition of abnormal proteins, oral ulceration and abnormal bleeding. [115] They therefore can impair host immune responses thus increasing the severity and extent of periodontitis. Moreover they increase the difficulties in periodontal management due to compromised immune responses and bleeding problems. The blood disorders include aplastic anaemia, neutropenia, leukemia, multiple myeloma and leukocyte adhesion deficiency, just to name a few.

Blood cells play a crucial role in systemic health and periodontal health. White blood cells or leukocytes are the major participants in immune and inflammatory system. Red blood cells have crucial roles in maintaining gas exchange and nutrient supply to the periodontium. Platelets are needed for efficient haemostasis of this well perfused tissue which, when inflamed, is commonly hyperaemic and haemorrhagic. These functions are not just vital to periodontium but to one's survival. Thus it is never an exaggeration to address their importance to systemic health and periodontal health.

In managing these patients, thorough medical history should be obtained prior to any treatment. Any abnormal inflammation or bleeding in periodontal disease patients requires special attention and blood tests.

Cancer Chemo- and Irradiation Therapy

Chemotherapy and radiotherapy are commonly used in head and neck cancer treatment and are well known to have negative impacts on normal head and neck structures surrounding tumor. Epstein et al. have studied the impact of head and neck radiation therapy on the progression of periodontal attachment loss in 10 patients who received unilateral radiation fields that included the dentition. They found that greater attachment loss and tooth loss occurred in the irradiated compared with the nonirradiated region. [116] Clinical attachment loss following head and neck radiation therapy has also been reported in another study in which 27 patients before and 6–8 months after radiotherapy treatment were monitored. [117] These preliminary studies indicate that individuals undergoing head and neck radiotherapy may be at greater risk for periodontitis progression. However contradictory finding has also been reported in a study in Hong Kong investigating oral health status of patients after radiotherapy for nasopharyngeal cancer, in which radiotherapy has been associated with root caries and candidiasis but not with periodontitis. [118] A systematic review summarizing studies from 1990 to 2008 about dental disease in patients undergoing cancer therapy, reported an overall prevalence of severe gingivitis in patients under or after chemotherapy as 20.3% and higher plaque index and gingival index than healthy controls. [119] However it also pointed out there is still a lack of studies to define the type of association between cancer therapy and periodontal disease. Further studies are required to illucidate the link between them.

Alcohol Consumption

Tezal et al. have investigated the relationship between alcohol consumption and severity of periodontitis in a cross-sectional study, and found alcohol consumption to be associated with increased severity of clinical attachment loss in a dose-dependent fashion. [120] The authors hence concluded that alcohol intake might be a mild risk indicator for periodontitis. [120] Another study however has failed to find an association between daily alcohol consumption and disease progression (additional attachment loss over 3 mm) over a 2-year period. [121] Although there is controversy among different studies on this topic, a recent systemic review based on 11 cross-sectional and 5 longitudinal observational studies reported that there was sound evidence to suggest alcohol consumption is a risk indicator for periodontitis. [122] However, the pattern of the association still needs further clarifications.

Human Immunodeficiency Virus (HIV) Infection

There are two types of periodontal diseases reported to be associated with HIV infections, i.e. necrotizing (ulcreative) gingivitis and necrotizing (ulcerative) periodontitis. [123] In addition to these two specific forms, marginal gingivitis and chronic periodontitis can occur in patients with HIV infection. Two longitudinal cohort studies documented an accelerated rate of attachment loss in HIV-seropositive patients. [124, 125] However, later studies have shown no differences in baseline attachment loss between HIV-seropositive patients and – seronegative controls. [126-128] Larger-scale longitudinal studies are required to determine how HIV infection influences periodontitis progression, but the advent of high activity anti-retroviral therapy (HAART) is likely to be a major confounder, at least in the western world, because of its impact on viral load and immune function. [129] Current evidence suggests that HIV seropositivity is not a predictor for progressive periodontitis. However, largerscale longitudinal studies in populations are needed to confirm these initial findings.

Medications

Immunosuppressant

Immunosuppressants are used for patients receiving transplants to prolong functional life of the transplanted organs. The commonly used immunosuppressants, for instance in patients with renal transplants, include cyclosporine A (CsA) and tacrolimus or FK506. CsA is thought to suppress interleukin 2 production, thus attenuates cell mediated immunity. [130] The common side effects of CsA include nephrotoxicity, hepatotoxicity, hypertrichosis and drug induced gingival enlargement (DIGE). The incidence of DIGE has been reported from 13 to 81%. [131, 132] FK506 is a relatively new immunosuppressant compared to CsA and is thought to induce less gingival overgrowth. A study in Hong Kong investigated DIGE due to CsA and FK506. [133] In this study, patients receiving CsA had a Gingival Growth Index of 45.2% while patients with FK506 had 25.1%. One year after non-surgical periodontal treatment, CsA patient's Gingival Growth Index dropped to 15.2%. [133] Such studies indicate that patients receiving immunosuppressant is a high-risk group for gingival enlargement although FK506 seems to exhibit lesser similar side effect compared to CsA. Periodontal treatment is effective in preventing and reducing the gingival enlargement. Hence, in patients receiving immunosuppressant for organ transplantation, adequate pre and post transplant oral health care is recommended.

Bisphosphonates

Bisphosphonates are widely used in the management of systemic metabolic bone diseases such as osteoporosis, hypercalcemia of multiple myeloma and bone metastases from cancers. They can partially inhibit bone resorption, increase osteoblastic differentiation and inhibit osteoclast recruitment and activity. [134] They have similar structure to pyrophosphate, a normal product of human metabolism presented in serum and urine that has calcium-chelating properties. [135]

Bisphosphonates have been shown to be an effective therapeutic agent for the management of osteoporosis by increasing bone mass and reducing fracture in the spine, hip and vertebral sites. [136, 137] They are also used for reducing bone pain from cancer bony metastasis through inhibiting osteoclastic activities. [138]

Studies have been carried out to investigate the possibility of using bisphosphonates to help managing periodontitis. Animal studies showed bisphosphonates could inhibit bone loss around affected teeth, [139] upregulate inflammatory processes, [140] stimulate alveolar bone growth [141] and increase bone formation around peri-implantitis defect. [142] Human clinical studies reported bisphosphonates could slow down alveoloar bone loss in periodontitis when systemically administered. [52, 53] However recent studies have shown that bisphophosnates are associated with osteonecrosis of the jaws (ONJ). ONJ is defined as "the presence of exposed bone in the maxillofacial region that does not heal within eight weeks after identification by a health care professional". [143] Since it was identified in 2003, it has been regarded as one of the important side effects of bisphosphonates causing numerous and often severe oral complications. Individuals receiving intravenous bisphosphonates are at significantly higher risk of ONJ than using oral bisphosphonates. At least 5% patietns receiving intravenous bisphosphonates develop ONJ. [144]

Based on the current findings it seems utilizing bisphosphonates as adjunct to periodontal treatment need cautious evaluation as the benefits from bisphosphonates can be outbalanced by its side effects. For periodontitis patients with osteoporosis or other situations that requires administration of bisphosphonates, dental practitioners shall evaluate presence of unhealing oral ulcers associated with pathologic bone changes in the maxillofacial area regularly.

Anti-epileptic Drugs

It has been reported that some degree of gingival enlargement is present in 36-67% of patients who take the anticonvulsant drug sodium 5,5-diphenylhydantoinate (DPH, phenytoin, Dilantin). It occurs primarily in young individuals and reportedly seen rarely in people over 40. The onset of gingival overgrowth is generally three months after the commencement of phenytoin therapy and approximately 50 per cent of phenytoin users develop these lesions. [145] Such effects can be reversed once the treatment has ceased. More importantly oral hygiene is crucial for controlling the severity of gingival enlargement. Thus oral health care shall be enhanced to those patients having anti-epileptic drugs.

Conclusion

This chapter summarizes the influence of some of the systemic diseases and conditions on periodontal health and related diagnosis and treatment considerations. Based on the literature review in the chapter, it can be concluded that periodontal status is influenced by systemic health. Many systemic diseases or conditions can affect periodontal status. It thus requires dental practitioners to carefully diagnose and manage periodontitis not only focusing on the periodontal symptoms within the oral cavities but also considering possible influences contributed by systemic diseases and related management. Consultation and collaboration with medical teams are recommended when managing periodontal disease patients compromised by systemic diseases or conditions.

References

[1] Page RC, Offenbacher S, Schroeder HE, Seymour GJ, Kornman KS. Advances in the pathogenesis of periodontitis: summary of developments, clinical implications and future directions. *Periodontol. 2000.* 1997;14:216-48.

[2] Schmidt AM, Weidman E, Lalla E, Yan SD, Hori O, Cao R et al. Advanced glycation endproducts (AGEs) induce oxidant stress in the gingiva: a potential mechanism underlying accelerated periodontal disease associated with diabetes. *J. Periodontal Res.* 1996;31:508-15.

[3] Leung WK, Movva LR, Wong MC, Corbet EF, Siu SC, Kawamura M. Health behaviour, metabolic control and periodontal status in medically treated Chinese with type 2 diabetes mellitus. *Ann. R. Australas Coll. Dent Surg*. 2008;19:102-10.

[4] Loe H. Periodontal disease. The sixth complication of diabetes mellitus. *Diabetes Care.* 1993;16:329-34.

[5] Mealey BL, Ocampo GL. Diabetes mellitus and periodontal disease. *Periodontol 2000.* 2007;44:127-53.

[6] Salvi GE, Carollo-Bittel B, Lang NP. Effects of diabetes mellitus on periodontal and peri-implant conditions: update on associations and risks. *J. Clin. Periodontol.* 2008; 35:398-409.

[7] Grundy SM, Cleeman JI, Daniels SR, Donato KA, Eckel RH, Franklin et al. Diagnosis and management of the metabolic syndrome: an American Heart Association/National Heart, Lung, and Blood Institute scientific statement. *Curr. Opin. Cardiol*. 2006;21:1-6.

[8] Bullon P, Morillo JM, Ramirez-Tortosa MC, Quiles JL, Newman HN, Battino M. Metabolic syndrome and periodontitis: is oxidative stress a common link? *J. Dent. Res.* 2009;88:503-18.

[9] Morita T, Ogawa Y, Takada K, Nishinoue N, Sasaki Y, Motohashi M et al. Association between periodontal disease and metabolic syndrome. *J. Public Health Dent.* 2009; 69:248-53.

[10] D'Aiuto F, Sabbah W, Netuveli G, Donos N, Hingorani AD, Deanfield J et al. Association of the metabolic syndrome with severe periodontitis in a large U.S. population-based survey. *J. Clin. Endocrinol. Metab.* 2008;93:3989-94.

[11] Li P, He L, Sha YQ, Luan QX. Relationship of metabolic syndrome to chronic periodontitis. *J. Periodontol.* 2009;80:541-9.

[12] Lockhart PB, Bolger AF, Papapanou PN, Osinbowale O, Trevisan M, Levison ME et al. Periodontal disease and atherosclerotic vascular disease: does the evidence support an independent association? A scientific statement from the American Heart Association. *Circulation*. 2012;125:2520-44.

[13] Rosamond W, Flegal K, Friday G, Furie K, Go A, Greenlund K et al. Heart disease and stroke statistics - 2007 update: a report from the American Heart Association Statistics Committee and Stroke Statistics Subcommittee. *Circulation*. 2007;115e:69-171.

[14] Otomo-Corgel J, Pucher JJ, Rethman MP, Reynolds MA. State of the science: chronic periodontitis and systemic health. *J. Evid. Based Dent. Pract.* 2012;12:20-8.

[15] Lim J, Perez Z, Guarda E, Fajuri A, Marchant E, Martinez A et al. Periodontal disease among patients with acute coronary syndrome. *Rev. Med. Chil.* 2005;133:183-9.

[16] Czerniuk MR, Gorska R, Filipiak KJ, Opolski G. Inflammatory response to acute coronary syndrome in patients with coexistent periodontal disease. *J. Periodontol.* 2004; 75:1020-6.

[17] Gotsman I, Lotan C, Soskolne WA, Rassovsky S, Pugatsch T, Lapidus L. Periodontal destruction is associated with coronary artery disease and periodontal infection with acute coronary syndrome. *J. Periodontol.* 2007;78:849-58.

[18] Pinho MM, Faria-Almeida R, Azevedo E, Conceicao Manso M, Martins L. Periodontitis and atherosclerosis: an observational study. *J. Periodontal Res.* 2013, doi:10.1111/jre.12026.

[19] Huck O, Saadi-Thiers K, Tenenbaum H, Davideau JL, Romagna C, Laurent Y et al. Evaluating periodontal risk for patients at risk of or suffering from atherosclerosis: recent biological hypotheses and therapeutic consequences. *Arch. Cardiovasc. Dis.* 2011;104:352-8.

[20] Firestein GS, Budd RC, Gabriel SE, McInnes IB, O'Dell JR. Aetiology and pathogenesis of rheumatoid arthritis, in Ruddy, S., E.D. Harris, Jr. and C.B. Sledge, editors, Kelly's Textbook of Rheumatology, MD Consult, LLC: St. Louis, Mo. 2013, pp. 1059-108.

[21] Liao F, Li Z, Wang Y, Shi B, Gong Z, Cheng X. *Porphyromonas gingivalis* may play an important role in the pathogenesis of periodontitis-associated rheumatoid arthritis. *Med. Hypotheses*. 2009;72:732-5.

[22] Pischon N, Pischon T, Kroger J, Gulmez E, Kleber BM, Bernimoulin JP et al. Association among rheumatoid arthritis, oral hygiene, and periodontitis. *J. Periodontol.* 2008;79:979-86.

[23] de Pablo P, Chapple IL, Buckley CD, Dietrich T. Periodontitis in systemic rheumatic diseases. *Nat. Rev. Rheumatol.* 2009;5:218-24.

[24] Marotte H, Farge P, Gaudin P, Alexandre C, Mougin B, Miossec P. The association between periodontal disease and joint destruction in rheumatoid arthritis extends the link between the HLA-DR shared epitope and severity of bone destruction. *Ann. Rheum. Dis.* 2006;65:905-9.

[25] National Institute of Health. (2010) Scleroderma fact sheet. National Institute of Health. http://report.nih.gov/nihfactsheets/Pdfs/Scleroderma%28NIAMS%29.pdf. (Accessed on Jan 15, 2013).

[26] American College of Rheumatology. (2010) Scleroderma (Systemic Sclerosis) http://www.rheumatology.org/practice/clinical/patients/diseases_and_conditions/scleroderma.asp (Accessed on Jan 15, 2013).
[27] Scully C. Medical Problems in Dentistry. 2010 6th Ed. Edinburgh: Churchill Livingstone Elsevier.
[28] Marmary Y, Glaiss R, Pisanty S. Scleroderma: oral manifestations. *Oral Surg. Oral Med. Oral Pathol.* 1981;52:32-7.
[29] Alexandridis C, White SC. Periodontal ligament changes in patients with progressive systemic sclerosis. *Oral Surg. Oral Med. Oral Pathol.* 1984;58:113-8.
[30] Eversole LR, Jacobsen PL, Stone CE. Oral and gingival changes in systemic sclerosis (scleroderma). *J. Periodontol.* 1984;55:175-8.
[31] Nagy G, Kovacs J, Zeher M, Czirjak L. Analysis of the oral manifestations of systemic sclerosis. *Oral Surg. Oral Med. Oral Pathol.* 1994;77:141-6.
[32] Rout PG, Hamburger J, Potts AJ. Orofacial radiological manifestations of systemic sclerosis. *Dentomaxillofac. Radiol.* 1996;25:193-6.
[33] Scardina GA, Messina P. Systemic sclerosis: description and diagnostic role of the oral phenomena. *Gen. Dent.* 2004;52:42-7.
[34] Poole JL, Brewer C, Rossie K, Good CC, Conte C, Steen V. Factors related to oral hygiene in persons with scleroderma. *Int. J. Dent. Hyg.* 2005;3:13-7.
[35] Vincent C, Agard C, Barbarot S, N'Guyen JM, Planchon B, Durant C et al. Orofacial manifestations of systemic sclerosis: a study of 30 consecutive patients. *Rev. Med. Interne.* 2009;30:5-11.
[36] Chu CH, Yeung CM, Lai IA, Leung WK, Mok MY. Oral health of Chinese people with systemic sclerosis. *Clin. Oral Investig.* 2011;15:931-9.
[37] Leung WK, Chu CH, Mok MY, Yeung KW, Ng SK. Periodontal status of adults with systemic sclerosis: case-control study. *J. Periodontol.* 2011;82:1140-5.
[38] Mavragani CP, Moutsopoulos NM, Moutsopoulos HM. The management of Sjögren's syndrome. *Nat. Clin. Pract. Rheumatol.* 2006;2:252-61.
[39] Boutsi EA, Paikos S, Dafni UG, Moutsopoulos HM, Skopouli FN. Dental and periodontal status of Sjögren's syndrome. *J. Clin. Periodontol.* 2000;27:231-5.
[40] Schiodt M, Christensen LB, Petersen PE, Thorn JJ. Periodontal disease in primary Sjögren's syndrome. *Oral Dis.* 2001;7:106-8.
[41] Kuru B, McCullough MJ, Yilmaz S, Porter SR. Clinical and microbiological studies of periodontal disease in Sjögren syndrome patients. *J. Clin. Periodontol.* 2002;29:92-102.
[42] Jorkjend L, Johansson A, Johansson AK, Bergenholtz A. Periodontitis, caries and salivary factors in Sjögren's syndrome patients compared to sex- and age-matched controls. *J. Oral Rehabil.* 2003;30:369-78.
[43] Antoniazzi RP, Miranda LA, Zanatta FB, Islabao AG, Gustafsson A, Chiapinotto GA et al. Periodontal conditions of individuals with Sjögren's syndrome. *J. Periodontol.* 2009;80:429-35.
[44] Ergun S, Cekici A, Topcuoglu N, Migliari DA, Kulekci G, Tanyeri H et al. Oral status and *Candida* colonization in patients with Sjögren's Syndrome. *Med. Oral Patol. Oral Cir. Bucal.* 2010;15 e:310-5.
[45] Consensus Development Panel. (2001) Osteoporosis Prevention, Diagnosis and Therapy. National Institute of Health.

http://consensus.nih.gov/2000/2000Osteoporosis111html.htm. (Accessed on Jan 15, 2013).

[46] Lerner UH. Inflammation-induced bone remodeling in periodontal disease and the influence of post-menopausal osteoporosis. *J. Dent. Res.* 2006;85:596-607.

[47] Geurs NC. Osteoporosis and periodontal disease. *Periodontol. 2000.* 2007;44:29-43.

[48] Jeffcoat MK, Lewis CE, Reddy MS, Wang CY, Redford M. Post-menopausal bone loss and its relationship to oral bone loss. *Periodontol. 2000.* 2000;23:94-102.

[49] Wactawski-Wende J, Hausmann E, Hovey K, Trevisan M, Grossi S, Genco RJ. The association between osteoporosis and alveolar crestal height in postmenopausal women. *J. Periodontol.* 2005;76:2116-24.

[50] Brennan RM, Genco RJ, Hovey KM, Trevisan M, Wactawski-Wende J. Clinical attachment loss, systemic bone density, and subgingival calculus in postmenopausal women. *J. Periodontol.* 2007;78:2104-11.

[51] Palomo L, Liu J, Bissada NF. Skeletal bone diseases impact the periodontium: a review of bisphosphonate therapy. *Expert Opin. Pharmacother.* 2007;8:309-15.

[52] El-Shinnawi UM, El-Tantawy SI. The effect of alendronate sodium on alveolar bone loss in periodontitis (clinical trial). *J. Int. Acad. Periodontol.* 2003;5:5-10.

[53] Rocha ML, Malacara JM, Sanchez-Marin FJ, Vazquez de la Torre CJ. Fajardo ME. Effect of alendronate on periodontal disease in postmenopausal women: a randomized placebo-controlled trial. *J. Periodontol.* 2004;75:1579-85.

[54] Lane N, Armitage GC, Loomer P, Hsieh S, Majumdar S, Wang HY et al. Bisphosphonate therapy improves the outcome of conventional periodontal treatment: results of a 12-month, randomized, placebo-controlled study. *J. Periodontol.* 2005; 76:1113-22.

[55] National Kidney Foundation. (2002) K/DOQI clinical practice guidelines for chronic kidney disease: evaluation, classification, and stratification. *Am. J. Kidney Dis.* 39, S1-266.

[56] Davidovich E, Schwarz Z, Davidovitch M, Eidelman E, Bimstein E. Oral findings and periodontal status in children, adolescents and young adults suffering from renal failure. *J. Clin. Periodontol.* 2005;32:1076-82.

[57] Proctor R, Kumar N, Stein A, Moles D, Porter S. Oral and dental aspects of chronic renal failure. *J. Dent. Res.* 2005;84:199-208.

[58] Craig RG. Interactions between chronic renal disease and periodontal disease. *Oral Dis.* 2008;14:1-7.

[59] Ioannidou E, Kao D, Chang N, Burleson J, Dongari-Bagtzoglou A. Elevated serum interleukin-6 (IL-6) in solid-organ transplant recipients is positively associated with tissue destruction and IL-6 gene expression in the periodontium. *J. Periodontol.* 2006;77:1871-8.

[60] Spolidorio LC, Spolidorio DM, Massucato EM, Neppelenbroek KH, Campanha NH, Sanches MH. Oral health in renal transplant recipients administered cyclosporin A or tacrolimus. *Oral Dis.* 2006;12:309-14.

[61] Ronderos M, Ryder MI. Risk assessment in clinical practice. *Periodontol 2000.* 2004;34:120-35.

[62] Linden GJ, Mullally BH, Freeman R. Stress and the progression of periodontal disease. *J. Clin. Periodontol.* 1996;23:675-80.

[63] Genco RJ, Ho AW, Grossi SG, Dunford RG, Tedesco LA. Relationship of stress, distress and inadequate coping behaviors to periodontal disease. *J. Periodontol.* 1999;70:711-23.

[64] Hugoson A, Ljungquist B, Breivik T. The relationship of some negative events and psychological factors to periodontal disease in an adult Swedish population 50 to 80 years of age. *J. Clin. Periodontol.* 2002;29:247-53.

[65] Anttila SS, Knuuttila ML, Sakki TK. Relationship of depressive symptoms to edentulousness, dental health, and dental health behavior. *Acta Odontol. Scand.* 2001; 59:406-12.

[66] Persson GR, Persson RE, MacEntee CI, Wyatt CC, Hollender LG, Kiyak HA. Periodontitis and perceived risk for periodontitis in elders with evidence of depression. *J. Clin. Periodontol.* 2003;30:691-6.

[67] Schneider G, Leyendecker SS. Correlation between psychosocial factors and periodontal disease--a systematic review of the literature. *Z. Psychosom. Med. Psychother.* 2005;51:277-96.

[68] Preeja C, Ambili R, Nisha KJ, Seba A, Archana V. Unveiling the role of stress in periodontal etiopathogenesis: an evidence-based review. *J. Investig. Clin. Dent.* 2013, doi:10.1111/jicd.12000.

[69] Alzheimer's Disease International. 2013, Media quick facts - dementia. The gobal impact of dementia. http://www.alz.co.uk/media/dementia.html. (Accessed on Jan 15, 2013).

[70] Akiyama H, Barger S, Barnum S, Bradt B, Bauer J, Cole GM et al. Inflammation and Alzheimer's disease. *Neurobiol. Aging.* 2000;21:383-421.

[71] Mamelak M. Alzheimer's disease, oxidative stress and gammahydroxybutyrate. *Neurobiol. Aging.* 2007;28:1340-60.

[72] Ghezzi EM, Ship JA. Dementia and oral health. *Oral Surg. Oral Med. Oral Pathol. Oral Radiol. Endod.* 2000;89:2-5.

[73] Chalmers JM, Carter KD, Spencer AJ. Oral diseases and conditions in community-living older adults with and without dementia. *Spec. Care Dentist.* 2003;23:7-17.

[74] Jones JA, Lavallee N, Alman J, Sinclair C, Garcia RI. Caries incidence in patients with dementia. *Gerodontol.* 1993;10:76-82.

[75] Ship JA, Puckett SA. Longitudinal study on oral health in subjects with Alzheimer's disease. *J. Am. Geriatr. Soc.* 1994;42:57-63.

[76] Guncu GN, Tozum TF, Caglayan F. Effects of endogenous sex hormones on the periodontium-review of literature. *Aust. Dent. J.* 2005;50:138-45.

[77] Armitage GC. Bi-directional relationship between pregnancy and periodontal disease. *Periodontol. 2000.* 2013;61:160-76.

[78] Loe H, Silness J. Periodontal disease in pregnancy. I. Prevalence and severity. *Acta Odontol. Scand.* 1963;21:533-51.

[79] Silness J, Loe H. Periodontal disease in pregnancy. II. Correlation between oral hygiene and periodontal condtion. *Acta Odontol. Scand.* 1964;22:121-35.

[80] Arafat AH. Periodontal status during pregnancy. *J. Periodontol.* 1974;45:641-3.

[81] Tilakaratne A, Soory M, Ranasinghe AW, Corea SM, Ekanayake SL, de Silva M. Periodontal disease status during pregnancy and 3 months post-partum, in a rural population of Sri-Lankan women. *J. Clin. Periodontol.* 2000;27:787-92.

[82] Gursoy M, Pajukanta R, Sorsa T, Könönen E. Clinical changes in periodontium during pregnancy and post-partum. *J. Clin. Periodontol.* 2008;35:576-83.

[83] Machtei EE, Mahler D, Sanduri H, Peled M. The effect of menstrual cycle on periodontal health. *J. Periodontol.* 2004;75:408-12.

[84] Mariotti A. Sex steroid hormones and cell dynamics in the periodontium. *Crit. Rev. Oral Biol. Med.* 1994;5:27-53.

[85] Bergstrom J. Tobacco smoking and chronic destructive periodontal disease. *Odontol.* 2004;92:1-8.

[86] Jansson L, Lavstedt S. Influence of smoking on marginal bone loss and tooth loss-a prospective study over 20 years. *J. Clin. Periodontol.* 2002;29:750-6.

[87] Preber H, Bergstrom J. Cigarette smoking in patients referred for periodontal treatment. *Scand. J. Dent. Res.* 1986;94:102-8.

[88] Hyman JJ, Reid BC. Epidemiologic risk factors for periodontal attachment loss among adults in the United States. *J. Clin. Periodontol.* 2003;30:230-7.

[89] Johnson GK, Slach NA. Impact of tobacco use on periodontal status. *J. Dent. Educ.* 2001;65:313-21.

[90] James JA, Sayers NM, Drucker DB, Hull PS. Effects of tobacco products on the attachment and growth of periodontal ligament fibroblasts. *J. Periodontol.* 1999;70:518-25.

[91] Machuca G, Rosales I, Lacalle JR, Machuca C, Bullon P. Effect of cigarette smoking on periodontal status of healthy young adults. *J. Periodontol.* 2000;71:73-8.

[92] Johnson NW, Bain CA. Tobacco and oral disease. EU-Working Group on Tobacco and Oral Health. *Br. Dent. J.* 2000;189:200-6.

[93] Bergstrom J, Bostrom L. Tobacco smoking and periodontal hemorrhagic responsiveness. *J. Clin. Periodontol.* 2001;28:680-5.

[94] Rezavandi K, Palmer RM, Odell EW, Scott DA, Wilson RF. Expression of ICAM-1 and E-selectin in gingival tissues of smokers and non-smokers with periodontitis. *J. Oral Pathol. Med.* 2002;31:59-64.

[95] Huttner EA, Machado DC, de Oliveira RB, Antunes AG, Hebling E. Effects of human aging on periodontal tissues. *Spec. Care Dentist.* 2009;29:149-55.

[96] Papapanou PN, Wennstrom JL, Grondahl K. A 10-year retrospective study of periodontal disease progression. *J. Clin. Periodontol.* 1989;16:403-11.

[97] Ismail AI, Morrison EC, Burt BA, Caffesse RG, Kavanagh MT. Natural history of periodontal disease in adults: findings from the Tecumseh Periodontal Disease Study, 1959-87. *J. Dent. Res.* 1990;69:430-5.

[98] Norderyd O, Hugoson A, Grusovin G. Risk of severe periodontal disease in a Swedish adult population. A longitudinal study. *J. Clin. Periodontol.* 1999;26:608-15.

[99] Brown LF, Beck JD, Rozier RG. Incidence of attachment loss in community-dwelling older adults. *J. Periodontol.* 1994;65:316-23.

[100] Baelum V, Luan WM, Chen X, Fejerskov O. A 10-year study of the progression of destructive periodontal disease in adult and elderly Chinese. *J. Periodontol.* 1997; 68:1033-42.

[101] Albandar JM. Global risk factors and risk indicators for periodontal diseases. *Periodontol. 2000.* 2002;29:177-206.

[102] Nunn ME. Understanding the etiology of periodontitis: an overview of periodontal risk factors. *Periodontol. 2000.* 2003;32:11-23.

[103] Stanford TW, Rees TD. Acquired immune suppression and other risk factors/indicators for periodontal disease progression. *Periodontol. 2000*. 2003;32:118-35.

[104] Heitz-Mayfield LJ. Disease progression: identification of high-risk groups and individuals for periodontitis. *J. Clin. Periodontol.* 2005;32(6);196-209.

[105] Cheng HW, Yiu KY, Leung WK. Oral health in individuals with Down Syndrome. In: Dey, S., ed. Prenatal Diagnosis and Screening for Down Syndrome. InTech - Open Access Publisher, Rijeka, Croatia. Part 2. Dentistry and Skeletal features. Chapter 5, 2011;pp. 59-76.

[106] Desai SS. Down syndrome: a review of the literature. *Oral Surg. Oral Med. Oral Pathol. Oral Radiol. Endod.* 1997;84:279-85.

[107] Skrinjaric T, Glavina D, Jukic J. Palatal and dental arch morphology in Down syndrome. *Coll. Antropol.* 2004;28:841-7.

[108] Shaw L, Saxby MS. Periodontal destruction in Down's syndrome and in juvenile periodontitis. How close a similarity? *J. Periodontol.* 1986;57:709-15.

[109] Lopez-Perez R, Borges-Yanez SA, Jimenez-Garcia G, Maupome G. Oral hygiene, gingivitis, and periodontitis in persons with Down syndrome. *Spec. Care Dentist.* 2002; 22:214-20.

[110] Bradley C, McAlister T. The oral health of children with Down syndrome in Ireland. *Spec. Care Dentist.* 2004;24:55-60.

[111] Cichon P, Crawford L. Grimm WD. Early-onset periodontitis associated with Down's syndrome--clinical interventional study. *Ann. Periodontol.* 1998;3:370-80.

[112] Sakellari D, Belibasakis G, Chadjipadelis T, Arapostathis K, Konstantinidis A. Supragingival and subgingival microbiota of adult patients with Down's syndrome. Changes after periodontal treatment. *Oral Microbiol. Immunol.* 2001;16:376-82.

[113] Yoshihara T, Morinushi T, Kinjyo S, Yamasaki Y. Effect of periodic preventive care on the progression of periodontal disease in young adults with Down's syndrome. *J. Clin. Periodontol.* 2005;32:556-60.

[114] Cheng RH, Leung WK, Corbet EF. Non-surgical periodontal therapy with adjunctive chlorhexidine use in adults with Down syndrome: a prospective case series. *J. Periodontol.* 2008;79:379-85.

[115] Schlosser BJ, Pirigyi M, Mirowski GW. Oral manifestations of hematologic and nutritional diseases. *Otolaryngol. Clin. North Am.* 2011;44:183-203.

[116] Epstein JB, Lunn R, Le N, Stevenson-Moore P. Periodontal attachment loss in patients after head and neck radiation therapy. *Oral Surg. Oral Med. Oral Pathol. Oral Radiol. Endod.* 1998.86:673-7.

[117] Marques MA, Dib LL. Periodontal changes in patients undergoing radiotherapy. *J. Periodontol.* 2004;75:1178-87.

[118] Schwarz E, Chiu GK, Leung WK. Oral health status of southern Chinese following head and neck irradiation therapy for nasopharyngeal carcinoma. *J. Dent.* 1999;27:21-8.

[119] Hong CH, Napenas JJ, Hodgson BD, Stokman MA, Mathers-Stauffer V, Elting LS et al. A systematic review of dental disease in patients undergoing cancer therapy. *Support Care Cancer.* 2010;18:1007-21.

[120] Tezal M, Grossi GS, Ho AW, Genco RJ. Alcohol consumption and periodontal disease. The Third National Health and Nutrition Examination Survey. *J. Clin. Periodontol.* 2004;31:484-8.

[121] Ogawa H, Yoshihara A, Hirotomi T, Ando Y, Miyazaki H. Risk factors for periodontal disease progression among elderly people. *J. Clin. Periodontol.* 2002;29:592-7.

[122] Shepherd S. Alcohol consumption a risk factor for periodontal disease. *Evid. Based Dent.* 2011;12:76.

[123] EC - Clearinghouse on Oral Problems Related to HIV Infection and WHO Collaborating Centre on Oral Manifestations of the Immunodeficiency Virus. Classification and diagnostic criteria for oral lesions in HIV infection. *J. Oral Pathol. Med.* 1993;22:289-91.

[124] Barr C, Lopez MR, Rua-Dobles A. Periodontal changes by HIV serostatus in a cohort of homosexual and bisexual men. *J. Clin. Periodontol.* 1992;19:794-801.

[125] Yeung SC, Stewart GJ, Cooper DA, Sindhusake D. Progression of periodontal disease in HIV seropositive patients. *J. Periodontol.* 1993;64:651-7.

[126] Smith GL, Cross DL, Wray D. Comparison of periodontal disease in HIV seropositive subjects and controls (I). Clinical features. *J. Clin. Periodontol.* 1995;22:558-68.

[127] Cross DL, Smith GL. Comparison of periodontal disease in HIV seropositive subjects and controls (II). Microbiology, immunology and predictors of disease progression. J. *Clin. Periodontol.* 1995;22:569-77.

[128] Robinson PG, Boulter A, Birnbaum W, Johnson NW. A controlled study of relative periodontal attachment loss in people with HIV infection. *J. Clin. Periodontol.* 2000;27:273-6.

[129] Chapple IL, Hamburger J. The significance of oral health in HIV disease. *Sex Transm. Infect.* 2000;76:236-43.

[130] Timmerman LA, Clipstone NA, Ho SN, Northrop JP, Crabtree GR. Rapid shuttling of NF-AT in discrimination of Ca^{2+} signals and immunosuppression. *Nature.* 1996;383:837-40.

[131] Friskopp J, Klintmalm G. Gingival enlargement. A comparison between cyclosporine and azathioprine treated renal allograft recipients. *Swed. Dent. J.* 1986;10:85-92.

[132] Wondimu B, Dahllof G, Berg U, Modeer T. Cyclosporin-A-induced gingival overgrowth in renal transplant children. *Scand. J. Dent. Res.* 1993;101:282-6.

[133] Chu FC, Tsang PC, Chan AW, Leung WK, Samaranayake LP, Chan TM. Oral health status, oral microflora, and non-surgical periodontal treatment of renal transplant patients receiving cyclosporin A and FK506. *Ann. R. Australas Coll. Dent. Surg.* 2000;15:286-91.

[134] Pilgram TK, Hildebolt CF, Yokoyama-Crothers N, Dotson M, Cohen SC, Hauser JF et al. Relationships between longitudinal changes in radiographic alveolar bone height and probing depth measurements: data from postmenopausal women. *J. Periodontol.* 1999;70:829-33.

[135] Rodan GA. Mechanisms of action of bisphosphonates. *Annu. Rev. Pharmacol. Toxicol.* 1998;38:375-88.

[136] Fleisch H. Mechanisms of action of the bisphosphonates. *Medicina* (B Aires). 1997;57(1):65-75.

[137] Chavassieux PM, Arlot ME, Reda C, Wei L, Yates AJ, Meunier PJ. Histomorphometric assessment of the long-term effects of alendronate on bone quality and remodeling in patients with osteoporosis. *J. Clin. Invest.* 1997;100:1475-80.

[138] Devogelaer JP, Broll H, Correa-Rotter R, Cumming DC, De Deuxchaisnes CN, Geusens P et al. Oral alendronate induces progressive increases in bone mass of the

spine, hip, and total body over 3 years in postmenopausal women with osteoporosis. *Bone*. 1996;18:141-50.

[139] Brunsvold MA, Chaves ES, Kornman KS, Aufdemorte TB, Wood R. Effects of a bisphosphonate on experimental periodontitis in monkeys. *J. Periodontol*. 1992;63:825-30.

[140] Weinreb M, Quartuccio H, Seedor JG, Aufdemorte TB, Brunsvold M, Chaves E et al. Histomorphometrical analysis of the effects of the bisphosphonate alendronate on bone loss caused by experimental periodontitis in monkeys. *J. Periodontal Res*. 1994;29:35-40.

[141] Yaffe A, Golomb G, Breuer E, Binderman I. The effect of topical delivery of novel bisacylphosphonates in reducing alveolar bone loss in the rat model. *J. Periodontol*. 2000;71:1607-12.

[142] Meraw SJ, Reeve CM, Wollan PC. Use of alendronate in peri-implant defect regeneration. *J. Periodontol*. 1999;70:151-8.

[143] Drake MT, Clarke BL, Khosla S. Bisphosphonates: mechanism of action and role in clinical practice. *Mayo Clin. Proc*. 2008;83:1032-45.

[144] Cartsos VM, Zhu S, Zavras AI. Bisphosphonate use and the risk of adverse jaw outcomes: a medical claims study of 714,217 people. *J. Am. Dent. Assoc*. 2008;139:23-30.

[145] Kinane DF, Marshall GJ. Periodontal manifestations of systemic disease. *Aust. Dent. J*. 2001:46:2-12.

In: Current Trends in Periodontics and Implant Dentistry ISBN: 978-1-62618-819-8
Editors: Vishal Anand and Minkle Gulati

Chapter III

Genetic and Behavioral Risk Factors Associated with Periodontal Disease

*Andre Paes B. da Silva** *and Nabil F. Bissada*
Department of Periodontics,
CWRU School of Dental Medicine, Cleveland, OH, US

Abstract

Substantial evidence indicates that susceptibility to periodontal disease varies among patients and is modulated by both acquired and intrinsic risk factors. Genetic, systemic, medication induced, behavioral, and tooth-related local factors have been reported in various scientific investigations to be related to periodontitis. The central intent of this chapter is to discuss the genetic and behavioral risk factors associated with periodontitis. Polymorphism of genes that affect the expression of the inflammatory mediators might be associated with severity of periodontal diseases. It appears that there is at least a weak association between polymorphisms in the interleukin-1 genes and chronic periodontitis. As is the case for the association of smoking and periodontitis, cross-sectional and longitudinal studies provide strong epidemiologic evidence of a positive association between the two (2-8-fold increased risk for periodontal attachment loss and/or bone loss). Certain micronutrients such as antioxidants might be beneficial in periodontitis by downregulating proinflammatory cascades. Antioxidants such as vitamin C, E, GSH, folic acid, catechin (green tea), and melatonin have been associated with periodontal health. Stress might be associated with more severe periodontal disease and a poorer healing response to periodontal therapy. Furthermore, low levels of physical activity might be associated with an elevated prevalence of periodontitis. However, up till now no evidence documents that improved physical activity could influence the periodontal condition.

Keywords: Behavioral, genetic, risk factor

* Correspondence: Andre Paes B. da Silva, Department of Periodontics, CWRU School of Dental Medicine, 2124 Cornell Road, Cleaveland, OH 44106-4905.

Introduction

Susceptibility to periodontal disease varies among patients and is modulated by both acquired and intrinsic risk factors. A risk factor is defined as "any characteristic, behavior or exposure with an association to a particular disease. The relationship is not necessarily causal in nature. Genetic, systemic, medication-induced, behavioral, and tooth-related local factors are related to periodontitis. Studies have linked specific genetic markers to susceptibility towards periodontitis. Besides smoking, behavioral factors such as life style, physical exercise, diet, and stress have been related to periodontitis. The intent of this chapter is to discuss the genetic and behavioral risk factors associated with periodontitis.

The Influence of Genetics in Periodontal Diseases

The risk for periodontitis is not identical for all individuals. [1] There are a few factors that amplify the host response making people susceptible to increased severity of periodontitis. Studies of untreated disease in a Sri Lankan population identified three forms of disease progression. [2] Approximately 10% to 15% of the general U.S. population develops severe, destructive forms of periodontal diseases. [3] Investigations of twins indicated that part of the clinical characteristics of periodontitis may be explained by genetic factors. [4, 5]

Michalowicz et al. (2000) [5] suggested that due to genetic variations in immunologic host defenses an inherited factor to periodontitis may exist. In this study, dizygotic and monozygotic pairs of adult twins were evaluated clinically. Monozygotic twins were more similar than dizygotic twins for all clinical parameters measured, with estimations of adult periodontitis reaching 50% heritability. It was concluded that approximately half the change in disease in the population is due to genetic variance and not due to behavioral factors. The effects that host genes and the early family environment have on subgingival plaque were not apparent in adulthood. [6]

Host genes have been suggested to be important determinants in periodontal diseases. Certain animal strains show variable susceptibility to periodontitis. [7] In humans, genetic mutations of single genes can greatly increase susceptibility to periodontitis, as demonstrated by the association of severe periodontitis with a variety of disease conditions. [8] Also, there is evidence for smaller contributions by genes that may modify periodontal disease expression. [9] In contrast to simple genetic diseases that may be caused by a single genetic mutation, it is hypothesized that the collective effect of multiple genes is a determinant of disease susceptibility in complex diseases such as chronic periodontitis. [10] These genetic factors may involve more subtle changes that might slightly alter expression or function of a gene product. These are referred to as functional variants. Genetic variants that occur with a population prevalence of greater than 1% are termed genetic "polymorphisms", which are relatively frequent. In contrast, genetic mutations usually are rare, occurring with a frequency of much less than 1%. Polymorphism may occur in any part of the gene. Many of these polymorphisms may be functionally neutral, but others could have direct functional significance by affecting gene transcription, RNA stability, or the coded protein itself. Complex genetic diseases may result from the combined effect of multiple functional genetic polymorphisms interacting with each other and with environmental factors to such an extent that over time, they modulate disease risk. However, these polymorphisms sometimes are found in individuals with no evidence of disease and who may not be at great risk for disease. The correlation between genetic polymorphisms and disease is generally much weaker than the relationship between a functional mutation and disease phenotype. [11]

In periodontitis, most of the tissue destruction is due to the innate and adaptive immune reactions against periodontopathogenic microorganisms, leading to an inflammatory response. Diseases associated with anomalies of leucocyte and neutrophil function are examples of how genetic disorders involving inflammatory cells can cause disease. That high levels of host response mediators such as IL-1, TNF and PGE2 are correlated with periodontal destruction [12] and that these mediators are able to aggravate the inflammatory response [13] led to the hypothesis that some individuals may be "high-responders" i.e. they will respond to periodontal infection with the production of high levels of inflammatory mediators, which leads to progression of periodontal disease. Some individuals when challenged with LPS, will consistently respond with high production of IL-1 and TNF, whereas others will not. [14] Consequently, polymorphisms that modify immune reactions could determine individual differences. Such genetic variations characterize patients at high risk for the development of abnormal and devastating inflammatory responses. Since certain cytokines are key regulators of the inflammatory response and are important in periodontitis, it appears that there is a relationship between genetic polymorphisms associated with cytokine production and periodontitis severity. Polymorphism of genes that affect the expression of interleukin-1, interleukin-6, tumor necrosis factor, interleukin-10, E-selectins, Fc-gamma receptor, CD14, toll-like receptors, caspase recruitment domain 15, and vitamin D receptor might be associated with the appearance or the severity of periodontitis. However, most studies show variable and inconclusive correlations between the presence of disease markers and the tested single nucleotide polymorphisms in both the aggressive and chronic forms of periodontitis (Loos et al., 2005). [15]

Among the more studied genetic associations with periodontal disease is that of the IL-1 genotype. In clinical studies of periodontitis, when two of these IL-1 polymorphisms are found together, they were reported to be associated with severe chronic periodontitis in a non-smoking Caucasian population (over 40 years old). [16] This specific genotype is characterized by the presence of allele 2 in the polymorphic gene clusters IL-1A (- 889) and IL-1B (+ 13953), also referred to as "genotype-positive". In this study cigarette smoking appeared to diminish the genetic predisposition to an exaggerated host response so that a positive IL-1 genotype status had an effect on attachment loss only in nonsmokers. Moreover, it was shown that this specific composite IL-1 polymorphism was associated to the expression of elevated levels of IL-1 in crevicular fluid and gingival tissue. [17] Furthermore, a positive composite IL-1 genotype was shown to have some prognostic value for periodontal disease progression, assessed as clinical attachment loss or tooth loss when included in a multilevel risk-assessment model. [18, 19] IL-1 genotype-positive smokers and IL-1 genotype-positive subjects harboring P. gingivalis displayed increased probing depths over a five years span. [20] Also, an association between the positive composite IL-1 genotype and clinical indicators of periodontal disease deterioration has been reported. [21], In this context, knowledge of the IL-1 genotype status may prove helpful in customizing the frequency of supportive periodontal therapy, thereby reducing the risk for future disease progression or tooth loss. [22] In contrast to investigations that found an association between a positive IL-1 genotype and periodontitis, there are various investigations that rejected the presence of an association between the positive IL-1 genotype status and periodontal disease progression. [23-27] A systematic review revealed that there is a lack of evidence to support the use of the composite IL-1 genotype to discriminate subjects at risk for periodontal disease progression and/or to predict treatment outcomes. [22] In a more recent meta-analysis, it was suggested that there is a weak association between single nucleotide polymorphisms in the interleukin-1 genes and chronic periodontitis. [28]

Another genetic polymorphism associated with periodontal disease is in the Fc-gamma receptor genes. It has been reported to be the only polymorphism that seemed to be associated with periodontitis in different ethnic groups. [15] In an unrelated study, as per polymorphism in the IL-10 gene, there was an association between the occurrence of a single nucleotide polymorphism in the interleukin-10 gene in both chronic and aggressive forms of periodontitis (Hu et al., 2009). [29] These single nucleotide polymorphisms are functional in that the ATA / ATA genotype is associated with the aggressive form of periodontitis, and is also correlated with low levels of the immune response cytokine interleukin-10. [22] However, the Fc-gamma receptor and IL-10 gene polymorphisms were found in both chronic periodontitis and aggressive periodontitis and no difference could be identified between the clinical manifestations of the two diseases. [30, 31]

Advances in genetics have had a great impact on the focus of many studies on the association between inflammatory mediator's gene polymorphisms and periodontal diseases. However, the approach of finding a "target gene" may neglect additional genes involved in the exacerbated inflammatory response to the bacterial challenge. Moreover, Reichert (2008) [31] suggested that genetic confounders should be considered when evaluating the results based on a single-gene method.

The Influence of Smoking on Periodontal Diseases

Cigarette smoking has emerged as a significant risk factor for various forms of periodontal disease. Second to bacterial plaque, smoking is the most modifiable risk factor. The topic has been extensively reviewed and highlighted by various studies (more than 330) that have shown a relationship between smoking and periodontitis. [32-43]

Both cross-sectional and longitudinal studies provide strong epidemiologic evidence of a positive association between smoking and clinical and radiographic signs of periodontitis. [44] Smoking is associated with a 2-8-fold increased risk for loss of periodontal attachment and/or loss of bone. [45-43] The number of cigarettes smoked per day is a major risk-determining factor, doubling the risk for those in the lowest consumption category and increasing it six-fold in the subgroup smoking more than thirty cigarettes per day. [48] Furthermore, smokers have a higher prevalence of tooth loss and edentulism. Studies comparing smokers with nonsmokers displaying similar plaque levels showed deeper probing depths, increased loss of clinical attachment, gingival recession, alveolar bone loss, and teeth loss among current smokers, whereas the clinical signs of gingival inflammation were significantly less among smokers. [3, 49, 47, 50]

The association of smoking with periodontitis is significant when considering possible confounding factors. In the National Health and Nutrition Examination Survey (NHANES) III survey, which included 12,329 U.S. adults 20 years and older, current smokers were four times as likely to have periodontitis (defined as one or more sites with concomitant 4-mm probing depth and clinical attachment loss) compared to nonsmokers after adjusting for age, race or ethnicity, income, and educational level. Heavy smokers (31 cigarettes or more per day) had a greater risk than light smokers (nine or fewer cigarettes per day), with estimated odds ratios of 5.6 and 2.8, respectively. [51] Moreover, multivariate analysis, which takes into account various known confounding factors, indicated that smokers tend to have poorer oral hygiene and a lower socioeconomic status. These factors only partly accounts for the increase in the prevalence of periodontitis in smokers. [43] Former smokers were more likely to have periodontitis than persons who had never smoked. However, former smokers have lower rates of periodontitis than current smokers. [52]

As per the progression of periodontal disease, longitudinal studies indicate that periodontal disease may progress faster in smokers in comparison to non-smokers. [53, 54] In dentally aware subjects with high standards of oral hygiene, the amount of crestal bone loss among smokers was approximately three times that of nonsmokers over a 10-year period. [55] In contrast, in the Sri Lankan tea laborer population, smoking was not associated with progressive attachment loss. This observation may be explained by a lack of quantification of smoking exposure and a lack of oral hygiene and professional dental care. Moreover, long-term studies have shown that smoking is associated with the recurrence of periodontitis during periodontal maintenance. [56] Furthermore, the negative effect of smoking has been shown to be particularly marked in younger individuals. [57, 58, 43]

The role of tobacco in the pathogenesis of periodontal diseases may be explained by the influence of tobacco products on the periodontal microflora and the host response. Tobacco smoking has widespread systemic effects, many of which may provide mechanisms for the increased susceptibility to chronic destructive periodontal disease and the poorer response to treatment. [59, 44, 60] The mechanisms by which tobacco smoking might affect periodontal tissues are not fully understood, but possible mechanisms have been discussed in various review papers and are beyond the scope of this chapter. [34-36, 61]

The Influence of Nutrition on Periodontal Disease

Role of nutrition has been implicated in a number of inflammatory diseases and conditions, including cardiovascular diseases, type 2 diabetes, rheumatoid arthritis, and inflammatory bowel disease, all of which have been associated with periodontitis. [62] In periodontal disease, most tissue destruction results from an abnormal inflammatory immune response in patients predisposed to the condition. [63] Since traditional management approaches have been unsuccessful to diminish disease prevalence, the research emphasis has changed toward managing host-mediated inflammatory response. This section is focused in the role of nutrition in the development and resolution of inflammatory diseases, such as periodontitis. It has been demonstrated that subtle shifts in nutritional status are significantly associated with the prevalence of periodontitis. The results of animal and human studies have demonstrated the role of specific micronutrients in the modulation of the host's inflammatory response by reducing inflammatory biomarkers and bone loss. [64]

There are six major classes of nutrients: carbohydrates, fats, minerals, proteins, vitamins, and water. These nutrient classes can be categorized as either macro or micro nutrients. Macronutrients are needed in relatively large amounts, whereas micronutrients [vitamins, minerals, trace elements, amino acids, polyunsaturated fatty acids (PUFA)] that are required in only small quantities and are essential for optimal health, proper growth, and metabolism. [62] Macronutrients and micronutrients modulate proinflammatory and anti-inflammatory cascades, [65] which influence baseline inflammatory status. Nutrients act as molecular signals that are capable of modulating gene and protein expression at the molecular level. Therefore, it is conceivable that the downregulation of proinflammatory cascades by certain micronutrients such as antioxidants may be beneficial in periodontitis. [66] Antioxidants counteract oxidative stress and proinflammatory events. Reactive oxygen species (ROS) have been associated with the inflammatory response in periodontitis; if not buffered by sufficient (vitamins C, E, selenium, zinc, and cooper), these could increase damage to the periodontal tissue. [67] Thus, ROS promotes the use of the antioxidant vitamins and minerals during periodontal disease. Antioxidant micronutrients (carotenoids, polyphenols, bilirubin, GSH, uric acid, and melatonin) and non-antioxidant micronutrients such as the vitamin B group (niacin, folic acid), and omega-3 PUFAs, vitamin D and calcium have also been investigated in relation to periodontal disease. [64]

The beneficial effects of vitamin C during periodontitis have been investigated. In early studies no relationship could be measured between vitamin C and the severity of periodontal disease. [68, 69, 70] However, in more recent investigations an association has been found between vitamin C and periodontitis. In the NHANES I study, there was a weak but significant negative correlation between dietary vitamin C intake and periodontal disease after controlling for potentially confounding variables such as age, gender, race, education, income, and oral hygiene status (Ismail et al., 1983). [71] Another study found that the intake of vitamin C showed an inverse relationship to periodontal disease in current and former smokers. [72] In the NHANES III study, was shown a strong inverse association between serum vitamin C concentrations and the prevalence of periodontitis in adjusted models. The results of the last named study also showed that serum levels of vitamin C were inversely associated with periodontitis prevalence, even among persons who never smoked. [66] Amarasena et al. (2005) [73] showed in an elderly population of Japanese subjects an inverse relationship between serum vitamin C levels and attachment loss regardless of the confounding factors (smoking, diabetes, oral hygiene, gender, or number of teeth present). Moreover, there are lower levels of plasma vitamin C in periodontitis patients compared with periodontally healthy controls. [74-76] Furthermore, Pussinen et al. (2003) [77] demonstrated an inverse relationship between plasma vitamin C values and serum antibody levels to P. gingivalis (linear regression analysis adjusted for age, number of teeth and dental fillings, serum carbohydrate-deficient transferrin concentrations, and number of cigarettes smoked per day). In addition, Panjamurthy et al. (2005) [75] demonstrated lower plasma levels of vitamin C, vitamin E, and reduced glutathione (GSH) in periodontitis patients compared with healthy controls.

GSH is the key intracellular antioxidant redox-regulator of NF-κB. The functions of GSH include antioxidant defense and immune regulation. [78] Inflammatory states promote a decrease in the amount of systemic GSH levels. Therefore, GSH levels appear depleted in periodontitis and methods of enhancing intracellular GSH may prove beneficial. [79] The vitamins pyridoxal phosphate (B6) and riboflavin (B2) are important in maintaining GSH status. [80] In addition, dietary intake of other antioxidants, such as folic acid, also is associated with periodontal health. Multiple regression analysis showed that dietary folic acid was significantly correlated with bleeding on probing. [81] Furthermore, Kushiyama et al. (2009) [82] showed that the intake of green tea, which contains among other polyphenols catechin, was inversely correlated with mean pocket depth, mean clinical attachment level, and bleeding on probing. In a matched case control study, Gomez-Moreno et al. (2007) [83] showed that plasma levels of melatonin, a powerful antioxidant, were increased in patients with an advanced periodontal condition. Srinath et al. (2010) [84] also showed that the amount of melatonin in gingival crevicular fluid (GCF) was reduced in periodontitis patients compared to controls.

As per the non-antioxidants micronutrients associated with periodontal health, dietary intake of omega-3 (n-3) polyunsaturated fatty acids (n-3 PUFAs) increases tissue concentrations of fatty acids, such as eicosapentaenoic acid and docosahexaenoic acid that downregulate inflammation. [85] Eicosapentaenoic acid (EPA) and docoshexaenoic acid (DHA) are the primary metabolites of omega-3 fish oils. It has been suggested that n-3 PUFA metabolites may prevent neutrophil-mediated tissue damage. [86, 87] n-3 PUFAs also inhibit lipid mediators of inflammation, such as prostaglandin E2, arachidonic acid, 5-lipoxygenase and cyclo-oxygenase, modulate lymphokine production and increase antioxidant capacity. [88] In a recent clinical study the control group was treated with scaling and root planning (SRP) and placebo while the test group received SRP followed by dietary supplementation of fish oil (900mg EPA + DHA) and 81mg aspirin daily. It showed a significant reduction in pocket depth and attachment gain after 3 and 6 months in the test group compared with baseline and control group. The frequency of pockets over 4 mm was also reduced in the test group. [89] Vitamin D has also been associated with improvement of periodontal conditions. Dietrich et al. (2005) [90] indicated that vitamin D also has immune-modulatory functions by which it may reduce periodontitis predisposition. They showed that serum levels of 25(OH) D were associated with gingivitis and periodontal disease. [90, 91] Low dietary calcium and dairy products intake are associated with increased levels of periodontal disease. [72, 92] A clinical trial of calcium and vitamin D supplementation showed increased tooth retention after 3 years in the elderly people. [93] Since vitamin D and calcium metabolism are interlinked, and low dietary intake of calcium results in more severe periodontal disease, it is advised to evaluate daily calcium intake by patients. [62]

As is the case for macronutrients, periodontitis risk decreases with higher whole-grain intake after the data has been adjusted for age, smoking, BMI, physical activity, and alcohol and energy intakes. [94] Whole grains (brown rice, dark breads, whole-grain breakfast cereal, cooked cereal, popcorn, wheat germ, bran, etc) slow digestion and absorption of carbohydrates from the gut, which results in lower serum concentrations of glucose that are maintained over a long period. [1] In addition, whole-grain intake is associated with greater insulin sensitivity, [95] which in turn is associated with a lesser production of advanced glycation end-products, and consequently less oxidative stress, cytokine production, and possibly less periodontitis. [96] Furthermore, whole grains contain a number of substances known to affect health, including antioxidants, fiber, lignans, and phytoestrogens. A diet rich in whole grains lowers inflammatory biomarkers, [97] and fiber intake is inversely related to C-reactive protein. [98]

Periodontitis as an inflammatory disease may lead to systemic inflammation, which alters utilization of various nutrients. Some of these nutrients, such as vitamins and minerals play a direct role in inflammation. Increasing number of studies is addressing these nutrients importance to periodontitis. However, there is insufficient evidence to support these nutrients as monotherapies for periodontal disease. Interventional studies are needed to address this important area.

The Influence of Psychological Stress on Periodontal Disease

The detrimental role of stress on systemic health and wound healing has been well documented. [43] A stressor is any stimulus, situation, or circumstance with the possibility of prompting stress responses. Whether or not a subject exhibits a stress reaction is influenced by numerous factors, including coping behaviors, genetic predisposition, concomitant stressors, levels of social support, and other lifestyle factors. [99] Emotional stress, depression, anxiety, social isolation, socio-economic status, and personality factors are possibly associated with periodontal disease. [100-104] An increasing number of studies have been addressing the effect of psychological stress on the periodontium, on periodontal disease progression and on periodontal response to treatment, so that psychological stress is currently classified as a risk indicator for periodontal disease. [105, 46] Studies on psychosocial stress and periodontal disease identify many problems: various studies are cross-sectional, which sometimes deal with a relatively small sample; varying methods are used to define both psychosocial factors and periodontitis; the demographic of the population (age, gender, education level, race) and control of potential confounding variables (smoking, oral hygiene status) differ distinctly across studies. The main mechanisms by which psychosocial factors promote periodontal disease development have been classified in two main categories: (i) health-impairing behaviors (e.g., poor oral hygiene, increased tobacco and alcohol consumption, and poor nutritional intake; and (ii) pathophysiological factors that lead to higher glucocorticoid and catecholamine levels that indirectly disturb hormonal, inflammatory, and immunological profiles, leading to increased susceptibility to periodontal disease. [99, 106] Consequently, interference with the relationship between psychosocial factors and periodontal disease needs to be approached cautiously.

Two pathways have been suggested for the pathophysiological factors that link psychosocial stress to periodontal disease. First is through the deregulation of the immune system. This impairment is mainly through the hypothalamic– pituitary–adrenal and the sympathetic–adrenal medullary axes. [107] Stimulation of the hypothalamic–pituitary–adrenal axis by stress leads to the secretion of increased amounts of corticotropin-releasing hormone from the hypothalamus. In turn, this hormone, acts on the anterior pituitary, leading to the release of adrenocorticotropic hormone (ACTH). The ACTH then acts on the adrenal cortex and causes the production and release of glucocorticoid hormones (mainly cortisol). Glucocorticoids such as cortisol have numerous effects in humans, such as altering cytokine and growth factors profiles, suppressing the inflammatory response, and increasing blood glucose levels. [108, 109] The second major pathway stimulated by stress is the sympathetic nervous system. Stress activates the nerve fibers of the autonomic nervous system (flight or fight response to potentially harmful stimuli). The release of catecholamines results in the hormonal secretion of norepinephrine and epinephrine from the adrenal medulla, which may lead to modulation of immune responses. Under stressful circumstances, catecholamines contribute to the development of hyperglycemia by directly stimulating glucose production and interfering with the tissue disposal of glucose. [108] Also, it has been reported that the sympathetic nervous system influences the regulation of immune cell activities. [110] Consequently, hypersecretion of these hormones occurs during stressful stimuli, especially when it is prolonged (e.g., chronic anxiety states and depression), which may contribute to the pathogenesis of periodontal diseases.

The ability to cope with stressful life events may be more important than the stressful event itself. In studies that evaluated the relationship of stress, distress and inadequate coping behaviors, individuals with periodontitis or attachment and bone loss were at greater risk for severe periodontitis. [102, 111-113] A study reported that lifestyle and psychosocial stress might affect the periodontal status of diabetic patients. [114] Studies that controlled the confounding factors (oral hygiene, age, gender and smoking), reported that stress might play a role in the progression of periodontal disease. [111, 115, 116] However, other studies reported no indication for such associations. [117, 118] As in aggressive periodontitis, Davies et al. (1985) [119] noted that in some patients the disease appeared to be associated with stress and / or depression. The possible importance of stress in relation to the time of onset and rate of progression of idiopathic and rapidly progressing periodontitis also was suggested. [120] Moreover, Kamma and Baehni (2003) [122] monitored 25 patients with aggressive periodontitis over a period of five years and found that periodontitis progression was significantly associated with a number of factors including smoking and stress. In a review of the literature, it was found that patients in the generalized aggressive periodontitis group exhibit significantly increased depression and loneliness compared to the patients in the chronic periodontitis and control groups. [43]

In a systematic review, despite the different methodologies used in the included studies, stress had a positive association with periodontal disease. [103] Stabholz et al. (2010) [43] indicated that the role of stress in periodontal disease has a sound pathophysiological basis, supporting the current evidence that stress might be associated with severe periodontal disease and a poorer healing response to periodontal therapy. The significance of stress and coping behaviors on periodontitis progression requires further investigation.

The Influence of Physical Activity on Periodontal Disease

The protective effects of performing regular physical activity on the risk of coronary heart disease, hypertension, high cholesterol, obesity, diabetes mellitus, colon cancer, breast cancer, osteoporosis, arthritis, anxiety and depression are well-documented. [122-126] Among older adults, regular physical activity improves the quality of sleep, reduces depressive symptoms, and reduces the age-associated decline in cognitive ability. [127-129] Furthermore, physical activity was suggested to contribute to the management of anxiety and stress. [130]

An increasing number of reports address the relationship between physical activity and periodontitis. Earlier cross-sectional studies reported no association. [131, 132] However, these studies had a small sample size and a limited questionnaire about physical activity. In contrast, in one prospective cohort study, lower levels of physical activity were associated with a higher prevalence of periodontitis in men. [94] This study consisted of 39,461 male health professionals who were free of periodontitis at baseline. The results of this study showed a 13% reduction in the risk for developing periodontitis for men in the highest quintiles of physical activity as compared to men in the lowest quintiles independent of known risk factors for periodontitis. They reported that increased physical activity improves insulin sensitivity and glucose metabolism and may therefore impede the onset of periodontal disease. [94] In a cross-sectional study, an inverse association between physical fitness and periodontitis was reported. [133] In another study, it was shown that long-term physical inactivity is associated with a higher need for periodontal treatment. [134] Furthermore, Al-Zahrani et al. (2005) [135] showed a significant association between an increased level of physical activity and lower periodontitis prevalence in never and former smokers, whereas among current smokers the association was non-significant. Never smokers who met the recommended level of physical activity, at the time of NHANES III survey and who had similar activity levels for the 10 years before the survey, were about 54% less likely to have periodontitis than never smokers who did not engage in any physical activity. For former smokers, the prevalence of periodontitis was 74% lower for physically active compared to inactive individuals. In agreement, a more recent cross-sectional study showed that a low level of physical activity was significantly associated with increased odds of periodontal disease. [136] However, up till now no studies have utilized improved physical activity to influence the periodontal condition. [137]

There are four main possible mechanisms by which physical activity might protect against periodontitis:

1. By increasing sensitivity to insulin with its subsequent prevention of progression of type II diabetes, a recognized risk factor for periodontitis. Physical exercise was suggested to have a synergistic effect with insulin in enhancing glucose uptake into the cells, related to both increased blood flow and enhanced glucose transport to the muscle cell. [78]
2. By reducing inflammation; it has been reported that there is an inverse association between physical activity and the plasma level of inflammatory markers such as IL-1β, C-reactive protein. [98] This may be related to the physical activity improving both blood flow and efficiency of oxygen exchange.
3. By protecting against development of obesity. [135]
4. By reducing stress, which has been associated with higher periodontitis prevalence [102]

Conclusion

This chapter explores the major intrinsic (genetic) and acquired (behavioral, environmental) risk modulators that are associated with periodontal diseases. The risk modulators discussed were genetics, smoking, nutrition, psychological stress, and physical activity:

1. Polymorphism of genes that affect the expression of the inflammatory mediators (interleukin-1, interleukin-6, tumor necrosis factor, interleukin-10, E selectins, Fc-gamma receptor, CD14, toll-like receptors, caspase recruitment domain 15, vitamin D receptor) might be associated with severity of periodontal diseases. Among one of the most studied genetic associations with periodontal disease is that of the IL-1 genotype. It appears that there is at least a weak association between polymorphisms in the interleukin-1 genes and chronic periodontitis. Another polymorphism that appears to be associated with periodontal disease is in the Fc-gamma receptor genes and in the IL-10 gene. However, the search for a specific gene may end up neglecting other genes that have a lesser, but important role in the pathogenesis of periodontitis.
2. As is the case for the association of smoking and periodontitis, cross-sectional and longitudinal studies provide strong epidemiologic evidence of a positive association between the two (2-8-fold increased risk for periodontal attachment loss and/or bone loss). The number of cigarettes smoked per day appears to be a major risk-determining factor.
3. Certain micronutrients such as antioxidants might be beneficial in periodontitis by downregulating proinflammatory cascades. Various studies have shown the beneficial effect of vitamin C to periodontitis. Other antioxidants such as vitamin E, GSH, folic acid, catechin (green tea), and melatonin have also been associated with periodontal health. Furthermore, dietary intake of n-3 PUFAs increases tissue concentrations of fatty acids that downregulate inflammation. At this point, there is insufficient evidence to support recommendations of these nutrients as monotherapies for periodontal disease.
4. The psychological factors involved in the development periodontal diseases operate mainly via two mechanisms: (a) health-impairing behaviors (eg. poor oral hygiene, increased tobacco and alcohol consumption, and poor nutrition; and (b) pathophysiological factors that lead to higher glucocorticoid and catecholamine levels, which indirectly disturb hormonal and immunological profiles. Stress might be associated with more severe periodontal disease and a poorer healing response to periodontal therapy. The significance of stress and coping behaviors on periodontitis progression requires further investigation.
5. Low levels of physical activity might be associated with an elevated prevalence of periodontitis. However, up till now no evidence documents that improved physical activity could influence the periodontal condition. Long-term physical inactivity is associated with a higher need for periodontal treatment. Possible mechanisms include (i) increasing sensitivity to insulin; (ii) reducing inflammation; (iii) protecting against development of obesity; (iv) reducing stress.

References

[1] Jenkins WM, Kinane DF. The 'high risk' group in periodontitis. *Br. Dent. J.* 1989; 167(5):168-171.

[2] Loe H, Anerud A, Boysen H, Smith M. The natural history of periodontal disease in man. the rate of periodontal destruction before 40 years of age. *J. Periodontol.* 1978; 49(12):607-620.

[3] Papapanou PN. Periodontal diseases: Epidemiology. *Ann. Periodontol.* 1996;1(1):1-36.

[4] Michalowicz BS, Aeppli D, Virag JG et al. Periodontal findings in adult twins. *J. Periodontol.* 1991;62(5):293-299.

[5] Michalowicz BS, Diehl SR, Gunsolley JC et al. Evidence of a substantial genetic basis for risk of adult periodontitis. *J. Periodontol.* 2000;71(11):1699-1707.

[6] Michalowicz BS, Wolff LF, Klump D, et al. Periodontal bacteria in adult twins. *J. Periodontol.* 1999;70(3):263-273.

[7] Breivik T, Sluyter F, Hof M, Cools A. Differential susceptibility to periodontitis in genetically selected wistar rat lines that differ in their behavioral and endocrinological response to stressors. *Behav. Genet.* 2000;30(2):123-130.

[8] Hart TC. Genetic considerations of risk in human periodontal disease. *Curr. Opin. Periodontol.* 1994:3-11.

[9] Schenkein HA. Inheritance as a determinant of susceptibility for periodontitis. *J. Dent. Educ.* 1998;62(10):840-851.

[10] Hart TC, Kornman KS. Genetic factors in the pathogenesis of periodontitis. *Periodontol.* 2000. 1997;14:202-215.

[11] Michalowicz BS. Genetic risk factors for the periodontal diseases. *Compendium.* 1994;15(8):1036, 1038, 1040 passim.

[12] Offenbacher S, Odle BM, Van Dyke TE. The use of crevicular fluid prostaglandin E2 levels as a predictor of periodontal attachment loss. *J. Periodontal Res.* 1986;21(2):101-112.

[13] Gemmell E, Seymour GJ. Immunoregulatory control of Th1/Th2 cytokine profiles in periodontal disease. *Periodontol.* 2000. 2004;35:21-41.

[14] Molvig J, Baek L, Christensen P, et al. Endotoxin-stimulated human monocyte secretion of interleukin 1, tumour necrosis factor alpha, and prostaglandin E2 shows stable interindividual differences. *Scand. J. Immunol.* 1988;27(6):705-716.

[15] Loos BG, John RP, Laine ML. Identification of genetic risk factors for periodontitis and possible mechanisms of action. *J. Clin. Periodontol.* 2005;32 Suppl 6:159-179.

[16] Page RC, Kornman KS. The pathogenesis of human periodontitis: An introduction. *Periodontol.* 2000. 1997;14:9-11.

[17] Engebretson SP, Lamster IB, Herrera-Abreu M, et al. The influence of interleukin gene polymorphism on expression of interleukin-1beta and tumor necrosis factor-alpha in periodontal tissue and gingival crevicular fluid. *J. Periodontol.* 1999;70(6):567-573.

[18] McGuire MK, Nunn ME. Prognosis versus actual outcome. IV. the effectiveness of clinical parameters and IL-1 genotype in accurately predicting prognoses and tooth survival. *J. Periodontol.* 1999;70(1):49-56.

[19] Nieri M, Muzzi L, Cattabriga M, Rotundo R, Cairo F, Pini Prato GP. The prognostic value of several periodontal factors measured as radiographic bone level variation: A 10-year retrospective multilevel analysis of treated and maintained periodontal patients. *J. Periodontol.* 2002;73(12):1485-1493.

[20] Cullinan MP, Westerman B, Hamlet SM, et al. A longitudinal study of interleukin-1 gene polymorphisms and periodontal disease in a general adult population. *J. Clin. Periodontol.* 2001;28(12):1137-1144.

[21] De Sanctis M, Zucchelli G. Interleukin-1 gene polymorphisms and long-term stability following guided tissue regeneration therapy. *J. Periodontol.* 2000;71(4):606-613.

[22] Huynh Ba G, Lang NP, Tonetti MS, Salvi GE. The association of the composite IL-1 genotype with periodontitis progression and/or treatment outcomes: A systematic review. *J. Clin. Periodontol.* 2007;34(4):305-317.

[23] Ehmke B, Kress W, Karch H, Grimm T, Klaiber B, Flemmig TF. Interleukin-1 haplotype and periodontal disease progression following therapy. *J. Clin. Periodontol.* 1999;26(12):810-813.

[24] Christgau M, Aslanidis C, Felden A, Hiller KA, Schmitz G, Schmalz G. Influence of interleukin-1 gene polymorphism on periodontal regeneration in intrabony defects. *J. Periodontal Res.* 2003;38(1):20-27.

[25] Cortellini P, Tonetti MS. Long-term tooth survival following regenerative treatment of intrabony defects. *J. Periodontol.* 2004;75(5):672-678.

[26] Weiss OI, Caton J, Blieden T, Fisher SG, Trafton S, Hart TC. Effect of the interleukin-1 genotype on outcomes of regenerative periodontal therapy with bone replacement grafts. *J. Periodontol.* 2004;75(10):1335-1342.

[27] Konig J, Ruhling A, Plagmann HC, Meisel P, Kocher T. Influence of interleukin (IL)-1 composite genotype on clinical variables in non-smoking, well-maintained compliant patients with chronic periodontitis. *Swed. Dent. J.* 2005;29(1):11-16.

[28] Nikolopoulos GK, Dimou NL, Hamodrakas SJ, Bagos PG. Cytokine gene polymorphisms in periodontal disease: A meta-analysis of 53 studies including 4178 cases and 4590 controls. *J. Clin. Periodontol.* 2008;35(9):754-767.

[29] Hu KF, Huang KC, Ho YP, et al. Interleukin-10 (-592 C/A) and interleukin-12B (+16974 A/C) gene polymorphisms and the interleukin-10 ATA haplotype are associated with periodontitis in a taiwanese population. *J. Periodontal Res.* 2009; 44(3):378-385.

[30] Yamamoto K, Kobayashi T, Grossi S, et al. Association of fcgamma receptor IIa genotype with chronic periodontitis in caucasians. *J. Periodontol.* 2004;75(4):517-522.

[31] Reichert S, Machulla HK, Klapproth J, et al. The interleukin-10 promoter haplotype ATA is a putative risk factor for aggressive periodontitis. *J. Periodontal Res.* 2008;43(1):40-47.

[32] Bergstrom J. Influence of tobacco smoking on periodontal bone height. long-term observations and a hypothesis. *J. Clin. Periodontol.* 2004;31(4):260-266.

[33] Johnson GK, Hill M. Cigarette smoking and the periodontal patient. *J. Periodontol.* 2004;75(2):196-209.

[34] Kinane DF, Chestnutt IG. Smoking and periodontal disease. *Crit. Rev. Oral Biol. Med.* 2000;11(3):356-365.

[35] Rivera-Hidalgo F. Smoking and periodontal disease. A review of the literature. *J. Periodontol.* 1986;57(10):617-624.

[36] Rivera-Hidalgo F. Smoking and periodontal disease. *Periodontol.* 2000. 2003;32:50-58.

[37] Gelskey SC. Cigarette smoking and periodontitis: Methodology to assess the strength of evidence in support of a causal association. *Community Dent. Oral Epidemiol.* 1999; 27(1):16-24.

[38] Gustafsson A, Asman B, Bergstrom K. Cigarette smoking as an aggravating factor in inflammatory tissue-destructive diseases. increase in tumor necrosis factor-alpha

priming of peripheral neutrophils measured as generation of oxygen radicals. *Int. J. Clin. Lab. Res*. 2000;30(4):187-190.

[39] Haber J. Cigarette smoking: A major risk factor for periodontitis. *Compendium*. 1994;15(8):1002, 1004-8 passim; quiz 1014.

[40] Heikkinen AM, Pajukanta R, Pitkaniemi J, et al. The effect of smoking on periodontal health of 15- to 16-year-old adolescents. *J. Periodontol*. 2008;79(11):2042-2047.

[41] Laxman VK, Annaji S. Tobacco use and its effects on the periodontium and periodontal therapy. *J. Contemp. Dent. Pract*. 2008;9(7):97-107.

[42] Preber H, Kant T, Bergstrom J. Cigarette smoking, oral hygiene and periodontal health in swedish army conscripts. *J. Clin. Periodontol*. 1980;7(2):106-113.

[43] Stabholz A, Soskolne WA, Shapira L. Genetic and environmental risk factors for chronic periodontitis and aggressive periodontitis. Periodontol 2000. 2010;53:138-153.

[44] Khan S. Effect of smoking on periodontal health. *Dis. Mon*. 2011;57(4):214-217.

[45] Grossi SG, Genco RJ, Machtei EE, et al. Assessment of risk for periodontal disease. II. risk indicators for alveolar bone loss. *J. Periodontol*. 1995;66(1):23-29.

[46] Grossi SG, Genco RJ. Periodontal disease and diabetes mellitus: A two-way relationship. *Ann. Periodontol*. 1998;3(1):51-61.

[47] Calsina G, Ramon JM, Echeverria JJ. Effects of smoking on periodontal tissues. *J. Clin. Periodontol*. 2002;29(8):771-776.

[48] Jacob V, Vellappally S, Smejkalova J. The influence of cigarette smoking on various aspects of periodontal health. *Acta Medica* (Hradec Kralove). 2007;50(1):3-5.

[49] Haffajee AD, Socransky SS. Relationship of cigarette smoking to attachment level profiles. *J. Clin. Periodontol*. 2001;28(4):283-295.

[50] Muller HP, Stadermann S, Heinecke A. Gingival recession in smokers and non-smokers with minimal periodontal disease. *J. Clin. Periodontol*. 2002;29(2):129-136.

[51] Tomar SL, Asma S. Smoking-attributable periodontitis in the united states: Findings from NHANES III. national health and nutrition examination survey. *J. Periodontol*. 2000;71(5):743-751.

[52] van Winkelhoff AJ, Bosch-Tijhof CJ, Winkel EG, van der Reijden WA. Smoking affects the subgingival microflora in periodontitis. *J. Periodontol*. 2001;72(5):666-671.

[53] Winn DM. Tobacco use and oral disease. *J. Dent. Educ*. 2001;65(4):306-312.

[54] Beck JD, Cusmano L, Green-Helms W, Koch GG, Offenbacher S. A 5-year study of attachment loss in community-dwelling older adults: Incidence density. *J. Periodontal Res*. 1997;32(6):506-515.

[55] Bergstrom J. Tobacco smoking and chronic destructive periodontal disease. *Odontology*. 2004;92(1):1-8.

[56] Rieder C, Joss A, Lang NP. Influence of compliance and smoking habits on the outcomes of supportive periodontal therapy (SPT) in a private practice. *Oral Health Prev. Dent*. 2004;2(2):89-94.

[57] Schenkein HA, Gunsolley JC, Koertge TE, Schenkein JG, Tew JG. Smoking and its effects on early-onset periodontitis. *J. Am. Dent. Assoc*. 1995;126(8):1107-1113.

[58] Machuca G, Rosales I, Lacalle JR, Machuca C, Bullon P. Effect of cigarette smoking on periodontal status of healthy young adults. *J. Periodontol*. 2000;71(1):73-78.

[59] Ryder MI. The influence of smoking on host responses in periodontal infections. *Periodontol*. 2000. 2007;43:267-277.

[60] Fumarulo R, Cassano A, Mariggio MA. Exogenous factors in the immunotoxicity of oral PMN. *Immunopharmacol. Immunotoxicol.* 2011;33(1):1-10.

[61] Palmer RM, Wilson RF, Hasan AS, Scott DA. Mechanisms of action of environmental factors--tobacco smoking. *J. Clin. Periodontol.* 2005;32(Suppl 6):180-195.

[62] Van der Velden U, Kuzmanova D, Chapple IL. Micronutritional approaches to periodontal therapy. *J. Clin. Periodontol.* 2011;38(Suppl 11):142-158.

[63] Page RC, Kornman KS. The pathogenesis of human periodontitis: An introduction. *Periodontol.* 2000. 1997;14:9-11.

[64] Chapple IL. Potential mechanisms underpinning the nutritional modulation of periodontal inflammation. *J. Am. Dent. Assoc.* 2009;140(2):178-184.

[65] O'Keefe JH, Gheewala NM, O'Keefe JO. Dietary strategies for improving post-prandial glucose, lipids, inflammation, and cardiovascular health. *J. Am. Coll. Cardiol.* 2008; 51(3):249-255.

[66] Chapple IL, Matthews JB. The role of reactive oxygen and antioxidant species in periodontal tissue destruction. *Periodontol.* 2000. 2007;43:160-232.

[67] Moynihan P. The interrelationship between diet and oral health. *Proc. Nutr. Soc.* 2005; 64(4):571-580.

[68] Barros L, Witkop CJ Jr. Oral and genetic study of chileans 1960. III. periodontal disease and nutritional factors. *Arch. Oral Biol.* 1963;8:195-206.

[69] Russell AL, Leatherwood EC, Consolazio CF, Vanreen R. Periodontal disease and nutrition in south vietnam. *J. Dent. Res.* 1965;44:775-782.

[70] Enwonwu CO, Edozien JC. Epidemiology of periodontal disease in western nigerians in relation to socio-economic status. *Arch. Oral Biol.* 1970;15(12):1231-1244.

[71] Ismail AI, Burt BA, Eklund SA. Relation between ascorbic acid intake and periodontal disease in the united states. *J. Am. Dent. Assoc.* 1983;107(6):927-931.

[72] Nishida M, Grossi SG, Dunford RG, Ho AW, Trevisan M, Genco RJ. Calcium and the risk for periodontal disease. *J. Periodontol.* 2000;71(7):1057-1066.

[73] Amarasena N, Ogawa H, Yoshihara A, Hanada N, Miyazaki H. Serum vitamin C-periodontal relationship in community-dwelling elderly japanese. *J. Clin. Periodontol.* 2005;32(1):93-97.

[74] Staudte H, Sigusch BW, Glockmann E. Grapefruit consumption improves vitamin C status in periodontitis patients. *Br. Dent. J.* 2005;199(4):213-7, discussion 210.

[75] Panjamurthy K, Manoharan S, Ramachandran CR. Lipid peroxidation and antioxidant status in patients with periodontitis. *Cell Mol. Biol. Lett.* 2005;10(2):255-264.

[76] Amaliya, Timmerman MF, Abbas F et al. Java project on periodontal diseases: The relationship between vitamin C and the severity of periodontitis. *J. Clin. Periodontol.* 2007;34(4):299-304.

[77] Pussinen PJ, Laatikainen T, Alfthan G, Asikainen S, Jousilahti P. Periodontitis is associated with a low concentration of vitamin C in plasma. *Clin. Diagn. Lab. Immunol.* 2003;10(5):897-902.

[78] Schmidt AM, Hori O, Brett J, Yan SD, Wautier JL, Stern D. Cellular receptors for advanced glycation end products. implications for induction of oxidant stress and cellular dysfunction in the pathogenesis of vascular lesions. *Arterioscler. Thromb.* 1994;14(10):1521-1528.

[79] Chapple IL, Brock G, Eftimiadi C, Matthews JB. Glutathione in gingival crevicular fluid and its relation to local antioxidant capacity in periodontal health and disease. *Mol. Pathol.* 2002;55(6):367-373.
[80] Grimble RF. Nutritional modulation of cytokine biology. *Nutrition.* 1998;14(7-8):634-640.
[81] Esaki M, Morita M, Akhter R, Akino K, Honda O. Relationship between folic acid intake and gingival health in non-smoking adults in japan. *Oral Dis.* 2010;16(1):96-101.
[82] Kushiyama M, Shimazaki Y, Murakami M, Yamashita Y. Relationship between intake of green tea and periodontal disease. *J. Periodontol.* 2009;80(3):372-377.
[83] Gomez-Moreno G, Cutando-Soriano A, Arana C et al. Melatonin expression in periodontal disease. *J. Periodontal Res.* 2007;42(6):536-540.
[84] Srinath R, Acharya AB, Thakur SL. Salivary and gingival crevicular fluid melatonin in periodontal health and disease. *J. Periodontol.* 2010;81(2):277-283.
[85] Ziboh VA, Miller CC, Cho Y. Metabolism of polyunsaturated fatty acids by skin epidermal enzymes: Generation of antiinflammatory and antiproliferative metabolites. *Am. J. Clin. Nutr.* 2000;71(1 Suppl):361S-6S.
[86] Van Dyke TE, Serhan CN. Resolution of inflammation: A new paradigm for the pathogenesis of periodontal diseases. *J. Dent. Res.* 2003;82(2):82-90.
[87] Mori TA, Beilin LJ. Omega-3 fatty acids and inflammation. *Curr. Atheroscler. Rep.* 2004;6(6):461-467.
[88] Alam SQ, Bergens BM, Alam BS. Arachidonic acid, prostaglandin E2 and leukotriene C4 levels in gingiva and submandibular salivary glands of rats fed diets containing n-3 fatty acids. *Lipids.* 1991;26(11):895-900.
[89] El-Sharkawy H, Aboelsaad N, Eliwa M, et al. Adjunctive treatment of chronic periodontitis with daily dietary supplementation with omega-3 fatty acids and low-dose aspirin. *J. Periodontol.* 2010;81(11):1635-1643.
[90] Dietrich T, Nunn M, Dawson-Hughes B, Bischoff-Ferrari HA. Association between serum concentrations of 25-hydroxyvitamin D and gingival inflammation. *Am. J. Clin. Nutr.* 2005;82(3):575-580.
[91] Dietrich T, Joshipura KJ, Dawson-Hughes B, Bischoff-Ferrari HA. Association between serum concentrations of 25-hydroxyvitamin D3 and periodontal disease in the US population. *Am. J. Clin. Nutr.* 2004;80(1):108-113.
[92] Al-Zahrani MS. Increased intake of dairy products is related to lower periodontitis prevalence. *J. Periodontol.* 2006;77(2):289-294.
[93] Krall EA, Wehler C, Garcia RI, Harris SS, Dawson-Hughes B. Calcium and vitamin D supplements reduce tooth loss in the elderly. *Am. J. Med.* 2001;111(6):452-456.
[94] Merchant AT, Pitiphat W, Franz M, Joshipura KJ. Whole-grain and fiber intakes and periodontitis risk in men. *Am. J. Clin. Nutr.* 2006;83(6):1395-1400.
[95] Jenkins DJ, Wolever TM, Jenkins AL, et al. Low glycemic response to traditionally processed wheat and rye products: Bulgur and pumpernickel bread. *Am. J. Clin. Nutr.* 1986;43(4):516-520.
[96] Lalla E, Lamster IB, Schmidt AM. Enhanced interaction of advanced glycation end products with their cellular receptor RAGE: Implications for the pathogenesis of accelerated periodontal disease in diabetes. *Ann. Periodontol.* 1998;3(1):13-19.

[97] Esposito K, Marfella R, Ciotola M, et al. Effect of a mediterranean-style diet on endothelial dysfunction and markers of vascular inflammation in the metabolic syndrome: A randomized trial. *JAMA*. 2004;292(12):1440-1446.

[98] Ajani UA, Ford ES, Mokdad AH. Dietary fiber and C-reactive protein: Findings from national health and nutrition examination survey data. *J. Nutr*. 2004;134(5):1181-1185.

[99] Boyapati L, Wang HL. The role of stress in periodontal disease and wound healing. *Periodontol*. 2000. 2007;44:195-210.

[100] Ronderos M, Ryder MI. Risk assessment in clinical practice. *Periodontol*. 2000. 2004;34:120-135.

[101] Genco RJ, Ho AW, Kopman J, Grossi SG, Dunford RG, Tedesco LA. Models to evaluate the role of stress in periodontal disease. *Ann. Periodontol*. 1998;3(1):288-302.

[102] Genco RJ, Ho AW, Grossi SG, Dunford RG, Tedesco LA. Relationship of stress, distress and inadequate coping behaviors to periodontal disease. *J. Periodontol*. 1999;70(7):711-723.

[103] Peruzzo DC, Benatti BB, Ambrosano GM, et al. A systematic review of stress and psychological factors as possible risk factors for periodontal disease. *J. Periodontol*. 2007;78(8):1491-1504.

[104] Dumitrescu AL. Psychological perspectives on the pathogenesis of periodontal disease. *Rom. J. Intern. Med*. 2006;44(3):241-260.

[105] Genco RJ. Current view of risk factors for periodontal diseases. *J. Periodontol*. 1996;67(10 Suppl):1041-1049.

[106] Wiebe DJ, McCallum DM. Health practices and hardiness as mediators in the stress-illness relationship. *Health Psychol*. 1986;5(5):425-438.

[107] Yang EV, Glaser R. Stress-induced immunomodulation and the implications for health. *Int. Immunopharmacol*. 2002;2(2-3):315-324.

[108] Miller DB, O'Callaghan JP. Neuroendocrine aspects of the response to stress. *Metabolism*. 2002;51(6 Suppl 1):5-10.

[109] Takada T, Yoshinari N, Sugiishi S, Kawase H, Yamane T, Noguchi T. Effect of restraint stress on the progression of experimental periodontitis in rats. *J. Periodontol*. 2004;75(2):306-315.

[110] Ader R, Cohen N, Felten D. Psychoneuroimmunology: Interactions between the nervous system and the immune system. *Lancet*. 1995;345(8942):99-103.

[111] Hugoson A, Ljungquist B, Breivik T. The relationship of some negative events and psychological factors to periodontal disease in an adult swedish population 50 to 80 years of age. *J. Clin. Periodontol*. 2002;29(3):247-253.

[112] Wimmer G, Janda M, Wieselmann Penkner K, Jakse N, Polansky R, Pertl C. Coping with stress: Its influence on periodontal disease. *J. Periodontol*. 2002;73(11):1343-1351.

[113] Pistorius A, Krahwinkel T, Willershausen B, Boekstegen C. Relationship between stress factors and periodontal disease. *Eur. J. Med. Res*. 2002;7(9):393-398.

[114] Negishi J, Kawanami M, Terada Y, et al. Effect of lifestyle on periodontal disease status in diabetic patients. *J. Int. Acad. Periodontol*. 2004;6(4):120-124.

[115] Vettore M, Quintanilha RS, Monteiro da Silva AM, Lamarca GA, Leao AT. The influence of stress and anxiety on the response of non-surgical periodontal treatment. *J. Clin. Periodontol*. 2005;32(12):1226-1235.

[116] Hilgert JB, Hugo FN, Bandeira DR, Bozzetti MC. Stress, cortisol, and periodontitis in a population aged 50 years and over. *J. Dent. Res*. 2006;85(4):324-328.
[117] Castro GD, Oppermann RV, Haas AN, Winter R, Alchieri JC. Association between psychosocial factors and periodontitis: A case-control study. *J. Clin. Periodontol*. 2006; 33(2):109-114.
[118] Solis AC, Lotufo RF, Pannuti CM, Brunheiro EC, Marques AH, Lotufo Neto F. Association of periodontal disease to anxiety and depression symptoms, and psychosocial stress factors. *J. Clin. Periodontol*. 2004;31(8):633-638.
[119] Davies RM, Smith RG, Porter SR. Destructive forms of periodontal disease in adolescents and young adults. *Br. Dent. J*. 1985;158(12):429-436.
[120] Monteiro da Silva AM, Oakley DA, Newman HN, Nohl FS, Lloyd HM. Psychosocial factors and adult onset rapidly progressive periodontitis. *J. Clin. Periodontol*. 1996; 23(8):789-794.
[121] Kamma JJ, Baehni PC. Five-year maintenance follow-up of early-onset periodontitis patients. *J. Clin. Periodontol*. 2003;30(6):562-572.
[122] Joshi SB. Exercise training in the management of cardiac failure and ischaemic heart disease. *Heart Lung Circ*. 2007;16(Suppl 3):S83-7.
[123] Wendel Vos GC, Schuit AJ, Feskens EJ et al. Physical activity and stroke. A meta-analysis of observational data. *Int. J. Epidemiol*. 2004;33(4):787-798.
[124] Lau H, Fang C, Yuen WK, Patil NG. Risk factors for inguinal hernia in adult males: A case-control study. *Surgery*. 2007;141(2):262-266.
[125] Thune I, Furberg AS. Physical activity and cancer risk: Dose-response and cancer, all sites and site-specific. *Med. Sci. Sports Exerc*. 2001;33(6 Suppl):S530-50; discussion S609-10.
[126] Mehta KM, Yaffe K, Brenes GA, et al. Anxiety symptoms and decline in physical function over 5 years in the health, aging and body composition study. *J. Am. Geriatr. Soc*. 2007;55(2):265-270.
[127] King AC, Oman RF, Brassington GS, Bliwise DL, Haskell WL. Moderate-intensity exercise and self-rated quality of sleep in older adults. A randomized controlled trial. *JAMA*. 1997;277(1):32-37.
[128] Singh NA, Clements KM, Fiatarone MA. A randomized controlled trial of the effect of exercise on sleep. *Sleep*. 1997;20(2):95-101.
[129] Yaffe K, Barnes D, Nevitt M, Lui LY, Covinsky K. A prospective study of physical activity and cognitive decline in elderly women: Women who walk. *Arch. Intern. Med*. 2001;161(14):1703-1708.
[130] Paluska SA, Schwenk TL. Physical activity and mental health: Current concepts. *Sports Med*. 2000;29(3):167-180.
[131] Sakki TK, Knuuttila ML, Vimpari SS, Hartikainen MS. Association of lifestyle with periodontal health. *Community Dent. Oral Epidemiol*. 1995;23(3):155-158.
[132] Shizukuishi S, Hayashi N, Tamagawa H, et al. Lifestyle and periodontal health status of japanese factory workers. *Ann. Periodontol*. 1998;3(1):303-311.
[133] Wakai K, Kawamura T, Umemura O, et al. Associations of medical status and physical fitness with periodontal disease. *J. Clin. Periodontol*. 1999;26(10):664-672.
[134] Karjalainen S, Vanhamaki M, Kanto D, Kossi L, Sewon L, Salo M. Long-term physical inactivity and oral health in finnish adults with intellectual disability. *Acta Odontol. Scand*. 2002;60(1):50-55.

[135] Al Zahrani MS, Borawski EA, Bissada NF. Increased physical activity reduces prevalence of periodontitis. *J. Dent.* 2005;33(9):703-710.
[136] Bawadi HA, Khader YS, Haroun TF, Al-Omari M, Tayyem RF. The association between periodontal disease, physical activity and healthy diet among adults in jordan. *J. Periodontal Res.* 2011;46(1):74-81.
[137] Ramseier CA. Potential impact of subject-based risk factor control on periodontitis. *J. Clin. Periodontol.* 2005;32(Suppl 6):283-290.

In: Current Trends in Periodontics and Implant Dentistry ISBN: 978-1-62618-819-8
Editors: Vishal Anand and Minkle Gulati

Chapter IV

Gingival and Periodontal Diseases in Children

Nilesh Deshpande and Suruchi Nilesh Deshpande
Senior Lecturer, Department of Pedodontics and Preventive Dentistry,
Chhattisgarh Dental College and Research Institute, Sundra,
Rajnandgaon, Chhattisgarh, India

Abstract

Gingiva forms an important part of oral mucosa as well as periodontium. The prevalence of gingivitis in children is as high as 99% but periodontal diseases are not common. The control of gingivitis in young children by its early detection, treatment and prevention may be a realistic approach to the reduction of the prevalence and severity of periodontal disease in adulthood. Components of periodontium are same in childhood, adolescence and adulthood. Clinical and radiographic images differ owing to the significant changes that take place during growth and development. "The periodontium during childhood and adolescence is in a constant state eruption of teeth. This makes a general description of the normal periodontium difficult because it varies with the age of the patient". The chapter would cover detailed description about periodontium stating the differences in adulthood and childhood and also various gingival and periodontal diseases in children.

Keywords: Gingival disease, periodontal disease, children

Introduction

The gingiva forms an important part of the periodontium, the supporting structure of the tooth. In the maintenance of the tooth in the oral cavity, the health of the periodontium as a whole is of paramount importance.

The prevalence of gingivitis in children has been reported to be as high as 99%. The gingivitis occurring in the primary dentition tends to remain confined to the marginal gingiva for reasons yet unexplained. The shorter life span of the deciduous teeth may be the reason why little attention is paid to periodontitis in children. Also the rate of periodontal destruction in children may be much slower to cause a substantial loss of attachment within the life span of deciduous teeth. [1]

The control of gingivitis in young children is by its early detection and treatment. Prevention may be a realistic approach to the reduction of the prevalence and severity of periodontal diseases in adults. [2]

Features of Normal Periodontium in Children

The oral mucosa is the lining which separates the interior of the oral cavity from the complex underlying organs. It serves to protect these organs and to receive and transmit stimuli from the environment.

Gingiva

It is a masticatory type of oral mucous membrane that forms the covering of the teeth. It is divided into three zones for descriptive purposes.

Marginal Gingiva

The marginal gingiva includes the gingival crevice or the sulcus and a free gingival margin. The free gingival margin is thicker and rounder around the primary teeth than in the permanent teeth.

Attached Gingiva

It is firm and resilient and tightly bound to the underlying periosteum of the alveolar bone. In children, it appears less dense and redder than in adults due to less keratinized epithelium with its greater vascularity.

The two unique characteristics of the attached gingiva in children are the interdental clefts and the retrocuspid papilla.

Interdental Gingiva

The interdental gingiva occupies the gingival embrasure, which is the interproximal space beneath the area of tooth contact. The interdental gingiva can be pyramidal or have a "col" shape in the adult dentition which is more susceptible to infection.

Alveolar Mucosa

The thin epithelium and an absence of keratin make the alveolar mucosa redder than the pink gingiva. This tissue has abundance of elastic fibers and is readily movable. Its width increases with age and eruption of teeth.

Gingival Sulcus

The gingival sulcus is the shallow crevice or space around the tooth bounded by the surface of the tooth on one side, and the epithelium lining the free margin of the gingiva on the other.

The sulcus depth around the primary teeth is comparatively greater than that found around the permanent teeth. The mean values range from 1.4mm to 2.1mm.

Gingival Fluid (Sulcular Fluid)

The gingival sulcus contains a fluid that seeps into it from the gingival connective tissue through the thin sulcular wall. The gingival fluid is believed to

1 Cleans material from the sulcus,
2 Contain plasma proteins that may improve adhesion of the epithelium to the tooth.
3 Possess antimicrobial properties.
4 Exert antibody activity in defense of the gingiva.

Correlation of the Normal Clinical and Microscopic Features

Colour

The colour of the attached and marginal gingiva is generally described as coral pink and is produced by the vascular supply, the thickness and degree of keratinization of the epithelium and the presence of pigment containing cells.

Contour

The contour or shape of the gingiva varies considerably and depends upon the shape of the teeth and their alignment in the arch, the location and size of the area of proximal contact and the dimensions of the facial and lingual gingival embrasures.

Shape

The shape of the interdental gingiva is governed by the contour of the proximal tooth surfaces and the location and shape of gingival embrasures. Interdental clefting is a common feature in the primary dentition.

Consistency

Around the primary dentition, the marginal and the attached gingiva in children are very flaccid and retractable.

The diminished rigidity and increased retractability of the marginal gingiva around the primary teeth have several causes.

1 Immature connective tissue composition
2 Immature gingival fibers system
3 Increased vascularization

Surface Texture

The gingiva presents a textured surface like that of an orange peel and is referred to as being stippled. Stippling is best viewed by drying the gingiva. The attached gingiva is stippled; the marginal gingiva is not. The central portion of the interdental papillae is usually stippled, but the marginal borders are smooth. Stippling varies with age. It is absent in infancy, appears in some children at about 5 years of age, increases until adulthood, and frequently begins to disappear in old age.

Position

The position of gingiva refers to the level at which the gingival margin is attached to the tooth. When the tooth erupts into the oral cavity, the margin and sulcus are at the tip of the crown; as eruption progresses. They are seen closer to the root.

Periodontal Ligament

The periodontal ligament is the connective tissue structure that surrounds the root and connects it with the bone. It is continuous with the connective tissue of the gingiva and communicates with the marrow spaces through vascular channels in the bone.

Cementum

Cementum is the calcified mesenchymal tissue that forms the outer covering of the anatomic root.

Normal Microscopic Features

There are two main forms of root cementum Acellular (primary) and cellular (secondary). Both consist of a calcified interfibrillar matrix and collagen fibrils.

The Alveolar Process

The alveolar process is the bone that forms and supports the tooth sockets (alveoli). It forms when the tooth erupts in order to provide the osseous attachment to the forming periodontal ligament; it disappears gradually when the tooth is lost. [5, 6]

Classification of Gingival and Periodontal Diseases in Children

Many classifications were given on this, the latest being that based on the deliberations of the International Workshop for a Classification of Periodontal Diseases and Conditions (1999). [7]

Gingivitis

a Puberty gingivitis (hormones)
b Gingival overgrowth (drug therapy)
c Necrotizing ulcerative gingivitis (stress, smoking and other factors)

Periodontitis

a Chronic periodontitis (old term -adult periodontitis: slow progression)
  1 Localized
  2 Generalized
b Aggressive periodontitis (old term early onset forms)
  1 Generalized aggressive periodontitis (new term for generalized juvenile periodontitis)
  2 Localized aggressive periodontitis (new term for localized juvenile periodontitis)
c Incidental attachment loss (localized periodontitis that does not fit into chronic or aggressive forms)
d Necrotising ulcerative periodontitis (stress, smoking and other factors)
e Systemic disease forms
  1 Leukocyte disorders
  2 Neutropenia
  3 Chediak-Higashi syndrome
  4 Leukocyte adhesion deficiency syndrome
  5 Papillon- Lefevre syndrome vi) Down's syndrome
  6 Diabetes mellitus
  7 Hypophosphatasia
  8 Histiocytosis syndromes xl Ehlers-Danlos syndrome
  9 Juvenile hyaline fibromatosis of gingiva
  10 Acquired immunodeficiency syndrome

11 Virus associated hemophagocytic syndrome
12 Malnutrition

Gingival Diseases in Childhood

The effects of periodontal disease observed in adults have their inception earlier in life. Gingival disease in the child may progress to jeopardize the periodontium of the adult.

The developing dentition and certain systemic metabolic patterns are peculiar to childhood. There are also gingival and periodontal disturbances that occur more frequently in childhood and are therefore identified with this period. [8]

Chronic Inflammatory Enlargement

Periodontal diseases are present in almost all persons with natural teeth. From an early age gingivitis increases in its severity to peak at the onset of puberty. Gingival enlargement may result from chronic or acute inflammatory changes. The former is by far the more common cause.

Chronic marginal gingivitis is the most prevalent type of gingival change in childhood. The gingiva exhibits all the changes in color, size, consistency, and surface texture characteristic of chronic inflammation. Gingival color change and swelling appear to be more common expressions of gingivitis in children than are bleeding and increased pocket depth. The characteristics of gingivitis in preschoolers can be summarized as follows: [9]

1 Children experience gingivitis in varying amounts
2 Gingivitis does not appear to have any irreversible effects on the primary periodontium
3 Gingivitis in children is largely reversible
4 The severity of gingivitis in children is less than compared with that in adults with similar levels of the plaque

Etiology

Chronic inflammatory gingival enlargement is caused by a prolonged exposure to the dental plaque. Factors that favour plaque accumulation and retention [10] include poor oral hygiene, abnormal relationships of the adjacent teeth and opposing teeth, lack of tooth function, cervical cavities, overhanging margins of dental restorations, improperly contoured dental restorations or pontics, impaction, irritation from clasps or saddle areas of removable prostheses, nasal obstruction, orthodontic therapy involving repositioning of the teeth, and habits such as mouth breathing and pressing the tongue against the gingiva.

Clinical Features

Chronic inflammatory gingival enlargement in children is usually limited to marginal and papillary gingiva. Chronic inflammatory gingival enlargement originates as a slight ballooning of the interdental papilla and/or the marginal gingiva.

In the early stages it produces a life preserver-like bulge around the involved teeth. The enlargement is generally papillary or marginal and may be localized or generalized. It progresses slowly and painlessly unless it is complicated by acute infection or trauma. [11]

Treatment

Treatment of gingivitis is accomplished through oral prophylaxis. Sound oral hygiene practices are to be followed to prevent its recurrence. When oral hygiene is suspended in humans, gingivitis develops in 15-21 days. [12. 13]

Prognosis

Periodontitis is a progressive process and epidemiologically speaking. There appears to be a transition from childhood gingivitis to adult periodontitis.

But no cause and effect relation relationship has been demonstrated yet in humans. Rarely gingivitis progresses to periodontitis in prepubertal children.

Acute Inflammatory Enlargement

Gingival Abscess

A gingival abscess is a localized, painful, rapidly expanding lesion that is usually of sudden onset. It is generally limited to the marginal gingiva or interdental papilla. In its early stages it appears as a red swelling with a smooth, shiny surface. The adjacent teeth are often sensitive to percussion. If permitted to progress, the lesion generally ruptures spontaneously.

Etiology

Acute inflammatory gingival enlargement result from bacteria carried deep into the tissues when foreign substance such as a toothbrush bristle, piece of apple core, or a lobster shell fragment is forcefully embedded into the gingiva. [13]

Histology

The gingival abscess consists of a purulent focus in the connective tissue surrounded by a diffuse infiltration of the polymorph nuclear leukocytes, edematous tissue and vascular engorgement. [14]

Treatment

The gingival abscess is a lesion of the marginal or interdental gingiva, usually produced by an impacted foreign object. It is treated as follows.

Under topical anesthesia the fluctuant area of the lesion in incised with a Bard-Parker blade. And the incision is gently widened to permit drainage. The area is cleansed with warm, water and covered with a gauze pad. After bleeding stops, the patient is dismissed for 24 hours and intimated to rinse every 2 hours with a glassful of warm water. [15]

When the patient returns after 24 hours, the lesion is generally reduced in size and symptom free. A topical anesthetic is applied, and the area is scaled. If the residual size of the lesion is too great, it is removed surgically.

Acute Necrotising Ulcerative Gingivitis

Acute necrotizing ulcerative gingivitis (ANUG) has been defined as an acute recurring gingival infection of complex etiology, characterized by necrosis of the tips of the gingival papillae, spontaneous bleeding, and pain. [16]

Several names have been assigned to it such as Trench mouth, acute ulcerative gingivitis, Vincent's stomatitis, Vincent's angina, Plaut-Vincent's stomatitis, Fusospirocheatal gingivitis, Necrotic gingivitis, putrid stomatitis.

Etiology

The precise etiology of acute necrotizing ulcerative gingivitis is not known, but a great increase in fusiform bacilli and spirochetes is seen in smears from the lesions and clinical signs of this disease have been attributed to this increase in Fusospirocheatal complexes and other bacilli.

Both humoral and cellular immune responses have been described in the tissues during the development of acute necrotising ulcerative gingivitis although the precise immunopathogenesis is still not clear. [17]

Local Predisposing Factors

Various local factors include erupting teeth, inadequate restoration margins, calculus accumulation, open contacts, occlusal trauma, poor oral hygiene, pre-existing gingivitis, and smoking, of which the last three seem to be the most commonly prevalent. [18]

Systemic Predisposing Factors

Reports have related ANUG to periods of psychic conflicts, emotional stress in college students, stress of drug addiction and certain personality types. [18, 19, 20] Other general predisposing factors include:

Nutritional Deficiency

Individual deficiency in vitamin B complex, vitamin C complex. [21]

Debilitating Diseases

Blood dyscrasias, malnutrition, Down's syndrome, Chediak-Higashi syndrome, diabetes, AIDS. [22]

Clinical Features

The 3 criteria sufficient for a reliable diagnosis are:

1 Acute necrosis and ulceration of interproximal papillae
2 Pain
3 Bleeding

The presence of pseudo membrane is not an essential diagnostic sign. Thus,

Primary diagnostic signs

1 Gingival Bleeding
2 Pain
3 Interdental ulceration and necrosis
4 Elevated temperature with resultant blunting and cratering of gingiv

Secondary diagnositic signs

1 Pseudomembrane
2 Fetid mouth odor
3 Bad taste especially in the mandibular anteriors
4 Wooden sensation of the teeth

Extraoral and Systemic Symptoms

Patients are usually ambulatory and have a minimum of systemic complications. Local lymphadenopathy and a slight elevation in temperature are common features of the mild and moderate stages of the disease.

In severe cases there are marked systemic complications such as high fever, increased pulse rate, leukocytosis, loss of appetite, and general lassitude.

Systemic reactions are more severe in children. Insomnia, constipation, gastrointestinal disorders, headache, and mental depression sometimes accompany the condition.

Clinical Course

The clinical course is indefinite. If untreated, ANUG may result in progressive destruction of the periodontium and denudation of the roots, accompanied by an increase in the severity of toxic systemic complications. The disease may subside spontaneously without treatment.

Such patients generally have a history of repeated remissions and exacerbations. Recurrence of the condition in previously treated patients is also frequent. [23]

Treatment of Acute Necrotizing Ulcerative Gingivitis

The treatment of ANUG consists of the following phases: [24]

1 Local: Alleviation of the acute inflammation plus treatment of the chronic disease either underlying the acute involvement or elsewhere in the oral cavity.
2 Systemic:
    a Supportive treatment: Alleviation of generalized toxic symptoms, such as fever and malaise
    b Etiotropic treatment: The correction of systemic conditions that contribute to the initiation or progress of the gingival changes

Antibiotics are administered systemically only in patients with toxic systemic complications or local adenopathy. They are not recommended in ANUG patients who do not have these complications. The antibiotic of choice is penicillin. Patients who are allergic to penicillin should be given erythromycin. Metronidazole may also be used. [25]

Supportive Systemic Treatment

In addition to systemic antibiotics, supportive treatment consists of copious fluid consumption and administration of analgesics for relief of pain.

Herpetic Gingivostomatitis

The herpes simplex virus (HSV) is probably more widely distributed and more constantly present in the man than any other virus over 60% of people are infected with this virus and remain carriers throughout life. Two types of HSV have been seen to commonly infect humans: HSV-1 causing infections in the upper part of the body, and HSV-2 causing infections in the lower part of the body. [26]

Clinical Features

The primary infection usually occurs in a children 5 years of age who has had no contact with HSV-I and who therefore has no neutralizing antibodies. It is believed that 99% of all primary infections are of the subclinical type.

The infection also occurs in susceptible adults who may not have the primary infection. A prodrome consisting of focal itching, bun or tingling sensations on the lips may precede herpes labialis the duration of which ranges from days to 7 days. This may be preceded by stress exhaustion, strain, oral trauma, menstruation upset, pharyngitis, sinusitis, fever, and myalgia.

Oral Signs

The condition appears as a diffuse, erythematous shiny involvement of the gingiva and the adjacent oral mucosa, with varying degrees of oedema and gingival bleeding.

The ulcers may be observed on any area of the mucous membrane, including the buccal and labial mucosa, tongue sub-lingual mucosa, hard and soft palate, pharynx, and tonsillar areas. [26, 27]

Oral Symptoms

The disease is accompanied by generalized "soreness" of tile oral cavity, which interferes with eating and drinking. The ruptured vesicles are the focal sites of pain and are particularly sensitive to touch. Thermal changes, foods such as condiments and fruit juices, and other foods of acid content

Extraoral and Systemic Signs and Symptoms

Herpetic involvement of the lips or face (herpes labial is, "cold sore", with vesicles and surface scab formation, may accompany the intraoral disease. Cervical adenitis, fever as high as 101 to 105° F (38.3 to 40.6° C) and generalized malaise are common. [28] The symptoms of the disease develop suddenly and include malaise, irritability and headache.

Diagnosis

The diagnosis is usually established from the patient's history and the clinical findings. Material may be obtained from the lesions and submitted to the laboratory for confirmatory tests. [28]

- Tzanck smear is a rapid, fairly sensitive and inexpensive diagnostic method
- The isolation of the virus can be done in tissue culture or in the chorioallantoic membrane of the cluck embryo
- Antibody titers are useful in the diagnosis of primary infections only as in reinfections there is a little change in the antibody titer
- Stained sections of the vesicles of acute herpetic gingivostomatitis reveal eosinophllic intranuclear inclusion bodies in the peripheral cells

Treatment

Treatment of acute herpetic gingivostomatitis in children, which runs a course of 10 to 14 days, should be directed toward the relief of the acute symptoms so that fluid and nutritional intake can be maintained.

Application of a mild topical anaesthetic. Such as dyclonine hydrochloride (0.5%) (Dyclone). Before meal time will temporarily relieve the pain and allow the child to take a soft diet.

A mixture of equal parts of diphenhydramine (Binaural) elixir and Kaopectate can also be used An antihistaminic drug will often make the child more comfortable and may produce drowsiness, which will encourage rest. Acyclovir 5% ointment (Zovirax), a medication recommended for the treatment of primary genital herpes and for RHL in immunocompromised patients has been found to be useful in otherwise healthy patients as well.

Prognosis

With a high incidence of infection and no effective treatment or prophylaxis, patients are concerned regarding infection, since recent reports have associated HSV-2 with cervical cancer.

It is the risk of physicians to help prevent new infections by advising individuals how long an active infection may be potentially contagious to another person. [26, 27, 28]

Drug Induced Gingival Hyperplasia

Phenytoin-induced gingival hyperplasia (PGH) has been recognized as a distinct pathological entity for more than 40 years and is a common side effect of phenytoin treatment.

Early research showed an increase in the number of fibroblast in patients receiving Dilantin; thus the condition,"as termed dilantin hyperplasia. Now the term phenytoin induced gingival overgrowth (PIGO) is preferred. [29]

Prevalence

Increasing severity of degree of PGH is associated with:

a Decreasing age
b Decreasing weight in all subgroups
c Increasing dose of phenytoin per unit body weight
d Increasing trough serum phenytoin levels
e Increasing serum vitamin B12 levels
f Decreasing degree of oral hygiene

Etiology

The etiology of the condition has not been well defined. Several mechanisms have been implicated but not fully substantiated, [30] including-

a Disturbance in adrenocortical function resulting in an exaggerated response to tissue injury
b Direct action of phenytoin on fibroblasts
c Local response to metabolic products of phenytoin in saliva
d The etiology of phenytoin hyperplasia is now felt to be multifactorial

Clinical Features

PIGO when it does develop begins to appear as early as 2 to 3 weeks after initiation of phenytoin therapy and peaks at 18 to 21 months. The initial clinical appearance is a painless enlargement of the interproximal gingiva. The buccal and anterior segments are more affected than the lingual and posterior segments. The gingiva appears pink and firm and does not bleed easily upon probing.

As the interdental lobulations grow, clefting becomes apparent at the midline of the tooth. With time the lobulations coalesce at the midline, forming pseudopockets and covering more of the crown tooth. The epithelial level usually remains constant.

Treatment

Unfortunately, no cure exists and treatment is often symptomatic in nature. Antihistamines, topical corticosteroids, ascorbic acid, folic acid supplements, topical antibiotics, and alkaline mouthwashes have been used with a limited success and are considered to be ineffective [31]. Conservative periodontal measures include a vigorous gingival massage coupled with efficient tooth brushing and gum stimulators.

Specific surgical approaches for PIGO include gingivectomy with periodontal knives, laser or electrosurgery, and internal bevel flap surgery. The use of periodontal knives allows the tissue to heal more quickly, but more operative and postoperative bleeding occurs. Also it requires more time and patient cooperation. Electrosurgery is less time consuming, decreases blood loss, improves visibility, and allows superior control for areas of limited access is self sterilizing, does not always require periodontal packs.

Disadvantages include its contraindication in cardiac pacemakers, unpleasant odour, delayed healing and potential for error in application that results in an undesired bone or tissue loss. Other drugs which cause the gingival enlargement are nifedipine and cyclosporine.

Combined Enlargement

Combined enlargement results when gingival hyperplasia is complicated by secondary inflammatory changes. Gingival hyperplasia produces conditions favorable for the accumulation of the plaque and materia-alba by accentuating the depth of the gingival sulcus. The secondary inflammatory changes increase the size of the pre-existing gingival hyperplasia and produce a combined gingival enlargement.

Conditioned Enlargement

Conditioned enlargement occurs when the systemic condition of the patient exaggerates or distorts the usual gingival response to the dental plaque, and a corresponding modification of the usual clinical features of chronic gingivitis occurs. There are three types of conditioned gingival enlargements: hormonal, nutritional, or allergic. Nonspecific conditioned enlargement is also seen. [32, 33, 34]

Hormonal (E.G. Pubertal Gingivitis)

Clinical Features

- Gingival enlargement is found in the circumpubertal period
- It occurs in both male and female adolescents and appears in areas of local irritation
- Hormonal changes are reported
- The microbiota may also react
- The size of gingival enlargement far exceeds
- After puberty the enlargement undergoes a spontaneous reduction but does not disappear unit local irritants are removed

Treatment

Removing all sources of irritation, and controlling the plaque by means of scaling and curettage.

Surgical removal may be required in severe cases. The problem in these patients is recurrence due to poor oral hygiene

Nutritional (E.G. Scurvy)

Clinical Features

- Gingiva is bluish red soft and friable and has a smooth shiny surface
- Spontaneous or hemorrhage on slight provocation and surface necrosis
- In infants the enlarged tissue may cover the clinical crowns of the teeth
- Typical foul breath with fusospirochetal stomatitis is present
- Swelling of the periodontal membranes and loss of bone and loosening of the teeth which eventually exfoliate
- Sometimes ulceration and necrosis of the papillae present.

Treatment

Treatment includes ingestion of vitamin C tablets and diet rich in Vitamin C like citrus fruits.

Treatment of gingivitis includes oral prophylaxis and later on maintenance of oral hygiene.

Non Specific Enlargement (E.G. Granuloma Pyogenicum)

Clinical Features

- The lesion varies from a discrete spherical, tumor-like mass with a pedunculated attachment to a flattened keloid like enlargement with a broad base
- It is bright red or purple and either friable or firm depending on its duration, in the majority of cases it presents with surface ulceration and purulent exudation
- The lesion tends to involve spontaneously to become a fibroepithelial papilloma or persists relatively unchanged for years

Treatment

Treatment consists of removal of lesions plus the elimination of irritating local factors. The recurrence rate is about 15%

Allergic (E.G. Plasma Cell Gingivitis)

Clinical Features

- The use of drugs may evoke an allergic response manifested as an inflammatory reaction
- May be associated with generalized allergic response

Treatment

The stoppage of the drug generally reverses this condition; anti-allergic drugs.

Leukemia (Leukemic Enlargement)

Leukemia is disease characterized by the progressive overproduction of white blood cells, which usually appear in the circulating blood in an immature form.

Oral Manifestations

Oral lesions occur in both acute and chronic forms of all types of leukemia; myeloid, lymphoid and monocytic. These manifestations are far more common, however, in the acute stage of the disease and are most common in monocytic leukemia.

These primary clinical manifestations of the disease may consist of gingivitis, gingival hyperplasia, hemorrhage, petechiae and ulceration of the mucosa. [35]

- True leukemic enlargement occurs commonly in acute leukemia, but may also be seen in subacute leukemia. It seldom occurs in chronic leukemia.
- Leukemic enlargement may be diffused or marginal, localized or generalized. The gingiva is generally bluish red and has a shiny surface cyanotic, with a rounding and tenseness of the gingival margin, and then it increases in size, most often in the interdental papilla and covering partially the crowns of the teeth.
- Gingival hemorrhage is a common finding in leukemic patients, even in absence of clinically detectable gingivitis. The gingival hemorrhage, which commonly occurs, is due to ulceration of the sulcus epithelium and necrosis of underlying tissue. [35]

Treatment

The most common form of leukemia in children, acute lymphocytic leukemia, once almost always fatal within a few months, now has a prolonged remission and probable cure rate approaching 50%. This area of treatment is changing so rapidly with the introduction of new drugs and new techniques.

Bleeding and clotting times and platelet count of the patient should be checked and the hematologist consulted before periodontal treatment is instituted. After the acute symptoms subside, remove the irritating factors to control the inflammatory component of the enlargement. The enlargement is treated by scaling and curettage carried out in stages under topical anesthesia. The initial treatment consists of gently removing all loose accumulations with cotton pellets, superficial scaling, and instructing the patient in oral hygiene for plaque control

Antibiotics are administered systemically, the evening before and for 48 hours after each treatment to reduce the risk of infection.

Gingival Cyst

Gingival cysts of microscopic proportions are common, but they seldom reach a clinically significant size. When they do, they appear as localized enlargements that may involve the marginal and attached gingiva. They occur in the mandibular canine and premolar areas, most often on the lingual surface. They are painless, but with expansion they may cause erosion of the surface of the alveolar bone. The cysts develop from odontogenic epithelium or from surface or sulcular epithelium traumatically implanted in area. Removal is followed by uneventful recovery. [36]

Gingival Recession

The prevalence of gingival recession in children varies from 1% to 19% depending on the criteria used to assess the lesion. gingival recession in children with mixed dentition is found most commonly on the facial aspect of mandibular incisors, whereas in young adults the recession occurs more frequently on the facial of maxillary and mandibular first molar premolars, and canines there is agreement that malpositions of the teeth such as labial displacement and rotation predispose to localized gingival recession in children in this situation aggravating factors such as excessive tooth brushing plaque accumulation orthodontic treatment high muscle attachments and frenal pull, may cause or aggravate gingival recession.

A conservative approach to treatment should primarily be adopted after professional cleaning. If the lesion persists reparative surgical treatment should be considered and if the tooth is malpositioned orthodontic treatment is indicated.

Periodontitis in Children

Juvenile Periodontitis

JP is relatively an uncommon form of severe periodontal disease belonging to a group termed as an early onset aggressive periodontal disease.

Three different types of diseases have been delineated such as a) chronic slowly progressive, b) fairly generalized, and c) an acute progressive and more general.

JP can be classified as

1 Those occurring in otherwise healthy individuals
2 Those associated with a variety of diseases of other systems. The term localized is used with reference to the first group, although some cases may show a generalized involvement. Cases of the second type are termed generalized juvenile periodontitis, because the whole dentition is usually involved

Etiology

The etiology of juvenile periodontitis is still not completely clarified. There is general agreement that the disease always comprises an element of infection, and recent research tends to lend support to the hypothesis of specific infection. Because of higher prevalence in females than in males, a genetic basis has been suggested and numerous family reports consistent with genetic transmission have been published. [37]

Clinical Features

Initially losses of attachment and alveolar bone are seen around the permanent incisors and first molars, but with much individual variation and differing combinations of involved teeth. The attack sequence appears to follow eruption chronology.

The most striking feature is lack of clinical inflammation despite the presence of deep pockets. The disease starts as a localized form in the first molars and or incisors, and develops, if not treated, to the generalized form of the same disease, which resembles an adult periodontitis.

Distribution of lesions in the mouth is characteristic and as yet unexplained. The classic distribution is in the region of the first molars and incisors teeth, the least destruction in the cuspid-premolar area. Three types of bone loss localization have been defined.

1 First molar and/or incisors
2 First molars, incisors and some additional teeth (total of less than 14 teeth)
3 Generalized involvement

Premature and excessive mobility of the maxillary and mandibular primary incisors and first primary molars is seen. Regional lymphadenopathy as a clinical finding in about the third of the JP patients examined. Clinically, there is a small amount of plaque, forming a thin film on the tooth and rarely mineralizing to become calculus.

The most common initial symptoms are the mobility and migration of the first molars and the incisors.

Classically, one sees a distolabial migration of the maxillary incisors, with diastema formation, Along with anterior tooth migration, an apparent increase in the size of the clinical crown, accumulation of plaque and calculus, and clinical inflammation also appear. The disease progresses rapidly, the rate of bone loss is 3-4 times more than in typical periodontitis.

As the disease progresses, other symptoms may arise. Denuded root surfaces become sensitive to thermal and tactile stimuli.

Deep, dull, radiating pain may occur with mastication and is probably due to irritation of the supporting structures by mobile teeth and impacted food. Periodontal abscesses may form at this stage. [38]

Radiographic Findings

Vertical loss of alveolar bone around the first molars and incisors in otherwise healthy teenagers is taken to be a diagnostic sign of classic juvenile periodontitis.

Roentgenographic findings include "an arc-shaped loss of alveolar bone extending from the distal surface of the second premolar to the mesial surface of the second molar. [38]

Microbiology

Lesion is characterized by a rather distinct microbial population of rod-shaped organisms located predominantly at the base of the defect. Gram-negative anaerobe, Actinobacillus actinomycetemcomitans appears to be primarily associated with the disease. [39]

Immunology

Defective production or function of circulating neutrophils is often associated with an increased frequency and severity of bacterial infections. [38, 39]

Differential Diagnosis

Conditions that could contribute to alveolar bone loss in the primary dentition and premature loss of primary teeth: Hypophosphates, Papillon Lefevere syndrome, Histiocytosis X, neutropenia and cyclic neutropenia.

Treatment

Induction of tooth eruption by occ/lusal adjustment or passive eruption, root resection. Subgingival irrigation with iodine and hydrogen peroxide has also been proposed. Augmentation of scaling and root planning with surgical therapy.

The rationale for antibiotic coverage is based upon the concept that JP is an infection of bacterial etiology and its use has appeared to enhance osseous repair in JP patients.

Tetracycline is considered the drug of choice, since it has been shown to be effective against A. actinomycetemcomitans and achieves a gingival fluid level 2 to 10 times greater than the blood serum.

Papillon Lefevre Syndrome

In 1924 Papillon and Lefevre first described a syndrome characterized by hyperkeratosis of the palms and soles combined with a precocious periodontal destruction and shedding of the deciduous and permanent dentitions.

Etiology

The etiology of this syndrome is not clearly understood. Papillon and Lefevre thought it to be an endocrinopathy and suggested the possibility of vitamin A deficiency.

Recently, two new aspects of PLS have been discovered [40]

1 Deep Subgingival flora associated with PLS periodontitis is composed of great numbers of motile, Gram- negative anaerobic rods, including Bacteroides gingivalis and Capnocytophaga, as well as of a large number of spirochetes.
2 Some PLS patients have exhibited either a cellular immune defect with a decreased PHA stimulation of lymphocytes or a deficient chemotaxis and phagocytic function of neutrophilic granulocytes.

Clinical Features

The signs and symptoms of the Papillon-Lefevre syndrome include the following triad: [40]

a Hyperkeratosis palmer-plantar
b Precocious periodontal destruction with loss or both dentitions
c Ectopic intracranial calcifications (not a constant finding).

A. Skin Lesions

The skin lesions usually start between the first and fourth year after birth and consist principally of well demarcated, hyperkeratotic lesions of the palms and soles bilaterally.

B. Dental Signs and Symptoms

The deciduous dentition is normal in development and age of emption. But many cases have been reported where the deciduous dentition is affected. As soon as the last deciduous tooth has erupted, several features are seen: swollen gingiva, migration and mobility of teeth, periodontal pockets, fetor-ex-oris and exfoliation in a rather painless sequence. By 3 1/2 to 4 1/2 years all of the deciduous teeth are lost.

The emption of the permanent teeth is enhanced and may even be completed by 5 years of age (except the third molars). The disease progresses then recycle, and by ages 13 to 14 usually all of the erupted permanent teeth are exfoliated, Extracted teeth generally show a few hard and soft deposits.

C. Ectopic Intracranial Calcifications

Ectopic intracranial calcifications of the tentorium, falx cerebri and choroid plexus often form the third sign.

A marked predisposition for infections has been noted and also low blood hemoglobin has also been reported.

Intraoral radiographs show a severe horizontal alveolar bone loss almost immediately after the last deciduous tooth erupts. The unerupted teeth tend to assume abnormal positions. Incomplete root formation has been noted.

Differential Diagnosis

Clinically similar lesions involving both the deciduous and permanent dentitions may be seen in immune deficiency states such as acatalasia, Chediak Higashi syndrome and neutropenia. [41]

Treatment

Before the advent of retinoids, antibiotic therapy was advised, but not much success was achieved. Vitamin A metabolites (Retinoids) are involved in the regulation of growth and differentiation of the epithelial cells.

Prognosis

Despite some evidence of an increased susceptibility to general infection in the Papillon Lefevre syndrome, no metabolic or immunological deficiency has been detected and life expectancy is normal.

Hypophosphatasia

Hypophosphatasia is a rather rare genetic disease manifested by bone pain with spontaneous fractures, rickets-like bone lesions during childhood which are resistant to treatment with vitamin D, and premature loss of the deciduous teeth.

Etiology

Hypophosphatasia is a familial disorder of the inborn error of metabolism. There is strong evidence that most cases of the disease result from an autosomal recessive trait, although in other instances dominant inheritance is indicated. [41]

Clinical Features

The disease occurs in severe and mild forms, and at least three types are recognized. The infantile type first appears between birth and 6 months of age.

The childhood type appears between the ages of 6 and 14 months, and the adult type manifests during childhood and radiographically osseous radiolucencies are seen.

The disease is characterized by abnormal mineralization of bone and dental tissues and is usually manifested by premature exfoliation of the primary teeth. Approximately 75% of patients with this disorder experience premature exfoliation of the primary teeth, which is frequently the first clinical symptom of the disease.

Diagnosis

Reference ranges for alkaline phosphatase are also age-related, children and adolescents having higher circulating alkaline phosphatase activity than adults. A diagnosis of hypophosphatasia can usually be made with confidence in subjects with a consistent clinical history and physical findings in whom serum ALP activity is low.

Treatment

A wide variety of treatments for hypophosphatasia have been attempted but without a proven success. Oral phosphate supplements have been attempted with a limited success and intravenous infusions of plasma from patients with Paget's disease and hyperphosphatemia was also of no clinical benefit.

Histiocytosis X

The langerhans cell histiocytosis is associated with a tumor-like proliferation but there is insufficient evidence to consider them as truly neoplastic. There is a general consensus to believe that they are reactive disorders in which the proliferation of Langerhans cells results from disturbances in immunoregulation.

In the past these diseases were referred to as histiocytosis X and were subdivided into three variants:

Eosinophilic granuloma, Hand-Schuller-Christian disease, and Letterer-Siwe disease. But many investigations have confirmed that they are separate entities. [42]

The oral manifestations of Histiocytosis·X are ulcerative necrotizing lesions of the gingiva, root exposure, increased mobility of teeth, halitosis, osteolytic areas of alveolar bone in the radiographic examination giving the appearance of "floating teeth".

Cyclic Neutropenia

Several forms of neutropenia [42] associated with periodontal disease have been described. The disappearance of neutrophils occurs periodically, approximately every 3 weeks. After 5 to 8 days, the neutrophils begin to reappear. It is inherited as an autosomal recessive disorder. [43]

Clinical Features

These patients have periodic symptoms including skin lesions and ear infections. Mucous membrane ulcerations, severe stomatitis and a profound neutropenia are reported to develop over recurrent periods of 14 to 24 days (average 21).

Normal cycling patterns of approximately 21 days may not be seen, but in some cyclic neutropenic patients, cycles may have become progressively shorter with periods of neutrophil elevation.

The attached, papillary and marginal gingivas are enlarged, edematous and erythematous and bleed easily on a gentle provocation. There is an extreme inflammation with proliferation of the marginal gingiva accompanied by a cleft formation, recession; antibiotics are ineffective and bone resorption progresses rapidly to the apex of the teeth.

Overall, the destruction exceeds repair and alveolar bone loss contributes to an early exfoliation of teeth.

Diagnosis

The absence of neutropenia on a hematological examination cannot completely exclude the possibility of it being present since the analysis may have been completed during a non-neutropenic cycle of the disease.

Prognosis

Prognosis, both medically and dentally is not encouraging. The patients are at a risk of an over whelming and fatal bacterial infection during the severe neutropenia cycles.

Etiology

Existing evidence indicates that prepubertal periodontitis tends to occur in families, and that it is considerably more common in females than in males. These observations suggest that the defect is based on an X-linked pattern of inheritance.

The defect might have been acquired and might have resulted from an inhibition of chemotaxis derived from the periodontal bacteria.

Clinical Features

The pattern of the disease is variable. The exact time of onset has not been established. The evidence indicates that the disease being around the age of 4 years or before, but it may not be diagnosed until 7 to 9 years.

Generalized Form

- Extremely acute inflammation is present, with proliferation of the gingiva
- There is a very rapid destruction of the alveolar bone and gingiva

- Profound functional defects of peripheral blood neutrophils and monocytes are seen; neutrophil are absent from the gingival tissue
- Peripheral blood white-cell count is marked elevated
- Otitis media and skin and upper respiratory infections are frequent findings
- Periodontitis may be refractory to antibiotic therapy
- All primary teeth are affected; the permanent dentition may or may not be affected

Localized Form

- Only some teeth are affected; pattern of involvement yet not determined
- Gingival tissues may exhibit little or no inflammation
- Destruction is not as rapid as in the generalized form
- Functional defects are present in either neutrophils or monocytes, but not both
- Recurrent otitis media is nota frequent finding and usually there is no history of frequent infections
- The disease is amenable to treatment by curettage and antibiotic therapy

Diagnosis

Analysis of the pocket flora, assessment of blood leukocyte chemotaxis and serum antibodies, combined with measurement of the serum and urinary biochemical markers for hypophosphatasia may provide a definitive diagnosis of the condition, as well as clarify the relationship between the two diseases.

Treatment

Curettage, antibiotic therapy, and improved oral hygiene arrest the progression of localized prepubertal periodontitis. Tetracycline is an important adjunct for a successful treatment of the early onset periodontitis, particularly for the non surgical management cases.

Success in resolving the inflammation by combining extraction of the hopeless molars with an aggressive plaque control can be obtained. [43, 44]

Prognosis

The final outcome of the generalized prepubertal periodontitis is not known. The presence of prepubertal periodontitis may or may not be a harbinger of periodontitis of the permanent dentition.

On the basis of cases described to date, it appears that prepubertal periodontitis may be followed either by a completely normal permanent dentition, or by periodontitis of the permanent first molars and incisors, or by a generalized severe periodontitis of the permanent teeth.

Risk Assessment

According to epidemiologic studies the most prevalent form of EOP among adolescents is characterized by minimal loss of attachment at one or two sites. Longitudinal clinical studies show that the initial alveolar bone loss is a predictor of future rate of bone loss.

Subgingival calculus has been shown to be the factor that is most strongly correlated to progression of alveolar bone loss in several studies. Children with subgingival calculus or early signs of alveolar bone loss should be considered as patents at risk for periodontal and involved in a preventive program.

Abnormalities in the host response, expressed as suppressed chemotaxis and phagocytosis of systemic disease such as neutropenia, Down syndrome and HIV infection are all conditions that are associated with an impairment of the host response and are risk factors for EOP.

It is important to take a complete medical history of the patient and assess if there is a hereditary trean within the family.

The dental team should perform the risk assessment of the child based on the patient's medical history as well as clinical and radiographic criteria of the disease. The assessment should include the occurrence of systemic disease, subgingival calculus andeanty sign of initial alveolar bone loss. [44]

Prevention

The basic content in the prevention strategy is to educate and motivate children to establish proper oral hygiene procedures tooth brushing at a frequency of twice a day introduced at a time point when the first tooth is erupted should be a routine already at the time but eruption of the primary molar. In preschool children the oral hygiene program should be focused on mechanical plaque removal by using a toothbrush.

Regarding interdental plaque removal the use of dental floss is recommended to be included in the daily oral hygiene procedure in teenagers. The patients have to be well instructed to avoid any harm to the gingival tissue including the dental papilla during flossing.

Adolescents have to be well educated about the cause of periodontal disease with special focus on supragingival and subgingival calculus formation and its importance as a risk factor for the initiation and progression of periodontal disease.

The well documented chemical antiplaque agent chlorhexadine can be used for a short time to reduce plaque accumulation and gingival inflammation for example in children undergoing orthodontic treatments.

The agent triclosan which is a nonionic phenol has been shown to have an inhibitory effect on genial inflammation in addition to what can be accounted for in the plaque reduction in 3 year double blind randomized controlled clinical trail conducted on adolescents it was shown that the use of a dentifrice containing triclosan(0.3%) reduced periodontal attachment loss significantly

Conclusion

The predominant form of periodontal disease in children and adolescents in gingivitis which is nonspecific inflammatory reaction of the marginal gingiva. The inflammatory reaction in the tissue initiated by dental plaque accumulation starts early during infancy and reflects the bacterial challenge to the host. In must children the process of gingival inflammation remains superficial.

Genetic factors that modify the host response to the bacterial challenge are major determinants of susceptibility to the development of EOP, and many systemic diseases have been reported to predispose children and adolescents to periodontal disease.

Dental professionally should rely on clinical and radiographic criteria of the disease for early identification of children at risk with special focus on the presence of subgingival calculus.

Children with overt gingival inflammation subgingival calculus or early signs of alveolar bone loss should be considered as periodontitis risk patients and should be included in a preventive program as early as possible.

References

[1] Hart, T. C., Kornman, K. S. Genetic factors in the pathogenesis of periodontitis. *Periodontol*. 2000. 2000;14:202-15.

[2] Moore, W., Holdeman, L., Smibert, R., et al. Bacteriology of experimental gingivitis in children. *Infect. Immun*. 1984;46:1-6.

[3] Van Dyke, T. E., Levine, M. J., Genco, R. J. Periodontal diseases and neutrophil abnormalities. In: Genco, R. J., Mergenhagen, S. E., eds. *Host-Parasite Interactions in Periodontal Diseases*. Washington, DC: American Society for Microbiology. 1982:235-45.

[4] Dennison, D. K., Van Dyke, T. E. The acute inflammatory response and the role of phagocytic cells in periodontal health and disease. *Periodontol*. 2000;14:54-78.

[5] Van Dyke, T. The role of neutrophils in host defence to periodontal infections. In: Hamada, S., Holt, S., McGhee, J., eds. *Periodontal Disease: Pathogens and Host Immune Responses*. Tokyo: Quintessence Publishing Co; 1991:251-61.

[6] Delaney, D. E., Kornman, K. S. Microbiology of subgingival plaque from children with localized prepubertal periodontitis. *Oral Microbiol. Immunol*. 1987;2:71-6.

[7] International Workshop for a Classification of Periodontal Diseases and Conditions. Papers. Oak Brook, Illinois, October 30-November 2, 1999. *Ann. Periodontol*. 1999;4(i):1-112.

[8] Harley, A. F., Floyd, P. D. Prevalence of juvenile periodontitis in school children in Lagos, Nigeria. *Community Dent. Oral Epidemiol*. 1988;16: 299-301.

[9] Brown, L. J., Löe, H. Prevalence, extent, severity and progression of periodontal disease. *Periodontol*. 2000. 1993;2:57-71.

[10] McHugh, W. D., McEwen, J. D., Hitchin, A. D. Dental disease and related factors in 13-year-old children in Dundee. *Br. Dent. J*. 1964;117: 246-53.

[11] Kelly, J. E., Sanchez, M. J. Periodontal disease and oral hygiene among children. United States. *Vital Health Stat*. 1972;11(117):1-28.

[12] Nakagawa, S., Fujii, H., Machida, Y., Okuda, K. A longitudinal study from prepuberty to puberty of gingivitis. Correla-tion between the occurrence of *Prevotella intermedia* and sex hormones. *J. Clin. Periodontol*. 1994;21:658-65.

[13] Slots, J., Moenbo, D., Langebaek, J., Frandsen, A. Microbiota of gingivitis in man. *Scand. J. Dent*. 1978;86:174-81.

[14] American Academy of Periodontology. "Parameter on acute periodontal diseases. American Academy of Periodontology". *J. Periodontol*. 2000; 71 (5 Suppl.):863–6.

[15] American Academy of Periodontology. "Consensus report: Abscesses of the Periodontium". *Ann. Periodontol*. 1999;4(1):83.

[16] Taiwo, J. O. Severity of necrotizing ulcerative gingivitis in Nigerian children. *Periodontal. Clin. Investig.* 1995;17:24-7.

[17] Contreras, A., Falkler, W. A. Jr, Enwonwu, C. O., et al. Human Herpes viridae in acute necrotizing ulcerative gingivitis in children in Nigeria. *Oral Microbiol. Immunol.* 1997;12:259-65.

[18] Loesche, W. J., Syed, S. A., Laughon, B. E., Stoll, J. The bacteriology of acute necrotizing ulcerative gingivitis. *J. Periodontol.* 1982;53:223-30.

[19] Listgarten, M. Electron microscopic observations on the bacterial flora of acute necrotizing ulcerative gingivitis. *J. Periodontol.* 1965;36:328-39.

[20] Horning, G., Cohen, M. Necrotizing ulcerative gingivitis, periodontitis, stomatitis: Clinical staging and predisposing factors. *J. Periodontol.* 1995;66:990-8.

[21] Enwonwu, C. O. Epidemiological and biochemical studies of necrotizing ulcerative gingivitis and noma (cancrum oris) in Nigerian children. *Arch. Oral Biol.* 1972;17:1357-71.

[22] Jimenez, L. M., Baer, P. N. Necrotizing ulcerative gingivitis in children: A 9-year clinical study. *J. Periodontol.* 1975;46:715-20.

[23] Pindborg, J. J., Bhat, M., Devanath, K. R., Narayana, H. R., Ramachandra, S. Occurrence of acute necrotizing gingivitis in South Indian children. *J. Periodontol.* 1966;37:14-9.

[24] Johnson, B., Engel, D. Acute necrotizing ulcerative gingivitis. A review of diagnosis, etiology and treatment. *J. Periodontol.* 1986;57:141-50.

[25] Van Winkelhoff, A. J., Rams, T. E., Slots, J. Systemic antibiotic therapy in periodontics. *Periodontol.* 2000. 1996;10:45-78.

[26] Slots, J. Herpes viruses in periodontal diseases. *Periiodontology* 2000. 2005;38:33-62.

[27] Scully, C. New aspects of oral viral diseases. In: Seifert, G., ed. *Oral Pathology: actual diagnostic and prognostic aspects*. Current Topics in Pathology, vol 90. Berlin: Springer Verlag, 1996:29-96.

[28] Porter, S. R., Mutlu, S., Scully, C. M. Viral infections affecting periodontal health. *Periodont. Clin. Invest.* 1993;15:17-24.

[29] Shafer, W. G., Hine, M. K., Levy, B. M. A *Textbook of Oral Pathology,* 4th edn. Philadelphia: WB Saunders, 1983: 760–800.

[30] Behjat, K. H. M., Gier, R. E. Common and less common gingival overgrowth conditions. *J. Periodontol.* 1995;56:46–48.

[31] Hassell, T. M., Hefti, A. F. Drug-induced gingival overgrowth: old problem, new problem. *Crit. Rev. Oral Biol. Med.* 1991;2:103-137.

[32] Sooriyamoorthy, M., Gower, D. B. Hormonal influences of gingival tissue: relationship to periodontal disease. *Journal of Clinical Periodontology.* 1989;16:201-08.

[33] Touyz, L. Z. Oral scurvy and periodontal disease. *J. Can. Dent. Assoc.* 1997;53:837-845.

[34] Neville, B. W., Damm, D. D., Allen, C. M., Bouquot, J. E. *Oral and maxillofacial pathology.* 2nd ed, 2002:WB Saunders, Philadelphia, 437-495

[35] Tjwa, E., Mattijssen, V. Images in clinical medicine. Gingival hypertrophy and leukemia. *N Engl. J. Med.* 2008;359:e21

[36] Kahn, Michael A. *Basic Oral and Maxillofacial Pathology.* Volume 1. 2001.

[37] Donly, K. J., Ashkenazi, M. Juvenile periodontitis: A review of pathogenesis, diagnosis, and treatment. *J. Clin. Pediatr. Dent.* 1992;16: 73-8.

[38] Kornman, K. S., Robertson, P. B. Clinical and microbiological evaluation of therapy for juvenile periodontitis. *J. Periodontol.* 1985;56: 443-6.

[39] Van Dyke, T., Levine, M., Tabak, L., Genco, R. Reduced chemotactic peptide binding in juvenile periodontitis: A model for neutrophil function. *Biochem. Biophys. Res. Commun.* 1981;100:1278-84.

[40] Gorlin, R. J., Sedano, H., Anderson, V. The syndrome palmar-plantar hyperkeratosis and premature periodontal destruction of teeth. A clinical and genetic analysis of the Papillon-Lefévre syndrome *J. Pediatr.* 1964; 65:895-908.

[41] Deasy, M. J., Vogel, R. I., Macedo-Sobrinho, B., Gertzman, G., Simon, B. Familial benign chronic neutropenia associated with periodontal disease. A case report. *J. Periodontol.* 1980;51:206-10.

[42] Moore, W., Moore, L. The bacteria of periodontal diseases. *Periodontol.* 2000. 1994;5:66-77.

[43] Baehini, P. C., Payot, T., Tsai, C. C., Cimasoni, G. Periodontal status associated with chronic neutropenia. *J. Clin. Periodontol.* 1983;10:222-30.

[44] Andrews, R. G., Benjamin, S., Shore, N., Canter, S. Chronic benign neutropenia of childhood with associated oral manifestations. *Oral Surg. Oral Med. Oral Pathol.* 1965;20:719-25.

In: Current Trends in Periodontics and Implant Dentistry
Editors: Vishal Anand and Minkle Gulati
ISBN: 978-1-62618-819-8

Chapter V

Periodontitis: Risk Factor for Systemic Diseases

Ana Pejcic and Draginja Kojovic
Periodontology and Oral Medicine, Medical Faculty, University of Nis, Serbia

Abstract

There is accumulating evidence that periodontal infections could influence overall health and the course of some systemic diseases. Periodontal disease is characterized by inflammation and bacterial infection of the gums surrounding the teeth.

The bacteria that are associated with periodontal disease can travel into the bloodstream and consequently to other parts of the body, and that puts health at risk. People think of gum disease in terms of their teeth, but they don't think about the fact that gum disease is a serious infection that can release bacteria into the bloodstream resulting in additional health risks in people whose health is already affected by other diseases or leading to serious complications like heart disease.

Periodontal medicine is a term used for different purposes in different parts of the world. In certain countries, it relates to the study of the dynamic relationship between periodontitis and systemic conditions, such as cardiovascular and cerebrovascular disease, pre-term labour and low-birth-weight babies, diabetes mellitus, osteoporosis and disorders of respiratory tract.

Such studies investigate the peripheral impacts of periodontal inflammation on systemic health and also the influence of systemic diseases on the progression of chronic periodontitis such as type II diabetes mellitus, where evidence exists for a bi-directional relationship with periodontitis.

In the other countries, “periodontal medicine” is a term used to describe the periodontal (and gingival) manifestations of medical conditions. This includes their investigation, diagnosis and therapeutic management and how management of the oral conditions integrates with the patient’s medical management as a part of a holistic approach within defined care pathways.

The text is a comprehensive analysis of research on periodontitis and its link to systemic conditions. It supports what many scientists have suspected for years-oral infections such as periodontal disease can adversely affect conditions outside the mouth.

The basis of periodontal medicine is treating periodontitis to preserve the structure, function and esthetics of the dentition, which will further prevent any untoward affects on a patient's over all health. Periodontology brought awareness and education to the public of the fact that infections in the mouth can cause health problems in other parts of the body as well.

Periodontal diseases have been linked to diabetes, heart disease, osteoporosis, preterm births, stroke, respiratory disease and renal disease.

Periodontal medicine is the emergence of a new branch of periodontology. The goal of the campaign will be to educate patients about periodontal infection and its associated general health risks. Oral health is often a good indicator of what is happening in the rest of the body. Therefore, a visit to a periodontist may benefit more than an older person's gums. It is important for patients to have regular oral check-ups to not only maintain oral health, but to identify possible risks for serious medical conditions.

Keywords: Periodontitis, systemic disease, risk factors

Introduction

The term "periodontal medicine" can be viewed as a term that defines a branch of periodontology focusing on a strong relationship between periodontal health or disease and systemic health or disease. For decades, physicians and dentists have paid close attention to their own respective fields, specializing in medicine pertaining to the body and in dentistry to the oral cavity, respectively. However, recent findings have strongly suggested that oral health may be indicative of systemic health. Currently, this gap between allopathic medicine and dental medicine is quickly closing, due to significant findings supporting the association between oral infections and systemic conditions such as cardiovascular disease, diabetes mellitus, adverse pregnancy outcomes, and osteoporosis. [1]

An association between oral infections and systemic diseases has been suspected for centuries. Over the past decade, a growing body of scientific evidence has suggested an exquisite association between periodontal disease and systemic diseases and also between systemic disease and periodontal diseases. [2] This means a two-way relationship in which periodontal disease in an individual may have a powerful influence on an individual's systemic health or disease as well as the role of systemic disease which may have influence on an individual's periodontal health or disease. [3]

The oral systemic connection is the phenomenon created by the fact that the most recent and compelling research demonstrates a clear, causal connection between periodontal disease and heart attack, stroke, pre-mature birth, diabetes and other serious health problems.

For a number of these conditions, identification and management of oral manifestation not only proactively addresses potential periodontal problems but also enhances patient's awareness of medical issues. Additionally, proper treatment of periodontal disease has been shown to reduce these risk factors.

While many different diseases affect the tooth-supporting structures, plaque-induced inflammatory lesions make up the vast majority of periodontal diseases and have traditionally been divided into two categories: gingivitis and periodontitis. [4] Gingivitis is a disease that refers to inflammation of the gums, in which the most apical portion of the junctional epithelium is on the enamel, or at or near the cemento-enamel junction.

While in some sites or individuals, gingivitis never progresses to periodontitis, data indicates that gingivitis always precedes periodontitis. [5]

Periodontal disease is a type of disease that affects one or more periodontal tissues: gingiva, alveolar bone, periodontal ligament and cementum. Periodontitis occurs when the periodontal ligament, the connective tissue that attaches the tooth to alveolar bone is destroyed by the inflammatory process. Periodontal disease often reflects serious health risks. Mild inflammation of the gums (gingivitis) can be prevented by regularly brushing and flossing teeth to remove plaque (build up of a film on teeth). This stops the development of calculus (hardened accumulation of plaque at the gum line), which can only be removed by dental cleaning.

More serious infection, called periodontitis, can cause not only disease of the gums, but loss of teeth and the bone structures that support the teeth.

Periodontitis, one of the most common diseases of humans, is an infectious condition that can result in the inflammatory destruction of periodontal ligament and alveolar bone. In light of the extensive microbial plaque associated with periodontal infections, the chronic nature of these diseases, and the exuberant local and systemic host response to microbial assault, it is reasonable to hypothesize that these infections may influence overall health and the course of some systemic diseases. [5]

Periodontal Disease and Cardiovascular Disease

Infectious disease can cause changes at distant body sites. The oral cavity is a portal of entry for microbial infections. So, the mouth can become a source of disease or pathological processes affecting other parts of the body and general health status.

Cardiovascular diseases (CVDs) are a great health problem in today's society of industrialized countries and they are highly prevalent among the adult population and constitute one of the first causes of mortality in men as well as women in the western world. According to the World Health Organization (WHO), cardiovascular disease is responsible for 20% of the world population mortality rate. [6]

The most common cause of cardiovascular diseases is coronary arterial obstruction, in most cases secondary to atherosclerosis. Atherosclerosis of the coronary arteries produces narrowing or occlusion of the vascular lumen, which in turn leads to deficient cardiac irrigation and an increased risk of anginal chest pain or acute myocardial infarction. [7]

Atherosclerosis is present in 90% of all cases of CVD. Atherosclerosis is hardening and thickening of the vascular wall and mainly affects the intimae layer of the thoracic or abdominal aorta and its branches, including the coronary arteries, together with the renal, cerebral and peripheral arteries of the lower limbs. [8]

The early atherosclerotic lesion consists of a yellowish and slightly elevated lipid striation composed of subendothelial accumulations of foam cells (macrophages filled mainly with cholesterol). These striations may either disappear spontaneously or evolve towards elevated fibrous plaques composed of a dense layer of hypertrophic smooth muscle cells and connective tissue surrounding a necrotic center or core of cell remains, cholesterol crystals and foam cells, macrophages and lymphocytes. [9]

The factors which favor the development of atherosclerosis include patient's age and sex, hypercholesterolemia, smoking, diabetes mellitus, a sedentary lifestyle and chronic infection. [10] The risk factors can be non modifiable such as the sex or age and other modifiable such as cholesterol levels, arterial hypertension, a smoking habit, educational level, chronic infections and others. Arterial hypertension is, together with a smoking habit and hypercholesterolema, one of the main risk factors in the development of ischemic heart diseases and the main risk factor for cerebrovascular events.

Interest has recently increased in the relationship between CVD and different infectious processes as triggering factors. Among the chronic infections which have been related to such risks are cytomegaloviruses (CMV), Helicobacter pylori and Chlamydia pneumoniae. [11] However, some patients develop no coronary complications despite the presence of such risk factors. This may be attributable to environmental or genetic factors which induce inter-individual variations in susceptibility to ischemic pathology.

Periodontitis is one of the most common chronic bacterial infection disease of the oral cavity which leads to local inflammation and cause the destruction of the supporting structures of the dentition. The oral cavity contains almost half of commensal bacteria in the human body-approximately six billion microbes representing 300 to 500 species. [12]

In certain conditions, some of these microorganisms may become opportunistic species that contribute to local or systemic infections. Periodontitis is initiated by Gram-negative pathogens organized as a biofilm, whose presence elicits a host inflammatory response. Acting as the prototypical endotoxin, lipopolysaccharides (LPS), a major component of the outer membrane of Gram-negative bacteria, initiate the cascade of events leading to periodontal tissue destruction. Briefly, LPS derived from plaque biofilms on the tooth root surface leads to the recruitment of polymorphonuclear leukocytes (PMNs) to the site. Monocytes and activated macrophages respond by releasing various proinflammatory cytokines, including interleukin 1β (IL-1β) and tumor necrosis factor- α (TNF-α), which, in turn, directs further destructive processes. [13]

Gingivitis represents the reversible inflammatory reaction to biofilms while periodontitis is the non-reversible destructive stage of a persistent bacterial infection. If left untreated, periodontitis results in soft tissue and progressive bone destruction and leads to tooth mobility and subsequent tooth loss.

The more severe form of the disease is present in approximately 10-15% of an adult population, whereas 35% exhibit moderate or mild signs of the disease. [14]

Periodontitis is believed to play an important role in different systemic disorders. It has been reported that the severity of periodontal pathology may be directly associated to the risk of coronary disease. [15]

It is strange to think that two such different groups of diseases such as the coronary and periodontal disease, without any apparent connection in their clinical and systemic severity pathogenesis, have been able to be related. Too much time has had to pass to understand that the mouth is not an isolated structure within the organism, and although the importance of the oral cavity is known in the field of human physiology and in certain groups of diseases, little is known about the relation of the characteristic infections of dental and periodontal tissues with other organs or systems in the human body. [16]

The mechanisms by which periodontitis contributes to cardiovascular disease have not been confirmed, but there are numerous working hypothesis that will be proved or disproved. [17]

A series of physiological or pathological conditions that relate closely to the development of cardiovascular disease (atherosclerotic complication) and periodontal disease share several common risk factors, including age, gender, hypertension , diabetes mellitus, smoking, low serum levels of high-density lipoprotein (HDL) cholesterol, obesity and other. [18, 19] These common risk factors are termed as confounding factors. This affirmation is based on the capacity of periodontal infection to alter the inflammatory response of an individual with cardiovascular disease in which there are common risk factors. [20] So, the explanation for this increase in risk is found in the fact that coronary disease and periodontal disease are multifactorial processes, in which the inflammatory mecanisms play an important role. [21] Males are more affected by CVD and periodontitis than females. [22]

Advanced age is a risk factor for both cardiovascular disease and periodontitis. The incidence and severity of CVD has been shown to increase with age in both sexes. [23, 24] Tobacco smoking is one of the principal risk factors of CVD and periodontitis. [25]

Periodontitis, as an infectious disease, worsens diabetes, and the latter in turn exerts a negative influence upon both periodontal disease and CVD. [26] It is clear, however, that high blood cholesterol is related to CVD risk. Many authors have confirmed a relation between periodontitis and hypercholesterolemia. [27-29]

It is well known that arterial hypertension is a risk factor for CVD; the relationship between periodontitis and arterial hypertesion has been described, too. [30]

Another mechanism that explains relationship between cardiovascular disease and periodontitis is infection. Infection is an acknowledged risk factor for atherosclerosis and for the development of cardiovascular disease. [31] The mechanisms by which chronic infections increase the likelihood of atherosclerosis are not clearly defined, but the prerequisite is believed to be the host response to a long-term systemic exposure to certain pathogens.

Data on the role of periodontitis in atherogenesis are based on detection of similar bacteria in subgingival plaque samples [32] and atheromatous plaques. [33] Presence of periodontal pathogens in atheromatous plaques supports a direct relationship of pathogens etiologically linked to periodontal disease with increased risk for subclinical, prevalent, and future CVD. Bacteria from the mouth directly infect blood vessel walls and contribute to the development of plaues and atherosclerosis.

Several periodontal microorganisms (*Porphyromonas gingivalis, Aggregatibacter actinomycetemcomitans, Tannerella forsythia*) have been detected within the atherosclerotic plaque lesion of the vessel wall. [34] The loss of epithelial integrity within the periodontal pocket creates direct bacterial translocation and bacteriemia. The presence of periodontal microorganisms may at least partially explain why consistent association was observed between periodontal status and cardiovascular disease.

The proposed etiological mechanism behind this association was attributed to the effect of oral bacteria on cells taking part in pathogenesis of atherosclerosis and thrombosis. These bacteria or the products derived from them, such as endotoxins (lipopolysaccharide) may alter vascular endothelial integrity. [35] They can accede to the vascular system of the underlying connective tissue, and pass to the general circulation, so providing high possibilities of interchange of bacterial toxic products between the periodontal pocket and the circulatory system. [36] Once in the circulation, these microorganisms and their products can cause systemic inflammation and proatherogenic responses: smooth muscle hyperplasia of the large arteries, with possible fatty degeneration of the latter, and increase the release of cytokines such as IL-1, TNF-α and C-reactive protein (CRP). This situation does not go unnoticed for the organism, being able to generate a greater immune response than expected.

These factors can favor the development and course of atherosclerosis. [37]

Furthermore, the inflammatory response may contribute to CVD and related periodontal disease. Both atherosclerosis and periodontitis are inflammatory conditions that commonly are chronic and asymptomatic in nature. The concept that inflammation plays important part in pathophysiology of atherosclerosis and its complication, coronary artery diseases have provided a new unifying hypothesis of the links between risk factors and the cellular and molecular alteration that underlie this disease. Inflammation can operate in all stages of this disease from initiation through progression to the thrombotic complication of atherosclerosis. [38] The hypothesis being that local periodontitis triggered by bacterial insult, is a chronic inflammatory disease and that production of circulating cytokines may contribute to the development of atherosclerosis and cardiovascular disease among patients with periodontitis. [39]

Moderate to severe periodontitis increases the level of systemic inflammation, a characteristic of all chronic inflammatory diseases, and periodontitis has been associated with increased systemic inflammation as measured by hsCRP (high-sensitivity CRP) and other proinflammatory cytokines such as prostaglandins and TNF-α. Bacterial products in the blood may stimulate liver production of proinflammatory or pro-coagulant molecules such as C-reactive protein and fibrinogen. [40] After the initial publication of Mattila et al. [41] reporting that patients with periodontal infections had significant elevations of plasma fibrinogen and white blood cell count, a subsequent study observed that periodontitis was also associated with other markers of activated inflammation and hemostasis, including CRP. Many systemic markers have been identified in different cardiac disorders, which are considered to be an independent risk factor for cardiac events. The presence of inflammatory markers (C-reactive protein, fibrinogen, IL-1, IL-6 and TNF) in peripheral blood among patients with periodontitis could increment the inflammatory activity present in coronary lesion, and thus predispose patients to cardiovascular disease.

Although periodontitis is chronic in nature, acute-phase elements are also a part of the innate immunity in periodontitis and confirm that in periodontitis a systemic inflammation is present. [42] So, periodontal infection might be one of the underdiagnosed chronic inflammations contributory to systemic inflammatory response, which in turn may increase the risk for cardiovascular diseases. [43] The association of periodontal disease and CRP levels appears to be independent of other contributing factors in patients with periodontal disease, and increased CRP levels has been associated significantly with the risk of ishemic stroke. [44]

On the other hand, high white cell counts and increased levels of fibrinogen have been found in certain individuals with periodontal disease and cardiovascular disease. [41] These elevated inflammatory factors may increase inflammatory activity in atherosclerotic lesions, potentially increasing the risk for cardiac or cerebrovascular events. Circulating inflammatory cytokines act as a systemic trigger that can activate complications associated with atherosclerosis.

Therefore, changes in this marker in periodontitis may be part of the explanation why periodontitis is associated with cardiovascular diseases. It is hypothesized that possibly daily episodes of a bacteremia originating from periodontal lesions are the cause for the changes in systemic markers in periodontitis, [45] resulting in the risk of cardiovascular disease.

Many studies suggest that periodontal disease may be a novel, modifiable risk factor for coronary heart disease.

Although these studies evaluated different populations and used different measures of periodontal and cardiovascular disease, the results are remarkably consistent, and the studies demonstrate that periodontal disease precedes coronary events. [46, 47]

In addition to "classical" risk factors for coronary heart disease "emerging" risk predictors include measures of chronic infection and low-grade inflammation in periodontitis. [48]

Increased inflammatory activity in atherosclerotic lesions, potentially increases the risk for cardiac or cerebrovascular events. [49] Another mechanism which has also received attention is the host immune response, since the reaction to periodontitis varies from one individual to another as a result of genetic differences, particularly in the case of monocyte secretory capacity. The genetic factors are very important in periodontal disease and must be taken into account not only at the time of diagnosis but also at the time of treatment.

Local macrophage activation in periodontium and in arterial intima plays a role in the inflammatory processes of both diseases. In this contex, a hyperinflammatory phenotype has been identified for monocytes which can release 3 to 10 fold more proinflammatory mediators such as PgE2, IL-1 and TNF-α than monocytes which lack this phenotype. [50] While the genes of interleukine -1 (IL-1) have been related to coronary diseases and osteoporosis, a specific association of polymorphisms IL-1α and IL-1β has been related to a serious periodontal disease in the adult. [51]

Different studies have been made to determine the relation between periodontitis and CVD.

A variety of methods are used to assess oral health, including the dental index, which quantifies the presence of caries, periodontal pocket probing, the presence of periapical lesions, gingival bleeding, the number of missing teeth, and the presence or absence of pericoronitis. A strong correlation has been observed between a periodontal pocket probe depth of over 5 mm and increase in the risk of CVD. Pejcic found an association between periodontitis and acute coronary syndrome, with the generalized presence of periodontal pockets measuring 5 mm in depth in patients with a history of infarction. [52]

Periodontal disease has also been linked to peripheral arterial disease and to stroke. [53] Stroke is a cerebrovascular disease that affects blood vessels supplying blood to the brain. It occurs when a blood vessel bringing oxygen and nutrients to the brain bursts or is clogged by local thrombus formation or by aggregates of bacteria and fibrin from other sources such as the heart. The inflamed periodontium releases inflammatory cytokines, LPS, and bacteria into the systemic circulation, and they may promote atherosclerosis and affect blood coagulation, and the function of platelets, thereby contributing to the onset of stroke. [54]

Many other authors found that patients with periodontitis are at a greater risk for developing CVD than patients without periodontitis. [24, 55, 56] In recent years, great attention of the world researchers has been focused on a possible association between oral health and systemic diseases, so contradictory results can also be found in the literature. [52, 54, 56] Although the mechanism responsible for the relationship between periodontal disease and cardiovascular events is not fully understood it is hypothesized that removal of the infections and inflammatory burden of periodontal disease through periodontal therapy would be accompanied by a decrease in the levels of the inflammatory markers and a decrease risk of coronary heart disease. [51, 57, 58]

Finding that periodontal therapy improves periodontal disease and decrease systemic inflammatory markers is consistent with a possible causative role for periodontal disease in the pathogenesis of atherosclerosis, perhaps mediated through systemic inflammation. A practical conclusion that can be drawn is that periodontal therapy may reduce other cardiovascular disease risk factors, and further provide systemic benefits. Therefore, treating inflammation may not only help manage periodontal diseases but may also help with the management of other chronic inflammatory conditions. [52]

Patients with CVD and those known to be at risk for CVD should be advised to have a comprehensive periodontal examination and to undergo appropriate periodontal treatment as indicated. The importance of long-term control of periodontal diseases should be part of comprehensive health education for such patients. Measures that can be implemented to improve oral health include definitive treatment of periodontitis, regular visits to a dental professional for tooth cleaning, and improved oral hygiene.

Periodontal Disease and Diabetes Mellitus

For many years, dentists have recognized the importance of dental health to general health. Recent research findings point to the possible association between chronic oral infections such as periodontitis and systemic health problems such as diabetes, heart and lung diseases, stroke, and low birth weight premature births. [59] Diabetes mellitus (DM) is the sixth leading cause of death in the world. More than 9% of the adult population has diabetes, and both the incidence and prevalence are increasing every year. Diabetes mellitus is a metabolic disorder characterized by hyperglycemia. The key hormonal disturbance causing diabetes mellitus can be either a defect in insulin secretion, insulin action, or both. [60]

Diabetes mellitus can be divided into three classifications according to signs and symptoms: type 1, type 2 and gestational. [61] Type 1 DM results from the destruction of beta- cells within the islets of Langerhans of the pancreas, which leads to complete insulin deficiency. A patient with type 1 DM must take exogenous insulin. Type 2 DM ranges from insulin resistance progressively leading to pancreatic beta-cell failure. Insulin resistance results in a decreased capacity to transfer glucose into target cells; thus, hyperglycemia develops. Lastly, gestational diabetes mellitus is a glucose intolerance that develops during pregnancy. [62] Many organs or systems are now recognized to be affected by diabetes. The long-term effect diabetes may include development of nephropathy, neuropathy, retinopathy, cardiovascular, peripheral, vascular, and cerebrovascular disease. [63]

Diabetes mellitus is a key example of a chronic medical condition with a significant impact on oral health. Diabetes has been associated with a number of oral complications, including periodontitis and gingivitis, dental caries, salivary gland dysfunction and xerostomia, burning mouth syndrome and increased susceptibility to oral infections. [64]

Effects of Diabetes on the Periodontium

Both diabetes and periodontitis are common chronic disorders prevelant in several parts of the world. The results of many studies have confirmed a strong interrelationship between

DM and periodontal disease. [65] In this interrelation diabetes is considered as a risk factor for periodontal disease and vice versa.

Both DM and periodontitis are inflammatory conditions that commonly are chronic and asymptomatic in nature. [66] Severe periodontal disease often coexists with severe DM. It has been known for years that patients with uncontrolled diabetes have a high risk for periodontal disease and that the disease severity is related to the duration of diabetes. [67]

Almost one third of individuals with diabetes have severe periodontal disease. [68] People with diabetes are more likely to have deeper periodontal pockets, significantly greater gingival bleeding and greater attachment loss than pople who do not have diabetes. [69, 70]

Numerous mechanisms have been elucidated to explain the impact of diabetes on the periodontium.

Researchers suggests that this association is similar to the association between glycemic control and the classic complications of diabetes such as retinopathy and nephropathy and others, such that periodontitis should be listed among the "classic" complications of diabetes. [71]

Although bacteria are necessary for periodontitis to occur and even though some of the earlier studies have reported higher proportions of several periodontal pathogens in diabetics, yet many later studies have also demonstrated that bacterial microflora at periodontal diseased sites of diabetics is similar to the microflora in non-diabetics. [72]

However, the apparent lack of significant differences in potential pathogens suggests that alterations in the host immuno-inflammatory response may have a major influence on the increased prevalence and severity of periodontal destruction seen in diabetes. It has been suggested that inflammation may be one mechanistic link between the two diseases. Evidence in the literature supports the role of inflammation as a major component in the pathogenesis of diabetes and diabetic complications. [73] Inflammation as a result of diabetes can also affect periodontal disease and therefore periodontitis is considered the sixth complication of diabetes. [74]

Macrophages and monocytes in inflammatory reactions elevate production of proinflammatory cytokines and mediators such as interleukin-1β (IL-1β) and tumor necrosis factors α (TNF-α) in subjects with diabetes.

Because gingival crevicular fluid is a serum transudate, elevated serum levels of inflammatory mediators associated with diabetes are also increased in gingival crevicular fluid. Also, because of the high vascularity of the inflamed periodontium, this inflamed tissue may serve as an endocrine-like source for TNF-α and other inflammatory mediators. [75]

The changes seen in the microvasculature of other organs in people with diabetes also occur in the periodontium. [76] Changes in collagen synthesis and homeostasis are common in diabetes and its can contribute to the pathogenesis of periodontal disease because collagen is the major structural protein in the periodontium. [77]

Diabetes also may contribute to the pathogenesis of periodontitis via associated vascular compromise, deficits in cell mediated immunity and the presence of a high glucose content in the blood, which enhances bacterial growth. [78] Evidence has consistently indicated that diabetes is a risk factor for increased severity of periodontitis because diabetes prolongs the inflammatory response to a bacterial stimulus through cytokine dysregulation. [79, 80]

The association between DM and periodontal disease is therefore, considered to be bidirectional: diabetes as a risk factor for periodontitis and periodontitis as a possible severity for diabetes. [81]

Although most research on the relationship between diabetes and periodontal disease has focused on how diabetes may affect periodontal status, a growing body of evidence also has examined the converse relationship of how periodontal diseases affect the metabolic state. So, worsening periodontal disease adversely affects glycemic control, increasing the risk for certain diabetes complications, and possibly increasing the risk for the development of diabetes. The converse possibility that periodontal disease either predisposes or exacerbates the diabetic condition has received more and more attention. These findings suggest that severe periodontitis may be an important risk factor in the progression of diabetes. Increasing scientific evidence shows that acute infections may alter the endocrinologic metabolic status of the host, thus leading to difficulty with glycemic control. [82]

Effects of Periodontitis on the Diabetes Mellitus

Periodontal diseases are infections that colonize the tooth surface at, or below the gingival margin. The bacteria that causes periodontal disease may enter the bloodstream and activate cytokines, (damaging immune system factors), which then destroy cells in the pancreas where insulin is produced. As a result, periodontitis may be a particular problem in patients with diabetes, especially those with uncontrolled diabetes. In patients with diabetes, host responses may be impaired, wound healing is delayed, and collagenolytic activity may be enhanced. [75]

Active inflammation characteristic of periodontitits generates compounds that may increase insulin resistance. [83] It seems that in individuals with diabetes, periodontitis elevates chronic systemic inflammatory state which may contribute to insulin resistance through certain mechanisms, worsening glycemic control, and making diabetic condition harder to control. [84]

Mechanisms underlying the association of periodontitis and DM are not clear. Within the oral cavity dwells a dynamic microbiologic ecosystem of approximately 6 billion microbes living in a delicate balance that can be altered by the health of the host and the integrity of its defenses. Protective barriers such as mucous membranes, immunologic defenses and high oxidation reduction potentials prevent easy penetration of bacteria. [85] In case of diabetic patients; concentration of oral microbial flora is increased due to higher concentration of glucose in saliva. It was found that diabetics have a higher than normal levels of periodontal pathogens. Bacterial and viral infections are known to increase insulin resistance and worsen glycemic control. [82] Because the pathogens associated with periodontitis do not appear to differ greatly in people with and without diabetes. Researchers have focused attention on potential differences in the immunoinflammatory response to bacteria. [87]

Systemic inflammation has been associated with DM. Periodontitis, a chronic infectious and inflammatory disease of the gingiva and supporting tissues, has been associated with systemic inflammation and conditions such as DM. [88] This evidence suggests that periodontitis have systemic effects that extend beyond the local periodontal environment. So, the effect of periodontitis on DM is believed to result from the nature of the inflammatory response in the periodontal tissues. Patients with periodontitis have significantly higher serum markers of inflammation. A number of proinflammatory cytokines produced in inflamed periodontal tissue, including tumor necrosis factor-α, interleukin-6 and interleukin-1, antagonize insulin.

These mediators via the periodontal microcirculation can affect tissuesand organs at distant sites. [89] The increased production of TNF-α and IL-6 in patients with periodontitis also increase insulin resistance. This could explain why periodontitis increases the risk of poor glycemic control in patients with diabetes. [90]

One of the mechanisms linking these two disease may be inhibition of cellular functions of inflammatory cells that are the first line of host's defense (neutrophils, monocytes and macrophages) which may further prevent destruction of bacteria in the periodontal pocket leading to increased periodontal destruction. [91] This destruction occurs due to toxic bacterial byproducts (lipopolysaccharides, peptidoglycans, hydrolytic enzymes); a mounted host response (cytokines, interleukins, and prostaglandins), [92] and systemic reaction via serum antibodies. [93, 94] It is, therefore, reasonable to hypothesize that periodontal infections may influence overall health and the course of some systemic diseases. Moreover, induced production of pro-inflammatory cytokines (such as TNF-α, IL-1β and IL-6, prostaglandin- PgE2) in periodontal disease also mediates insulin resistance and reduces insulin action. [95] Furthermore, obesity is associated with high plasma levels of TNF-α and its soluble receptors, which in turn may lead to a hyperinflammatory state increasing the risk for periodontal disease and also accounting in part for insulin resistance. [96] Obesity is an important risk factor for diabetes, cardiovascular disease, and periodontal disease. Adipocytes appear to secrete proinflammatory cytokines which may be the molecules linking the pathogenesis of these diseases. Obesity is a significant predictor of periodontal disease and insulin resistance and appears to mediate this relationship. [90, 97]

Like diabetic control improves the prognosis of periodontitis as seen in patients with controlled diabetes exhibiting periodontal conditions similar to those of the healthy population, similarly periodontal treatment may help decrease inflammation and inflammatory mediators in the serum that are associated with insulin resistence, thereby improving glycemic control in people with diabetes. [98] It has been shown that periodontal treatment directed at elimination of pathogenic species and controlling inflammation may have a positive impact on glycemic control by restoring insulin sensitivity in patients with poorly controlled diabetes, possibly by suppressing glycosylation of proteins as well as suppressing formation of advanced glycation end-products, and activities of matrixmetalloproteinases and other inflammatory mediators. [99-101]

Physicians should recognize periodontitis as a complication of DM and as a condition that, if left unresolved, can complicate the management of DM. Patients with diabetes, especially those for whom control of the disease proves to be difficult and those at risk of developing the disease, should be advised for a comprehensive periodontal examination and should undergo appropriate periodontal treatment as indicated.

In this regard, prevention of periodontal diseases and control of established periodontal diseases should be considered an integral part of diabetes control.

Periodontal Disease and Pre-Term Low Birth Weight

The term periodontal medicine encompasses the study of the contribution of periodontal infections on several systemic conditions including premature delivery. The evidence continues to suggest that maternal periodontitis may be an important risk factor or risk indicator for pregnancies culminating in preterm low birth-weight deliveries. [102]

Preterm low birth weight (PLBW) is a problem encountered in most world communities and a significant cause of perinatal morbidity and mortality. The international definition of low birth weight adopted by the 29th World Health assembly in 1976 is defined as delivery at < 37 weeks and low birth weight <2500 g.103 Over 60% of perinatal mortality (except for anatomic and genetic abnormalities) is caused by pre-term birth (PTB) and low birth weight. The World Health Organization reported that the incidence of low birth weight ranges to 8% in Europe. [104] Preterm births account for two thirds of all infant mortality in developed countries. The specific etiologies and pathogenesis of this adverse pregnancy outcome are still unclear. During normal pregnancy, maternal hormones and locally acting cytokines play a key role in regulating the onset of labour, cervical ripening, uterine contraction, and delivery.

PLBW is multifactorial in nature. Multiple factors are known to contribute to preterm low birth weight, including poor prenatal care, a mother older than 34 or younger than 17. Traditional risk factors are also smoking, genetics, the use of alcohol, prenatal care, poor maternal nutrition, hypertension, diabetes, multiple pregnancies, drug abuse, gestational diabetes, and low socio-economic status, educational disadvantages and, infection of the reproductive and urinary organs. As mentioned earlier, both generalized and localized infections have been associated with PLBW deliveries. [105]

While various factors have been found to predispose mothers to PLBW deliveries, the inability of medical intervention to resolve such occurrences is probably due to presence of other unidentified contributing factors. [106] These risk factors are not present in approximately 50% of cases. Consequently, the search continues for other causes for PB and LBW, including the presence of chronic infectious diseases to distant organs. Maternal infection during pregnancy have been demonstrated to perturb normal cytokine and hormone-related gestation, sometimes resulting in preterm labour, preterm premature rupture of membranes, and preterm low birth weight. This suggests that distant sites of infection or sepsis may be targeting the placental membranes. [107] Besides genitourinary infection and other infections, possibly periodontal, may adversely affect pregnancy outcomes. [108]

Many studies indicate that bacterial infections that cause moderate to severe periodontal disease in pregnant women increased the risk of premature delivery and low birth weight infants. The more severe infection, the greater risk to the baby. [109-111]

Both preterm delivery and low birth weight put infant at risk of experiencing increased medical complications. [112]

Recently, the impact of periodontal disease on adverse pregnancy outcome has received much attention. There is emerging interest and increasing evidence that support the interrelationship between periodontitis and systemic conditions. [113]

Periodontal disease is a Gram-negative infection and may become a source of subclinical and persistent infection, which induce systemic inflammatory responses that increase the risk of adverse pregnancy outcomes. [114]

The biological mechanisms by which periodontal disease act on PLBW is numerous but three hypothesis are the most important. That hypothesis may explain the relationship between periodontal infection and PLB.

Infection is a key factor in adverse pregnancy outcome. It has been suggested that spontaneous pre-term labour is commonly associated with bacterial vaginitis, a vaginal condition characterized by a prevalence of anaerobes.

Researchers indicates that the bacteria from gum disease, and from tooth decay, may trigger the same factors in the immune system as genital and urinary tract infections. [115]

Periodontal bacteria can directly cause infections both of the uteroplacenta and the fetus because they disseminate systemically within the mother and gain access to the fetal compartment. Potential mechanisms involve bacterially induced activation of cell-mediated immunity leading to cytokine production and the ensuing synthesis and release of prostaglandins, which appears to trigger preterm labour. [116]

The toxins produced by bacteria attack the gums, ligaments and bone surrounding the teeth to produce infected pockets that act similar to large infected wounds in mouth. The infected pockets provide access to the bloodstream allowing bacteria to travel throughout the body. [117]

Periodontal pathogens, being Gram-negative anaerobic bacterial species, cause direct contamination of the fetoplacental unit and may cause inflammation of the placental membrane. Among the microbacterial factors, only *P. gingivalis* had slightly different distribution in the PLBW case. The oral inflammatory burden index based on the clinical findings of gingival bleeding on probing, probing depth, and the presence of dental calculus and mouth ulcers has been significantly associated with PTB. [118] Hence, it can be assumed that severe periodontal disease with increased bacterial load, such as *P. gingivalis*, is related with preterm delivery. [119-121]

Another mechanism stresses that periodontitis as local infection may be due to an indirect action of translocated bacterial products such as lipopolysaccharide. Lipopolysaccharide, a bacterial endotoxin normally found in infected periodontal tissue, is released and acts on the fetoplacental unit through the blood. Bacterial lipopolysaccharide triggers release of a variety of biologically active mediators (interleukin-1β, tumor necrosis factor-α, prostaglandin E2) which may contribute to premature labour. [122]

Systemic inflammatory changes induced by periodontal diseases also can activate responses at the maternal fetal interface. Inflammatory mediators from an infected periodontal reservoir provoke problems in the fetoplacental unit. [123] New inflammatory reaction within the placental tissues of a pregnant woman (as a result of periodontal infection) may occur, the physiological levels of prostaglandin E2 (PgE2) and tumor necrosis factor-α (TNF-α) in the amniotic fluid may increase and eventually lead to premature delivery. Body reacts to the infections in gums by producing prostaglandins, a natural fatty acid that's involved with inflammation control and smooth muscle (uterine) contraction. During pregnancy the level of prostaglandins gradually increases, peaking when the pregnant woman goes into labour. One theory is that, if extra prostaglandins are produced as a reaction to the bacterial infection in gums, body may interpret it as a signal to go into labour and baby can be born too early or too small. This has also been shown to elicit an inflammatory burden resulting in placental damage and distress and, hence, fetal growth restriction. In addition, the cascade of disordered cytokine response can lead to the stimulation of prostaglandin synthesis and the release of matrix metalloproteinases, which account for the uterine contractions and membrane rupture leading to the induction of labour. [124]

Prostaglandin E2, and TNF-α are normal biologically active molecules during childbirth. They may be raised to high levels with infection and induce premature labour.

In a case-control study, preterm low-birth-weight infants had mothers with significantly more periodontal attachment loss than the control group with normal-weight infants at birth. [125]

Women whose periodontal condition worsens during pregnancy have an even higher risk of having a premature baby. Hence, periodontal disease has the potential to influence preterm low birth weight through an indirect mechanism involving inflammatory mediators or a direct bacterial assault on the amnion. [126]

A Spanish study, however, reported that there is no significant relationship between gestational age and periodontal parameters or between low-weight delivery and plaque index. [108] At the same time, Lunardelli and Peres [126] showed that the condition of the periodontal pocket is not significantly associated with low birth weight or PTB after controlling maternal health variables. A Brazilian study advocated that determinants other than periodontal disease and health conditions may explain the lack of significance. [128]

In light of the possible link between periodontal infection and adverse pregnancy outcomes, the dental/periodontal clinicians will need to educate the pregnant patient on the latest research and the implications. This may be due to alterations in the composition of subgingival plaque, altered immunoresponse, and increases in sex hormone concentrations during pregnancy. More frequent periodontal maintenance visits in order to maintain periodontal health during pregnancy is paramount. [129] The second trimester is the safest time to treat the pregnant patient because most organ systems have been formed. The third trimester is also safe, however, the clinicians should be aware of the pressure of the gravid uterus on the inferior vena cava creating a risk for postural hypotension. In light of the new research, however, it is apparent that the patient should have closer monitoring and management of periodontium and oral infections. [130] Periodontitis is preventable and treatable. Integration of periodontal care into obstetric management may improve pregnancy outcomes as early intervention may reduce the microbial challenge to oral tissues already altered due to hormonal changes. Successful periodontal therapy in pregnant women suffering from periodontitis is a protective factor promoting the birth of children with normal weight. [131] Experts recommend that women should have a periodontal examination before becoming pregnant or as soon as possible thereafter because periodontal treatment is safe for pregnant women. [132]

Appropriate periodontal treatment at a suitable stage of pregnancy should be delivered to pregnant women with active periodontitis to reduce the risks of adverse pregnancy outcomes.

Periodontal therapy, phase I, results in a reduction in PLBW incidence rate. The application of such a simple method among periodontally diseased pregnant women is recommended. [133] Periodontitis of the patient during pregnancy can be regarded as an important risk factor for PB and mothers should be advised to have a comprehensive periodontal examination prior to pregnancy.

Periodontal Disease and Respiratory Disease

Recent research indicated that periodontal infection might worsen systemic diseases, including respiratory diseases. [134] The respiratory diseases are a group of diseases caused by a wide variety of infectious agents, including bacteria, mycoplasma, fungi, parasites, and viruses, resulting in infection of the pulmonary parenchyma. Chronic obstructive pulmonary disease and pneumonia are a major cause of death in the world. [135]

Accumulating evidence suggests that oral disorders, particularly periodontal disease, may influence the course of respiratory infection. [136] Pneumonia can be a life-threatening infection, especially in the elderly and immunocompromised patient and it is a significant cause of morbidity and mortality in patients of all ages.

It is possible that this disease may be adversely influenced by oral conditions. Chronic bronchitis is an inflammatory condition associated with excessive tracheobronchial mucous production sufficient to cause cough with expectoration for at least 3 months of the year for 2 or 3 successive years. Emphysema is the destruction of the air spaces distal to the terminal bronchiole with destruction of the alveolar septa. [60] Chronic obstructive pulmonary disease (COPD) is characterized by chronic obstruction to airflow due to chronic bronchitis and/or emphysema. [137]

It is known that one of the most common routes of infection for respiratory diseases is aspiration of oropharyngeal contents. [138] Oral bacteria have been implicated in the pathogenesis of these diseases and, in this regard, dental plaque might be an important reservoir for these potential pathogens. [139] There is an increasing evidence that oral bacteria that reside in the mouth, especially periodontal pathogens, may alter the course of respiratory infections.

Also, it is known that the lower airway can be contaminated by microorganisms through aspiration of oropharyngeal contents, inhalation of infectious aerosols, hematogenous spread, or spread from contigous sites. [140] Oral bacteria, poor oral hygiene, and periodontitis seems to influence the incidence of pulmonal infection. It appears that oral colonization by potential respiratory pathogens; possibly fostered by periodontitis, and possibly by bacteria specific to the oral cavity or by periodontal diseases contribute to pulmonary infections. [141]

Increasing evidence has linked the anaerobic bacteria forming periodontopathic biofilms with aspiration pneumonia in elderly persons. The oral cavity, including dental plaque, can act as a reservoir of respiratory pathogens in patients in intensive care units, hospitalized patients with chronic lung diseases and nursing home residents. [142] In experiments designed to eliminate the potent respiratory pathogens forming biofilms in the oral cavity, it has been shown that the mechanical and chemical oral cleansing effectively reduces *Staphylococcus* species, *Streptococcus pneumoniae*, and *Haemophilus influenzae* in patients requiring endotracheal intubation. [143]

Several mechanisms can help to explain how oral infection can participate in the pathogenesis of respiratory infection. These are: oral pathogens, periodontal disease and enzymes in saliva that allow colonization by respiratory pathogens and cytokines originating from periodontal tissues.

The first hypothesis explains how oral bacteria may participate in the pathogenesis of respiratory infection. Resident bacteria in oral secretions are likely aspirated along with respiratory pathogens and may affect the adhesion of the later organisms to the respiratory epithelium. Studies suggest that oral bacteria may modulate the adhesion of respiratory pathogens to epithelial cell lines. In addition, oral bacterial products or cytokines in oral/pharyngeal aspirates may stimulate cytokine production from respiratory epithelial cells, resulting in recruitment of inflammatory cells. The resulting inflamed epithelium may be more susceptible to respiratory infection. [144]

In periodontal disease, oral pathogens stimulate the cells of the periodontium to release a wide variety of cytokines and other biologically active molecules. Cytokines produced by cells in response to these bacteria include interleukin-1α, IL-1β, IL-6, IL-8 and TNF-α. These cytokines originating from the oral tissue contaminate respiratory cells that release other cytokines that damage epithelium that may become more susceptible to colonization by respiratory pathogens. [145] These findings support the association between respiratory and periodontal disease. [146]

Perhaps aspiration of saliva into which oral bacterial antigens, lipopolysaccharide and enzymes have been released promotes inflammation and infection of the lower airway.

It is also possible that host-derived mediators such as cytokines and prostaglandins, which are elevated in the saliva of subjects with periodontal disease, promote lung inflammation and infection if aspirated into the lower airway. [142]

Individuals with normal pulmonary functions had significantly better periodontal scores than with airway obstruction. All periodontal indices were elevated in patients with respiratory diseases. [147]

The possibility that bacteria in oral biofilms influence respiratory infection suggests that good oral hygiene may prevent the aspiration of large numbers of oral bacteria into the lower airway and thus prevent initiation or progression of respiratory infection in susceptible individuals. [148] Patients at risk of developing such diseases should be advised to have a comprehensive periodontal examination and to undergo appropriate periodontal treatment as indicated.

Recommendations for the dental clinicians include: reducing levels of periodontopathic flora by maintaining good home care and frequent periodontal maintenance; rinsing with chlorhexidine prior to dental/ periodontal therapy and performing required periodontal therapies to stabilize the periodontium.

Periodontal Disease and Other Systemic Disease

Rheumatoid Arthritis

Periodontitis and rheumatoid arthritis (RA) appear to share many pathologic features. Emerging evidence now suggests a strong relationship between the extent and severity of periodontal disease and RA.

While this relationship is unlikely to be causal, it is clear that individuals with advanced RA are more likely to experience more significant periodontal problems compared to their non-RA counterparts. A case is made that these two diseases could be very closely related through common underlying dysfunction of fundamental inflammatory mechanisms. Nonetheless, both conditions manifest as a result of an imbalance between proinflammatory and anti-inflammatory cytokines. [149]

Bartold and colleagues hypothesized that there is a common dysregulation of proinflammatory pathways for both arthritis and periodontitis, and they strongly suggested evaluating patients who have arthritis for periodontitis. [150] As a result, new treatment strategies are expected to emerge for both diseases that may target the inhibition of proinflammatory cytokines and destructive proteases. [151]

Severe arthritis also can diminish quality of life for patients, and alveolar bone loss has been associated with arthritis. [152] Since arthritis often limits manual dexterity and oral hygiene is key in preventing PD in patients with arthritis, the use of powered rotating-oscillating toothbrushes and antiseptic or fluoride mouth-rinses has been recommended to improve oral hygiene. However, clinicians need to emphasize to patients the importance of achieving good mechanical plaque control using appropriate aids.

Periodontitis has been implicated as a risk factor for rheumatoid arthritis. Infection with periodontal pathogens (*P. gingivalis*) may play a role in disease risk and progression in rheumatoid arthritis. [153] *P. gingivalis* possesses a unique microbial enzyme that leads to the production of a rheumatoid factor-containing immune complex and provoke local inflammation, both in gingiva and synovia. [154]

In addition, gingivitis and periodontitis are related to high levels of circulating TNF-α in patient with rheumatoid arthritis, contributing to the deterioration of the disease. [151, 155]

Osteoporosis

Over the past two decades, an ever-increasing number of studies have reported an association between destructive periodontal diseases and osteoporosis. [156] Osteoporosis is a physiologic, gender, and age related condition resulting from bone mineral content loss. It is a disease characterized by low bone mass and fragility, which in turn may lead to increase in fractures. Osteoporosis and periodontitis are very prevalent diseases and are most common in middle-aged and elderly women. Both osteoporosis and periodontal disease are chronic multifactorial diseases with many genetic and behavioral risk factors and determinants. Clinical data suggests a link between osteoporosis and periodontitis, as many common risk factors have been detected in the etiology of both these diseases. [157]

These diseases are also related, as both damage bone tissue along with sharing common risk factors. A hypothesis was raised that systemic imbalance in bone resorption and deposition might manifest itself in the alveolar bone loss earlier than in other bones. [158] While analyzing systemic and local changes in bone density, a number of issues were investigated and attempted to answer the question of whether dental osteopenia is a local manifestation of osteoporosis having similar etiology and risk factors, or is it an independent process depending primarily on factors that cause periodontal disease. There is a strong and consistent association between measured bone density and alveolar crestal height in postmenopausal women. [159] Periodontal disease is associated significantly with alveolar bone loss and osteoporosis. [160, 161] It had been suggested that stimulation of inflammatory mediators during the menopause period could promote an exacerbation of a coexisting periodontal inflammation cascade, thereby reducing alveolar bone and increasing tooth loss. These mediators probably represent the common biological mechanisms that inter-relate these two diseases. [162]

Alzheimer's Disease

Inflammation is now known to play a critical role in diseases that are not usually classified as inflammatory diseases, such as Alzheimer's disease. Although this conclusion is the result of many years of research, much of the knowledge has crystallized into coherent concepts only very recently. Inflammatory mechanisms appear to be critical factors in the development and progression of most of the chronic diseases of aging.

Diet and genetic variations interact to control differences in inflammation among individuals. Possibly Alzheimer's signpost and gum inflammation may be linked to increase risk of the brain disorders. [163] Periodontal disease may be a marker for chronic exposure to disease that provokes an inflammatory response. Chronic inflammation can damage tissue, including the brain, which may contribute to the development of the disease. [164]

Pancreatic Cancer

Patients who have cancer and who undergo chemotherapy and radiation therapy may experience significant deleterious oral complications, including oral mucositis, xerostomia, radiation-induced dental caries and even osteo-radionecrosis.

Opportunistic infections such as Candida albicans have been shown to increase in frequency with mucositis and immunosuppression, and infection may occur months or years after treatment. [165]

A new study has found that periodontal disease may be associated with an increased risk of cancer of the pancreas. Individuals with periodontal disease have elevated serum biomarkers of systemic inflammation, such as C-reactive protein, and these somehow contribute to the promotion of cancer cells. [157]

Another explanation is that periodontal disease could lead to increased pancreatic carcinogenesis because individual with periodontal disease have higher levels of oral bacteria and higher levels of nitrosamines, which are carcinogens, in oral cavity. [166]

Conclusion

Periodontal medicine will promote a strong collaboration of dental professionals and medical professionals for better diagnosis and treatment across specialities. Further integration of dental and general medicine requires a better communication between dentists and medical doctors, and more responsibilities and effective team approaches in the clinical management of their shared patients for better oral health and general health.

The promotion of health and management of disease should require interdisciplinary education and treatment strategies. With medical doctors and dentists working closely together, more patients with systemic diseases are likely to be successfully treated, and patients will benefit from predictable treatment regiments to save and rehabilitate their dentition.

The possibility that morbidity and mortality from systemic diseases may be reduced by improving periodontal health makes it imperative that this relationship be examined more closely.

The terms oral health and general health should not be interpreted as separate entities. Oral health is integral to general health; this chapter provides important reminders that oral health means more than healthy teeth and there cannot be general health without oral health.

References

[1] Kim, J., Amar, S. Periodontal disease and systemic conditions: a bidirectional relationship. *Odontology*. 2006;94(1):10-21.

[2] Pizzo, G., Guiglia, R., LoRusso, L., Campisi, D. Dentistry and internal medicine: from the focal infection theory to the periodontal medicine concept. *Eur. J. Intern. Med.* 2010; 21(6): 495-502.

[3] Williams, R. C., Offenbacher, S. Periodontal medicine: the emergence of a new branch of periodontology. *Periodontol*. 2000. 2000;23:9-12.

[4] Armitrage, G. C. Development of a classification system for periodontal diseases and condition. *Ann. Periodontol*. 1999; 4: 1-6.

[5] Djajic, D., Djukanovic, D. *Parodontologija*. 2006. Draslar Partner, Beograd.

[6] Beck, J., Offenbacher, S. Oral health systemic disease: periodontitis and cardiovascular disease. *J. Dent. Educ*. 1998;62:859-870.

[7] Mendez, M., Scott, T., LaMorte, W., Boconas, P., Menzoian, J., Garcia, R. An association between periodontal disease and peripheral vascular disease. *Am. J. Surg*. 1998; 176:153-157.

[8] D'Aiuto, F., Graziani, F., Tete' S., et al. Periodontitis: from local infection to systemic diseases. *Int. J. Immunopathol. Pharmacol*. 2005; 18(3 Suppl.):1-12.

[9] Chiu, B. Multiple infection in carotid atherosclerotic plaques. *Am. Heart J.* 1999;138: S534-S536.

[10] Haraszthy, V., Zambon, J., Trevisan, M., Genco, R. Identification of periodontal pathogens in atheromatous plaques. *J. Periodontol*. 2000; 71:1554-60.

[11] Loos, B., Craandijk, J., Hoek, F., Wertheim-van, P., van der Velden, U. Elevation of systemic markers related to cardiovascular diseases in peripheral blood of periodontitis patients. *J. Periodontol*. 2000;71:1528-1534.

[12] Jin, L., Chiu, G. K. C., Corbet, E. F. Are periodontal diseases risk factors for certain systemic disorders-what matters to medical practitioners? *Hong Kong Med. J.* 2003;9: 31-37.

[13] Newman, G. M., Takei, H. H., Carranza, A. *Carranza's Clinical periodontology*. W. B. Saunders company- 9th ed. 2002.

[14] Papapanos, P. Periodontal diseases: Epidemiology. *Ann. Periodontol*. 1996;1:1-36.

[15] Lopez, R., Oyarzun, M., Naranjo, C., Cumsille, F., Ortiz, M., Baelum, V. Coronary heart disease and periodontitis-a case control study in Chilean adults. *J. Clin. Periodontol*. 2002;29:468-473.

[16] Friedewald, V. E., Kornman, K. S., Beck, J. D., Genco, R., Goldfine, A., et al. The American Journal of Cardiology and Journal of Periodontology Editors' Consensus: Periodontitis and Atherosclerotic Cardiovascular Disease. *J. Periodontol*. 2009;80: 1021-1032.

[17] Sanz, M., D'Aiuto, F., Deanfield, J., Fernandez-Aviles, F. European workshop in periodontal health and cardiovascular disease - scientific evidence on the association between periodontal and cardiovascular diseases: a review of the literature. *Eur. Heart J.* 2010;12(suppl. B):B3-B12.

[18] Cairo, F., Castellani, S., Gorri, A. M., et al. Severe periodontitis in young adults is associated with sub-clinical atherosclerosis. *J. Clin. Periodontol.* 2008;35:465-472.

[19] Chobanian, A. V., Bakris, G. L., Black, H. R., et al. Seventh report of the Join National Committee on prevention, detection, evaluation, and treatment of high blood pressure. *Hypertension*. 2003;42:1206-1252.

[20] Buhlin, K., Hultin, M. K., Norderyd, O., Persson, L., Pockley, G. A., Rabe, P., et al. Risk factors for atherosclerosis in cases with severe periodontitis. *J. Clin. Periodontol.* 2009;36(7):541-549.

[21] Haffajee, A. D., Sockransky, S. S. Microbial etiology of destructive periodontal disease. An overview. *Periodontology* 2000. 1994;5:78-111.

[22] Garcia, R. I., Henshaw, M. M., Krall, E. A. Relationship between periodontal disease and systemic health. *Periodontol.* 2000. 2001;25:21-36.

[23] Mattila, K. J., Asikainen, S., Walf, J., Jousimies, S. H., et al. Age, dental infection and coronary heart disease. *J. Dent. Res.* 2000;79(2):756-760.

[24] Joesche, J. W., Schork, A., Terpenning, S. M., Chen, Y-M., Dominguez, L., Drossman, N. Assessing the relationship between dental disease and coronary heart disease in eldery US veterans. *JADA*. 1998;129:301-311.

[25] Buhlin, K., Gustafsson, A., Pockley, A. G., Frostegard, J., Klinge, B. Risk factors for cardiovascular disease in patients with periodontitis. *Eur. Heart J.* 2003;24:2099-2107.

[26] Loesche, W., Karapetov, F., Pohl, C. Plasma lipid and blood glucosa levels in patients with destructive periodontal disease. *J. Clin. Periodontol.* 2000;27:537-541.

[27] Taylor, G. W., Borgnakke, W. S. Periodontal disease: Associations with diabetes, glycemic control and complicacions. *Oral Dis*. 2008;14:191-203.

[28] Valenticiene, G., Paipaliene, P., Nedzelskiene, I., Zilinskas Jand Vide, O. The relationship betveen blood serum lipids and periodontal condition. *Infection and Immunity*. 2003;71(10):6012-6018.

[29] Pejcic, A., Kesic, L. J., Ilic, S., Pesic, Z., Mirkovic, D. Association between chronic periodontitis and serum lipid levels. *Military Medical J.* 2012;69(9):771-777.

[30] Saxlin, T., Suominen-Taipale, L., Kattainen, A., et al. Association between serum lipid levels and periodontal infection. *J. Clin. Periodontol.* 2008;35:1040-1047.

[31] Angeli, E., Verdecchia, P., Pellegrino, C., et al. Association between periodontal disease and left ventricle mass in essential hypertension. *Hypertension*. 2003;41:488-492.

[32] Pejcic, A., Kesić, L. j., Ilić, S., Obradović, R., Mirković, D. Investigation of risk factors for cardiovascular disease in periodontitis patients: C-reactive protein, fibrinogen and white blood cells. *Stom. Inform.* 2010; 16(27):5-10.

[33] Pejcic, A., Kesic, L. j., Milasin, J. C-reactive protein as systemic marker of inflammation in periodontitis. *Eur. J. Clin. Microbiol. Infect. Dis.* 2011; 30(3):407-414.

[34] Haraszthy, V. I., Zambon, J. J., Trevisan, M., Zeid, M., Genco, R. J. Identification of periodontal pathogens in atheromatous plaques. *J. Periodontal.* 2000;71:1554-1556.

[35] Beck, J. D., Eke, P., Heiss, G., Madianos, P., Couper, D. Periodontal disease and coronary heart disease. A peappraisal of the exposure. *Circulation*. 2005;112:19-24.

[36] Desvarieux, M., Demmer, R. T., Rundek, T., Boden-Albala, B., et al. Periodontal microbiota and carotid intima- media thickness. *Circulation*. 2005;11:576-582.

[37] Marcus, A. J., Hajar, D. R. Vascular transcellular signalling. *J. Lipid Res.* 1993;34: 2017-2031.

[38] Geert, So, Nys, M., De Mol, P., Charpentier, J. Systemic release of endotoxins induced by gentle mastication: Association with periodontitis severity. *J. Periodontol.* 2002;73 (1):73-78.
[39] Libby, P., Ridker, P. M. Inflammation and Atherothrombosis From Population Biology and Bench research to Clinical Practic. *J. Am. Coll. Cardiol.* 2006;48:33-46.
[40] Loos, B. G. Systemic markers of inflammation in periodontitis. *J. Periodontol.* 2005; 76:2106-2115.
[41] Mattila, K., Nieminen, M., Voltonen, V. Association between dental health and acute myocardial infarction. *BMJ.* 1989;289:779-782.
[42] Renuka Devi, R., Sarayan, R., Vijaya Kumar, N. Estimation of C-reactive protein level in the peripheral blood of patient with chronic periodontitis. *JIADS.* 2011;2(2):168-173.
[43] Pejcic, A., Kesic, L. J., Milasin, J., Brkic, Z., Mirkovic, D. Association between periodontopathogens and CRP levels in patients with periodontitis in Serbia. *J. Dent. Res. Dent. Clin. Dent. Prospect.* 2011;5 (1):10-16.
[44] Pejcic, A., Kesić, L. j, Pešić, Z., Mirković, D., Stojanović, M. White blood cell count in different stage of chronic periodontitis. *Acta Clin. Croat.* 2011;50(2):159-167.
[45] Ridker, P. M., Cushman, M., Stampfer, M. J., et al. Inflammation, aspirin, and the risk of cardiovascular disease in apparently healthy men. *N Engl. J. Med.* 1997;336:973-979.
[46] De Nardin, E. The role of inflammatory and immunological mediators in periodontitis and cardiovascular disease. *Ann. Periodontol.* 2001;6:30-40.
[47] Hung, H. C., Willett, W., Merchant, A., et al. Oral health and peripheral arterial disease. *Circulation.* 2003;107:1152-1157.
[48] Tuominen, R., Reunanen, A., Paunio, M., et al. Oral health indicators poorly predict coronary heart disease deaths. *J. Dent. res.* 2003;82:713-718.
[49] Pearson, T. A., Mensah, G. A., Alexander, R. W. Markers of inflammation and cardiovascular disease: application to clinical and public health practice: a statement for healthcare professionals from the Centers for Disease Control and Prevention and the American Heart Association. *Circulation.* 2003;107:499-511.
[50] Pejcic, A., Kesic, L. j, Brkic, Z., Pesic, Z., Mirkovic, D. Effect of Periodontal Treatment on Lipoproteins Levels in Plasma in Patients with Periodontitis. *South Med. J.* 2011;104(8):547-552.
[51] Beck, J., Garcia, R., Heiss, G., Vokonas, P., Offenbacher, S. Periodontal disease and cardiovascular disease. *J. Periodontol.* 1996;67:1123-37.
[52] Pejcic, A. *Effect of periodontal therapy on inflammatory markers in patients both with and without acute coronary syndrome.* Medical faculty, University of Nis. 2012.
[53] Shapira, L., Soskolne, W. A., Sela, M. N., Offenbacher, S., Barak, V. The secretion of PgE2, IL-1, IL-6, TNF-alfa by monocytes from early onset periodontitis patients. *J. Periodontol.* 1994;65:139-146.
[54] Chen, Y. W., Umeda, M., Nagasawa, T., et al. Periodontitis may increase the risk of peripheral arterial disease. *Eur. J. Vasc. Endovasc. Surg.* 2008;35:153-158.
[55] Peltola, J., Valtonen, V., Iivanainen, M., Kaste, M., Huttunen, J. K. Dental infections in association with cerebral infarction in young and middle aged men. *J. Intern. Med.* 1989;225:179-184.

[56] D'Aiuto, F., Parker, M., Nibali, I., Suvan, J., Lessem, J., Tonetti, M. S. Periodontal infections cause changes in traditional and novel cardiovascular risk factor: results from a randomized controlled clinical trial. *Amer. Heart J.* 2006;151:977-984.

[57] Pejcic, A., Peševska, S., Grigorov, I., Bojović, M. Periodontitis as a Risk Factor for General Disorders. *Acta Fac. Med. Naiss.* 2006;23(1):59-65.

[58] Hujoel, P. P., Drangshilt, M., Spiekerman, C., DeRouen, T. A. Periodontal disease and coronary heart disease risk. *JAMA*. 2000;37:445-450.

[59] Ramamoorthy, R. D., Nallasamy, V., Reddy, R., Esther, N., Maruthappan, Y. A review of C- reactive protein: A diagnostic indicator in periodontal medicine. *J. Pharm. Bioall. Sci*. 2012;4:422-426.

[60] Barnett, M. L. The oral systemic disease connection. An update for the practicing dentist. *JADA*. 2006;137:5S-6S.

[61] Ilic, S. (ed.). *Internal medicine*. Prosveta, Nis. 2004.

[62] American Diabetes Association. Diagnosis and classification of diabetes mellitus: position statement. *Diabetes Care*. 2005;28(supplement 1): S37-S42.

[63] Rose, L. F., Genco, R. J., Cohen, D. W., Mealey, B. L., (Eds.) *Periodontal medicine*. BC Decker, Inc., Hamiltom, Ontario 2000.

[64] Sadijot, S. M., Nigam, A., Das, S., Bajaj, S., Zargar, A. H., Prasannakumar, K. M., et al. The burden of diabetes and impaired glucose tolerance in India using the WHO 1999 criteria: Prevalence of diabetes in India study (PODIS). *Diabetes Res. Clin. Pract.* 2004; 66: 301-307.

[65] Al-Khabbaz, K. A., Al-Shammari, F. K., Al-Saleh, A. N. Knowledge About the Association Between Periodontal Diseases and Diabetes Mellitus: Contrasting Dentists and Physicians. *J. Periodontol*. 2011;82 (3):360-366.

[66] Campus, G., Salem, A., Uzzau, S., Baldoni, E., Tonolo, G. Diabetes and periodontal disease: A case-control study. *J. Periodontol*. 2005;75:418-425.

[67] Iacopino, M. A. Periodontitis and Diabetes Interrelationships: Role of Inflammation. *Annals of Periodontology*. 2011;6(1):125-137.

[68] Matthews, D. C. The relationship between diabetes and periodontal disease. *J. Can. Dent. Assoc.* 2002;68:161-164.

[69] Taylor, G. W., Manz, M. C., Borgnakke, W. S. Diabetes, periodontal diseases, dental caries and tooth loss: A review of the literature. *Compend. Contin. Educ. Dent*. 2004; 25:179-184.

[70] Taylor, G. W., Borgnakke, W. S. Periodontal disease: Associations with diabetes, glycemic control and complication. *Oral Dis*. 2008;14:191-203.

[71] Lalla, E., Cheng, B., Lal, S., Tucker, S., et al. Periodontal changes in children and adolescents with diabetes: a case-control study. *Diabetes Care*. 2006;29(2):295-299.

[72] King, L. G. The role of inflammatory cytokines in diabetes and its complication. *J. Periodontol*. 2008; 79(8s):1527-1534.

[73] Lalla, E., Cheng, B., Lal, S., et al. Diabetes mellitus promotes periodontal destruction in children. *J. Clin. Periodontol.* 2007;34(4): 294-298.

[74] American Academy of Periodontology. Diabetes and periodontal diseases (position paper) *J. Periodontol*. 1999;70:935-949.

[75] Loe, H. Periodontal disease. The sixth complication of diabetes mellitus. *Diabetes care*. 1993;16(Suppl. 1):329-334.

[76] Salvi, G. E., Yalda, B., Collins, J. G., Jones, B. H., Smith, F. W., Arnold, R. R., et al. Inflammatory mediator response as a potential risk marker for periodontal diseases in Insulin- dependent diabetes mellitus patients. *J. Periodontol.* 1997;68:127-35.
[77] Seppala, B., Sorsa, T., Ainamo, J. Morphometric analysis of cellular and vascular changes in gingival connective tissue in long-term insulin dependent diabetes. *J. Periodontol.* 1997;68:1237-1245.
[78] Ryan, M., Ramamurthy, N. S., et al. MMP-mediated events in diabetes *Ann. NY Acid. Sci.* 1999;878:311-334.
[79] Nagasawa, T., Noda, M., Katagiri, S., et al. Relationship between Periodontitis and Diabetes - Importance of a Clinical Study to Prove the Vicious Cycle. *Internal Medicine*. 2010;49(10):881-885.
[80] Naguib, G., Al-Mashat, H., Desta, T., Graves, D. Diabetes prolong the inflammatory response to a bacterial stimulus through cytokine dysregulation. *J. Invest. Dermatol.* 2004; 123:87-92.
[81] Salvi, G. E., Carollo-Bittel, B., Lang, N. P. Effects of diabetes mellitus on periodontal and peri-implant conditions. Update on association and risk. *J. Clin. Periodontol.* 2008;35(S8):398-409.
[82] Grossi, S. G., Genco, R. J. Periodontal disease and diabetes mellitus: A two-way relationship. *Ann. Periodopntol.* 1998;3(1):52-61.
[83] Lalla, E., Cheng, B., Lal, S., et al. Diabetes-related parameters and periodontal conditions in children. *J. Perio Res.* 2007;42:345-349.
[84] Bandyopadhyay, D., Marlow, M. N., Leite, S. R. Periodontal disease progression and glycaemic control among Gullah African Americans with type-2 diabetes. *J. Clin. Periodontol.* 2010;37(6):501-509.
[85] Mealey, B. L., Rose, L. F. Diabetes mellitus and inflammatory periodontal diseases. *Cur. Opion. Endocrinol. Diabetes Obes.* 2008;15: 135-141.
[86] Socransky, S. S., Haffajee, A. D., Cugini, M. A., Smith, C., Kent, R. L. Jr. Microbial complexes in subgingival plaque. *J. Clin. Periodontol.* 1998; 25:134-144.
[87] Mealey, B. L., Oates, T. W. Diabetes mellitus and periodontal diseases. *J. Periodontol.* 2006; 77: 1289-1303.
[88] Nishimura, F., Iwamoto, Y., Soga, Y. The periodontal host response with diabetes. *Periodontol.* 2000. 2007;43:245-253.
[89] Mealey, B. Diabetes and periodontal diseases. *J. Periodontol.* 1999;70 (8):935-949.
[90] Tilg, H., Moschen, A. R. Inflammatory mehanisma in the regulation of insulin resistence. *Mol. Med.* 2008;14(3-4):222-231.
[91] Genco, R. J., Grossi, S. G., Ho, A., Nishimura, F., Murayama, Y. A proposed model linkin inflammation to obesity, diabetes and periodontal infection. *J. Periodontol.* 2005; 76:2075-2084.
[92] Hussain, A. M. The relationship between diabetes mellitus and periodontitis. *AJMS.* 2011;4(1):84-86.
[93] Chen, L., Wei, B., Li, J., et al. Association of Periodontal Parameters With Metabolic Level and Systemic Inflammatory Markers in Patients With Type 2 Diabetes. *J. Periodontol.* 2010;81(3):364-371.
[94] American Academy of Periodontology. International Workshop for a classification of periodontal diseases and conditions. *Ann. Periodontol.* 1999;4:1-112.

[95] Slots, J., Ashimoto, A., Flynn, M. J., Li, G., Chen, C. Detection of putative periodontal pathogens in subgingival specimens by 16S ribosomal DNA amplification with the polymerase chain reaction. *Clin. Infect. Dis.* 1995;20(Suppl.):S304-S307.

[96] Page, R. C. The pathobiology of periodontal diseases may affect systemic diseases: inversion of a paradigm. *Ann. Periodontol.* 1998;3: 108-120.

[97] Pischon, N., Heng, N., Bernimoulin, J. P., Kleber, B. M., et al. Obesity, Inflammation, and Periodontal disease. *J. Dent. Res.* 2007;86(5):400-409.

[98] Zelkha, S. A., Freilich, R. W., Amar, S. Periodontal innate immune mechanisms relevant to atherosclerosis and obesity. *Periodontol.* 2000. 2010;54(1):207-221.

[99] Kiran, M., Arpak, N., Unsal, E., Erdoan, M. F. The effect of improved periodontal health on metabolic control in tip 2 diabetes mellitus *J. Clin. periodontol.* 2005;32:266-272.

[100] Sun, W. L., Chen, L. L., Zhang, Z. S., Wu, M. Y., Ren, Y., Qin, M. G. Inflammatory Cytokines, Adiponectin, Insulin Resistance and Metabolic Control after Periodontal Intervention in Patients with Type 2 Diabetes and Chronic Periodontitis. *Internal Medicine.* 2009;50(15):1569-1574.

[101] Darre, L., Vergnes, J. N., Gourdy, P., Sixou, M. Efficacy of periodontal treatment on glycemic control in diabetic patients: A meta –analysis of interventional studies. *Diabetes Metab.* 2008;34:497-506.

[102] Faria-Almeda, R., Navarro, A., Bescones, A. Clinical and metabolic changes after conventional tretment of type 2 diabetic patients with chronic periodontitis. *J. Periodontol.* 2006;77:591-598.

[103] Offenbacher, S., Katz, V., Fertik, G., et al. Periodontal infection as a possible risk factor for preterm low birth weight. *J. Periodontol.* 1999; 67(10s):1103-1113.

[104] World Health Organization. The incidence of low birth weight: an update. *Wkly Epidemiol. Res.* 1984;59:205-211.

[105] United Nation's Children's Fund, World Health Organization. Low Birthweight: Country, Regional and Global Estimates. New York: UNICEF. 2004;7-9.

[106] Berkowitz, G. S., Papiemik, E. Epidemiology of preterm birth. *Epidemiol. Rev.* 1993; 15:414-443.

[107] Scannapieco, F. A., Bush, R. B., Paju, S. Periodontal disease as a risk factor for adverse pregnancy outcomes. A systematic review. *Ann. Periodontol.* 2003;8:70-78.

[108] Moreu, G., Tellez, L., Gonzales–Jaranay, M. Relationship between maternal periodontal disease and low birth weight preterm infants. *J. Clin. Periodontol.* 2005; 32:622-627.

[109] Offenbacher, S., Lieff, S., Boggess, K. A., et al. Effects of periodontal therapy during pregnancy on periodontal status, biologic perameters, and pregnancy outcome: a pilot study. *J. Periodontol.* 2006b;77:2011-2024.

[110] Moliterno, L. F., Monteiro, B., Figueredo, C. M., Fischer, R. G. Association between periodontitis and low birth weight: A case-control study. *J. Clin. Periodontol.* 2005; 32: 886-890.

[111] Moore, S., Randhawa, M., Ide, M. A case-control study to investigate as association between adverse pregnancy outcome and periodontal disease. *J. Clin. Periodontol.* 2005;32:1-5.

[112] Jarjoura, K., Devine, P. C., Perez-Decboy, A., et al. Markers of periodontal infection and preterm birth. *Am. J. Obstet. Gynecol.* 2005; 192:512-519.

[113] Guimaraes, N. A., Silva-Mato, A., Siqueira, M. F., et al. Periodontal infection as a risk factor for preterm low birth weight. *J. Clin. Periodontol.* 2012;39(11):1024-1031.

[114] Reddy, P., Phulambrikar, T., Wanjan, P. V., Srivastava, R. Correlation of periodontitis during pregnancy and incidence of low birth weight babies. *J. Indian Aca Oral Med. radiol.* 2012,24(2):95-97.

[115] McGaw, T. Periodontal disease and preterm delivery of low birth - weight infants. *J. Can. Dent. Assoc.* 2002;68:165-169.

[116] Gibbs, R. S. The relationship between infection and adverse pregnancy outcomes: an overview. *Ann. Periodontol.* 2001;6:153-163.

[117] Minkoff, H. Prematurity: infection as an etiologic factor. *Obstet. Gynecol.* 1983;62:137-144.

[118] Nabet, C., Lelong, N., et al. Maternal periodontitis and the causes of preterm birth: the case-control EPIPAP study. *J. Clin. Periodontol.* 2010; 37(1):37-45.

[119] Heimonen, A., Janket, S. J., Kaaja, R., Ackerson, L. K., Muthukrishnan, P., Meurman, J. H. Oral inflammatory burden and preterm birth. *J. Periodontol.* 2009;80:884-891.

[120] Lin, D., Moss, K., Beck, J. D., Hefti, A., Offenbacher, S. Persistently high levels of periodontal pathogens associated with preterm pregnancy outcome. *J. Periodontol.* 2007; 78:833-841.

[121] Katz, J., Chegini, N., Shiverick, K. T., Lamont, R. J. Localization of P. gingivalis in preterm delivery placenta. *J. Dent. Res.* 2009;88:575-578.

[122] Buduneli, N., Baylas, H., Buduneli, E., Turkoglu, O., Kose, T., Dahlen, G. Periodontal infections and pre-term low birth weight: A case-control study. *J. Clin. Periodontol.* 2005; 32:174-1812.

[123] Lopez, N. J., Smith, P. C., Gutierrez, J. Higher risk of preterm birth and low birth weight in women with periodontal disease. *J. Dent Res.* 2002; 81:58-63.

[124] Hasegawa, K., Furuichi, Y., Shimotsu, A., et al. Associations between systemic status, periodontal status, serum cytokine levels, and delivery outcomes in pregnant women with a diagnosis of threatened premature labor. *J. Periodontol.* 2003;74:1764-1770.

[125] Tanaka, Y., Narahara, H., Takai, N., Yoshimatusu, J., Anai, T., Miyakawa, I. Interleukin-1β and interleukin-8 in cervicovaginal fluid during pregnancy. *Am. J. Obstet. Gynecol.* 1998;79:644-649.

[126] Canakci, V., Canakci, F. C., Yildirim, A., Ingec, M., Eltas, A., Erturk, A. Periodontal disease increases the risk of severe pre-eclampsia among pregnant women. *J. Clin. Periodontol.* 2007;34(8):639-645.

[127] Davenport, E. S., William, C. E. C. S., Sterne, J. A. C., Murad, S., Sivapathasundram, V., Curtis, M. A. Maternal periodontal disease and preterm low birth weight: Case-control study. *J. Dent. Res.* 2002;81 (5): 313-318.

[128] Lunardelli, A. N., Peres, M. A. Is there an association between periodontal disease, prematurity and low birth weight? A population-based study. *J. Clin. Periodontol.* 2005;32:938-946.

[129] Bassani, D. G., Olinto, M. T., Kreiger, N. Periodontal disease and perinatal outcomes: A case-control study. *J. Clin. Periodontol.* 2007;34: 31-39.

[130] Lopez, J. N., Da Silva, I., Ipinza, J., Gutierrez, J. Periodontal therapy reduces the rate of preterm low birth weight in women with pregnancy – associated gingivitis. *J. Periodontol.* 2005; 76(11): 2144-2153.

[131] Offenbacher, S., Beck, J. D., Jared, H. L., et al. Effects of periodontal therapy on rate of preterm delivery: A randomized controlled trial. *Obstet. Gynecol.* 2009;114:551-559.

[132] M. Jeffcoat, S. Parry, M. Sammel, B. Clothier, A. Catlin, G. Macones. Periodontal infection and preterm birth: successful periodontal therapy reduces the risk of preterm birth: Successful periodontal treatment reduces preterm birth BJOG. *An. Inter. J. Obstetr. Gynaecol.* 2011;118 (2):250-256.

[133] Gomes-Filho, S. I., Cruz, S. S., Costa, N. C. M., et al Preliminary results from an alternative methodological strategy. *J. Periodontol.* 2010; 81 (12):1725-1733.

[134] Forey, A. B., Thornton, J. A., Lee, N. P. Systematic review with meta-analysis of the epidemiological evidence relating smoking to COPD, chronic bromchitis and emphysema. *BMC Pulmonary Med.* 2011; 11(1): 36-41.

[135] Kim, J. A., Lo, J. A., Pullin, A. D., Thornton-Johnson, S. D., Karimbux, Y. N. Scaling and root planing treatment for periodontitis to reduce preterm birth and low birth weight: A systematic review and meta-analysis of rondomized controlled trials. *J. Periodontol.* 2012;83 (12): 1508-1519.

[136] Sharma, N., Shamsuddin, H. Association between respiratory disease in hospitalized patients and periodontal disease: A cross-sectional study. *J. Periodontol.* 2011; 82 (8): 1155-1160.

[137] Scannapieco, F. A. Role of oral bacteria in respiratory infection. *J. Periodontol.* 1999;70(7):793-802.

[138] Garcia, I. R. Epidemiologic associations between periodontal disease and chronic obstructive pulmonary disease. *Ann. Periodontol.* 2001;6(1): 71-77.

[139] Sinclair, D. G., Evans, T. W. Nosocomial pneumonia in the intensive care unit. *Br. J. Hosp. Med.* 1994;51:177-189.

[140] Scannapieco, F. A., Stewart, E. M., Mylotte, J. M. Colonization of dental plaque by rerspiratory pathogens in medical intensive care patients. *Crit. Care Med.* 1992;20:740-745.

[141] Paju, S., Scannapieco, F. A. Oral biofilms, periodontitis, and pulmonary infections. *Oral Diseases.* 2007;13(6):508-512.

[142] Si, Y., Fan, H., Song, Z., Zhou, Zhang, J., Wang, Z. Association Between Periodontitis and Chronic Obstructive Pulmonary Disease in a Chinese Population. *J. Periodontol.* 2012; 83(10):1288-1296.

[143] Raghavendran, K., Mylotte, J. M., Scannapieco, F. A. Nursing home-associated pneumonia, hospital-acquired pneumonia and ventilator-assisted pneumonia: the contribution of dental biofilms and periodontal inflammation. *Periodontol.* 2000. 2007; 44:164–177.

[144] Okuda, K., Kimizuka, R., Abe, S., Kato, T., Ishuhara, F. Involvement of Periodontopathic Anaerobes in Aspiration Pneumonia. *J. Periodontol.* 2005; 76(11s): 2154-2160.

[145] Reddi, K., Wilson, M., Nair, S., et al. Comparison of the pro-inflammatory cytokines-stimulating active of the surface-associated proteins of periodontopathic bacteria. *J. Periodont. Res.* 1996;31:120-130.

[146] Fiddian-Green, R. G., Baker, S. Nosocomial pneumonia in the critically ill: product of aspiration or translocation? *Crit. Care Med.* 1991;19:763–769.

[147] Costerton, J. W., Lewandowski, Z., Caldwell, D. E., et al. Microbial biofilms. *Ann. Rev. Microbiol.* 1995;49:711-745.

[148] Katancik, A. J., Kritchevsky, S., Weyant, J. R., et al. Periodontitis and Airway Obstruction. *J. Periodontol.* 2005;76(11s):2161-2167.

[149] Zuomin Wang, Z., Zhou, X., Zhang, J., et al. Periodontal health, oral health behaviors, and chronic obstructive pulmonary disease issue. *J. Clin. Periodontol.* 2009;36(9):750-755.

[150] Abou-Raya, S., Abou-Raya, A., Naim, A., Abuelkheir, H. Rheumatoid arthritis, periodontal disease and coronary artery disease. *Clin. Rheumatol.* 2008;27(4):421-427.

[151] Bartold, P. M., Marshall, R. I., Haynes, D. R. Periodontitis and rheumatoid arthritis: a review. *J. Periodontol.* 2005;76(11):2066–2074.

[152] Burcu Cetinkaya, Esra Guzeldemir, Ersin Ogus, Sule Bulut. Proinflammatory and Anti-Inflammatory Cytokines in Gingival Crevicular Fluid and Serum of Patients With Rheumatoid Arthritis and Patients With Chronic Periodontitis. *J. Periodontol.* 2013; 84 (1):84-93.

[153] Al-Emadi, A., Bissada, N., Farah, C., Siegel, B., Al-Zaharani, M. Systemic diseases among patients with and without alveolar bone loss. *Quintessence Int.* 2006;37(10): 761–765.

[154] Kobayashi, T., Yokoyama, T., Ishida, K., et al. Serum Cytokine and periodontal profiles in relation to disease activity of rheumatoid arthritis in Japanese adults. *J. Periodontol.* 2010; 81(5): 650-657.

[155] Mikuls, R. T., Payne, B. J., Reinhardt, A. R., et al. Antibody responses to Porphyromonas gingivalis (P.gingivalis) in subjects with rheumatoid arthritis and periodontitis. *Inter. immunopatharmacol.* 2009;9(1):38-42.

[156] Rosenstein, D. E., Greenwald, A. R., Kusher, J. L., Weismann, G. Hypothesis: The humoral immune response to oral bacteria provides a stimulus for the development of rheumatoid arthritis. *Inflammation* 2004; 28(6):311-318.

[157] Passos, J. S., Gomes-Filho, S. I., Vianna, P. I. M., et al. Outcome Measurements in Studies on the Association Between Osteoporosis and Periodontal Disease. *J. Periodontol.* 2010;81(12):1773-1780.

[158] Wactwski-Wende, J., Hausmann, E., Hovey, K., et al. The association between osteoporosis and alveolar crestal height in postmenopausal women. *J. Periodontol.* 2005; 76(1): 2116-2124.

[159] Gera, I. Osteoporosis: a risk factor for periodontal disease (literature review). *Fogorv. Sz.* 2002;95(2):49-54.

[160] Wactawski-Wende, J., Hausmann, F., Hovey, K., Trevisan, M., Grossi, S., Genco, R. J. The Association Between Osteoporosis and Alveolar Crestal Height in Postmenopausal Women. *J. Periodontol.* 2005;76 (11s):2116-2124.

[161] Persson, R. E., Hollender, L. G., Powell, L. V., et al. Assessment of periodontal conditions an systemic disease in older subjects. part II: focus on osteoporosis. *J. Clin. Periodontol.* 2002;29(9):796–802.

[162] Pejčić, A., Kojović, D., Grigorov, I., Stamenković, B. Periodontitis and Osteoporosis. *Facta Universitatis - Series Medicine and Biology.* 2005; 12 (2):100-103.

[163] Jabbar, S., Drury, J., Fordham, J., Data, H. K., Francis, R. M., Tuck, S. R. Plasma vitamin D and cytokines in periodontal disease and postmenopausal osteoporosis. *J. Periodontal.* 2011;73:298-301.

[164] Ship, J. A., Puckett, S. A. Longitudinal study on oral health in subjects with Alzheimer's disease. *J. Am. Geriatr. Soc.* 1994;42(1):57–63.

[165] Kamer, A. R., Craig, R. G., et al. Inflammation and Alzheimer's disease: Possible role of periodontal diseases. *Alzheimer's and Dementia*. 2008;4 (4):242-250.
[166] Orlov, S., Mirkovic, B., Kojovic, D., Kesic, L. j, Petrovic, D., Pesic, Z. *Oralna medicina*. 2006. Sitomehanika, Niš.
[167] Risch, H. A. Etiology of pancreatic cancer, with a hypothesis concerning the role of N-nitroso compounds and excess gastric acidity. *J. Natl. Cancer Inst.* 2003;95(13):948-960

In: Current Trends in Periodontics and Implant Dentistry ISBN: 978-1-62618-819-8
Editors: Vishal Anand and Minkle Gulati

Chapter VI

Modulation of the Host Response: Broadening Horizons in the Management of Periodontal Disease

***Minkle Gulati*[1] *and Vishal Anand*[2]**
[1]Department of Periodontics, BBDCODS, Uttar Pradesh, India
[2]Department of Periodontics, Faculty of Dental Sciences, KGMU, Uttar Pradesh, India

Abstract

Though bacteria are the primary etiologic factor of periodontal diseases, yet the extent and severity of tissue destruction seen in periodontal diseases is determined by the host immuno-inflammatory response to these bacteria. This increasing awareness and knowledge of the host-microbial interaction in periodontal pathogenesis has presented the opportunity for exploiting new therapeutic strategies for periodontitis by means of targeting host response via host modulating agents. Host modulation means supplementing the natural inherent defense mechanisms of the host by modifying or modulating destructive or damaging aspects of the inflammatory host response that develops in the periodontal tissues as a result of the chronic challenge presented by the subgingival bacterial. This chapter discusses the host-modulating role of various systemically delivered (Tetracycline analogues, NSAIDs, lipoxins, resolvins, protectins, maresin, anti-cytokines, bisphosphonates, probiotics, periodontal vaccine and certain nutrients) and locally delivered agents (Enamel matrix proteins, bone morphogenetic protein, platelet derived growth factor, hypochlorous acid and taurine-N-monochloramine and cimetidine). These host-modulating agents are potentially non-invasive, have fewer side effects, do not require complicated application method and tip the balance between periodontal health and disease progression in the direction of a healing response, when combined with conventional treatments aimed at reducing the bacterial burden.

Keywords: Periodontitis, host modulation, locally delivered, systemically delivered, NSAIDs, bisphosphonate, tetracycline

Introduction

Although microbial plaque has been recognized as the primary etiologic agent for the development of periodontal disease. [1] Yet the severity, pattern and progression of this disease cannot be solely explained by the amount of plaque present. [2] Periodontal pathogens present within the microbial biofilms initiate the periodontal disease by producing harmful by-products and enzymes (e.g. hyaluronidases, collagenases, proteases) that break down extracellular matrices, such as collagen, as well as host cell membranes, in order to produce nutrients for their growth and possibly subsequent tissue invasion. [3] This results in a host immune-inflammatory response in the periodontal tissues characterized by the production of inflammatory cytokines (e.g. interleukins, tumor necrosis factor-a), prostanoids (e.g. prostaglandin E2) and enzymes [including the matrix metalloproteinases (MMPs). [4, 5] The level of these inflammatory mediators in the periodontal tissues is usually balanced by the anti-inflammatory cytokines and enzymes [4] of the host immune system which ultimately functions to eliminate microbial pathogens and protect the host. [3] However, an improper or exuberate immune response in certain individuals directly leads towards overproduction of destructive enzymes and inflammatory mediators. [3] This immune-inflammatory response that develops in the periodontal tissues following chronic exposure to bacterial plaque largely determines the susceptibility of individuals to periodontal disease. [4]

The increased susceptibility of certain individuals to periodontal disease is due to the variability in the host response as a result of environmental and acquired risk factors such as diabetes mellitus, psychological stress, smoking, genetic factors [such as interleukin-1 (IL-1) gene polymorphisms] etc. which can accentuate the host inflammatory response [6] and create an imbalance between the pro-inflammatory and anti-inflammatory activities in the periodontal tissues that result in the tissue destruction. [4] Several studies have shown that the biological activity of these inflammatory cytokines may be significantly related to the extent of severity of periodontal destruction observed clinically. [7, 8] The host immune-inflammatory response against bacterial plaque can thus be viewed as a "dual-edged sword", i.e. the response is protective by intent, yet in susceptible patients who exhibit exaggerated inflammatory response to plaque, it ultimately is responsible for perpetuating destruction of periodontium. [3]

In 1992 Socransky and Haffajee [9] identified several factors that must be present for a periodontal disease to result from a pathogen which includes

1 Presence of pathogen in a virulent clonal form possessing the chromosomal and extra-chromosomal genetic factors to initiate disease; and in a number sufficient to exceed the host threshold
2 Presence of other bacterial species that must foster, or at least not inhibit, the disease process i.e. absence of beneficial species which may modify the effects of a known pathogen and
3 Lastly, the presence of susceptible host. [9]

The differences in the host response to plaque is essentially the basis for the existence of two types of population i.e. *periodontal disease resistant* -wherein inspite of the presence of abundant plaque and calculus there is minimal tissue destruction; and *periodontal disease susceptible*- wherein despite maintaining a high standard of plaque control, patients succumb to aggressive forms of periodontitis, with deep pocketing, tooth mobility and early tooth loss. [10] In 1985, research began to concentrate very closely on bacterial-host interaction, which marked the beginning of the "host-bacterial interrelationship" era. [11]

Also in recent years, the role of the host response as the agent responsible for periodontal destruction has been focused, highlighting a changing paradigm in the etiology and pathogenesis of periodontitis. [12-14] This improved understanding of the pathogenesis of periodontal disease has to a large extent led to the emergence of host response modulation as a treatment concept. [4]

"Host response in the periodontium" is the defense mechanisms in periodontal tissues against bacterial infections [15] and host modulation means modifying or modulating destructive or damaging aspects of the inflammatory host response that develops in the periodontal tissues as a result of the chronic challenge presented by the subgingival bacterial plaque [4] i.e. host modulation means treating the host side of the host bacterial interaction. [10] The rationale behind this approach is to aid the host in its fight against infectious agents by supplementing the natural inherent defense mechanisms or to modify its response by changing the course of inflammatory systems. [15] The concept of host modulation was first introduced to dentistry by Williams in 1990 [16] and Golub et al. in 1992 [17] and later on expanded by many researchers. Indeed, in 1990 Williams stated that "there are compelling data from studies in animals and human trials indicating that pharmacologic agents that modulate the host responses believed to be involved in the pathogenesis of periodontal destruction, may be efficacious in slowing the progression of disease". [16] This shift in paradigms, with emphasis on host response, has led to the development of Host Modulatory Therapies (HMT) which can improve therapeutic outcomes, slow the progression of disease, allow for more predictable management of patients, and possibly even work as preventive agents against the development of periodontitis. [18, 19] The purpose of host modulatory therapy is to restore balance between, on the one hand, pro-inflammatory mediators and destructive enzymes, and, on the other hand, anti-inflammatory mediators and enzyme inhibitors. [4] Periodontal disease can be viewed as a balance between (i) a persisting bacterial burden and pro-inflammatory destructive events in the tissues, and (ii) resolution of inflammation and downregulation of destructive processes. Historically, periodontal treatment has focused on reducing the bacterial bioburden by root surface instrumentation, which targets only one aspect of the pathogenic process by reducing the antigenic challenge but often leads to recolonisation by putative pathogens due to incomplete elimination of all pathogenic subgingival bacteria after conventional treatment of this chronic disease. [4] Host response modulation especially targets host response mechanism and therefore, offers the potential for downregulating destructive aspects of the host response to enhance opportunities for wound healing and periodontal stability. HMT does not "switch off" normal defense mechanisms or inflammation [10] Instead it ameliorates excessive or pathologically elevated host inflammatory processes so that the balance between health (characterized by resolution of inflammation and wound healing) and disease progression (characterized by continued pro-inflammatory, destructive events) is tipped in the direction of a healing response, when combined with conventional treatments aimed at reducing the bacterial burden. [4] It has been recognized that the severity of periodontal disease, its rate of progression, and its response to therapy vary from patient to patient, which in turn is determined by the host susceptibility that is further governed by the patient's risk factors. [20] Though some of the risk factors can be modified to reduce patient's susceptibility, yet, HMT is a key to addressing many of the risk factors that have adverse outcome on the host response but are either not easily managed (e.g. smoking, diabetes) or cannot be changed (e.g. genetic susceptibility). [2] When considering a risk-based approach to therapy, the practitioner proceeds with caution with regard to invasive surgical procedures but may aggressively use pharmacologic adjuncts such as antimicrobials and host modulatory therapy in addition to mechanical therapy. [20]

Therefore, the best chance for clinical improvement may come from implementing complementary treatment strategies for each patient that targets different aspect of the periodontal balance. This includes reduction of bacterial burden, risk factor modification and host modulation, [21] along with patient motivation (Figure 1). Manipulation of the immune response to suppress unwanted reactions is also desirable in conditions such as autoimmunity, allergy, or graft rejection. It is also required in the cases of infectious disease to stimulate the protective processes. [15] Host modulators that are used to manage periodontal disease may also have additional beneficial effects on systemic diseases that have been linked to periodontal disease, such as cardiovascular disease, diabetes, premature birth etc. [2] Compared to other therapeutic modalities employed against infection, host response modulation, potentially is non-invasive, has fewer side-effects, and does not require complicated application method. [22, 23]

The current chapter highlights various host modulatory therapeutic agents for the treatment and management of periodontal diseases including nonsteroidal anti-inflammatory drugs, cytokine receptor antagonists, bone-sparing agents and other novel pharmacotherapeutics, which are used as an adjunct to the traditional periodontal therapies.

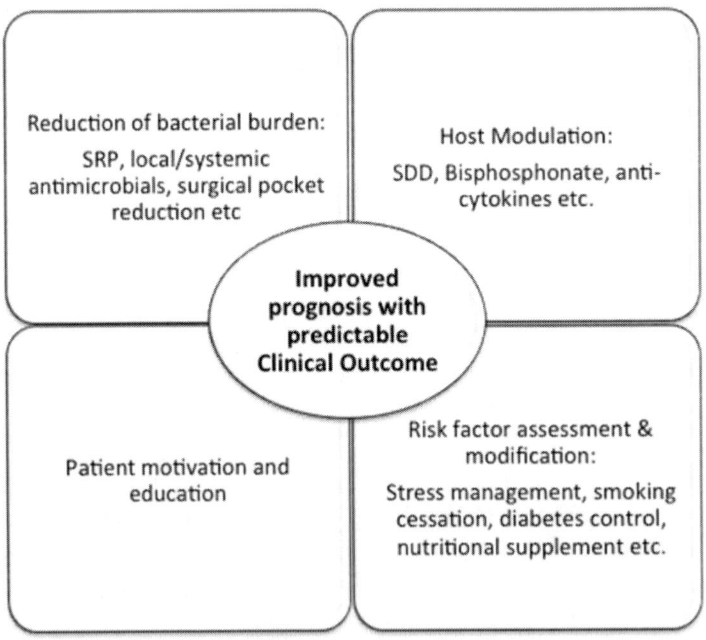

Figure 1. Complementary treatment strategies that target different aspects of the periodontal balance.

Locating potential targets for host modulatory agents to act upon has been made possible, based on the understanding of the host-microbial interaction in the pathogenesis of periodontal diseases. Hence, in order to understand the mechanism and site of action of these host modulators it is very essential to have a precise knowledge of the host microbial interactions.

Host Microbial Interaction in the Pathogenesis of Periodontal Diseases

Periodontitis is initiated and propagated by a group of predominantly gram-negative, anaerobic or microaerophilic bacteria that form a biofilm and also colonize the subgingival area, yet, although the microbial challenge comprising antigens and various other virulence factors, and in some cases invading bacteria are essential, they are insufficient for the disease to occur. [12]

There is increasing evidence that it is the microbially stimulated mobilization of the host tissues leading to the activation of monocytes, lymphocytes, fibroblasts, and other host cells and further production of inflammatory mediators including cytokines, matrix metalloproteinases, arachidonic acid metabolites and other enzymes, which are responsible for the bulk of tissue destruction seen in established periodontitis lesions. [18]

It is enigmatic that activation of the host immune-inflammatory system to achieve protection and defense virtually always results in some degree of destruction. Thus, immune-inflammatory host response is considered as a double-edged sword phenomenon in periodontitis in which the originally protective host response may lead to severe host tissue destruction on becoming exuberant due to factors like hyperresponsive host factors, both intrinsic (genetic) and induced (such as smoking) risk factors, or due to increased bacterial challenge within the tissues as a result of compromised bacterial control mechanisms at the gingival sulcus. Thus, the clinical picture observed is a result of the sum of these events, influenced by disease modifiers and risk factors. [12]

Inflammatory mediators released by host cells in turn stimulate more host cells to release additional quantities of inflammatory mediators in positive feedback cycles. [2] The severity and rate of progression of disease also feeds back to influence the nature and magnitude of the microbial challenge by, for example, influencing the pH and availability of oxygen and various nutrients in the periodontal pocket. [12] The adjunctive use of host modulatory therapy are used to interrupt these positive - feedback loops and slow down the progression of the disease and prevent and/or minimize the destruction. [2, 6]

However, a more recent approach to host modulation is targeting cell signaling pathways which affect expression of more than one inflammatory mediator and alter the whole cytokine network. For this reason, it is also important to understand the role of individual signaling pathways in inflammation and tissue destruction in periodontal disease, as modulation of these pathways will probably prove more effective than current treatment strategies.

In periodontal disease the most important pathways include the mitogen activated protein kinase (MAPK), nuclear factor kappa b (NFκβ) and janus tyrosine kinase-signal transducer and activator of transcription (JAK/ STAT). [24]

Some of the intermediate signaling molecules of these pathways, which can be targeted by HMT, are extracellular regulated kinases (ERK), c-Jun N-terminal activated kinases (JNK) and p38 of MAPK pathway; and interleukin-1-receptor associated kinase (IRAK), TNF-receptor associated factor-6 (TRAF-6) and Iκβ kinase complex (IKK) of NFκβ pathway. [16] Another pathway that can be targeted by HMT is the RANK/RANKL/OPG (receptor activator of nuclear factor kappa β/receptor activator of nuclear factor kappa β ligand/ osteoprotegrin) pathway.

RANKL, a membrane-bound protein is a member of the tumor necrosis factor superfamily, which is normally expressed by osteoblasts but at inflammatory sites can also be expressed by immune cells like T-cells.

The binding of RANKL to its receptor RANK on the surface of pre-osteoblasts results in the activation of c-jun terminal kinase and the subsequent activation of nuclear factor-kappaB, leading to osteoclast formation. This RANK-RANKL binding can however be naturally blocked by OPG, a soluble tumor necrosis factor receptor-like molecule that acts as a decoy and thus prevents osteoclastogenesis. [24]

Host Modulatory Therapy

Host modulatory therapies include systemically or locally delivered pharmaceuticals that are prescribed as adjuncts to other forms of periodontal treatment. [4] A number of host modulatory agents have been investigated in clinical trials for their potential use as adjuncts to mechanical nonsurgical periodontal therapy.

These include the systemic (flurbiprofen) and topical (ketoprofen) use of nonsteroidal anti-inflammatory drugs, the systemic use of subantimicrobial-dose doxycycline (SDD; Periostat [Colla- Genex Pharmaceuticals, Newtown, Pennsylvania]), the systemic use of bisphosphonates (Fosamax) etc. [20]

Yet, among the systemically delivered HMT, low-dose doxycycline (20 mg orally two times daily), is the only drug, which has received regulatory approval from FDA (US Food and Drug Administration) for its adjunctive use in conjunction with nonsurgical periodontal procedures for treating periodontitis. [25]

However, among the locally delivered HMT, FDA has approved Enamel matrix derivative (EMD - Emdogain®, Biora AB, Malmö, Sweden), PDGF combined with a resorbable synthetic bone matrix growth-factor enhanced matrix (GEM 21S®, Osteohealth, Shirley, NY) and as well as recombinant human bone morphogenetic protein-2 (rhBMP-2; INFUSE® Bone Graft, Medtronic, Minneapolis, MN, US) for adjunctive use during surgery to assist with clinical attachment gain and wound healing and to assist in regenerative procedures. [26, 27]

With an increasing understanding of the characteristics of the host's immune-inflammatory response to plaque and the mechanisms of tissue destruction that lead to periodontitis, novel approaches to modulating the immune response have been explored in humans. [5]

Systemically Administered HMT

Host Modulating Agents Acting against MMPs

MMPs are zinc- and calcium-dependent endopeptidases, which are secreted by a variety of host cells (such as polymorphonuclear leukocytes, macrophages, fibroblasts, bone, epithelial and endothelial cells) and play key roles in the degradation of the extracellular matrix, basement membrane and modify the action of cytokines as well as activation of osteoclasts. [28] Over 25 MMPs have been identified which have been categorized as collagenases, gelatinases, matrilysins, stromelysins, membrane-type MMPs, metalloelastase and others. [29, 30]

The activities of these MMPs are naturally regulated in the host by endogenous MMP inhibitors that includes a family of tissue-inhibitors of metalloproteinases (TIMPs: TIMP-1, TIMP-2, TIMP-3 and TIMP-4) as well as by liver-derived, serum borne α2-macroglobulin. [31] However, during active periodontal diseases, the host's immune response towards microbial attack leads to excessive production as well as activity of these MMPs which if not adequately controlled by the endogenous metalloproteinases inhibitors, results in enormous tissue destruction. To impede this destruction of host tissues many agents modulating the host response by inhibiting these MMPs have been developed. These Synthetic inhibitors of MMP generally contain a chelating group, which inhibits MMPs by binding to the catalytic zinc atom at its active site. In the medical field, recent advances have taken place in the synthetic MMP inhibitor designs that are based on the recognition of different zinc chelating groups. These include hydroxamate, carboxylate, thiol, pyrimidine, hydroxpyrone, phosphorus and tetracycline based MMP inhibitor. [32, 33] Though numerous MMP inhibitors have been investigated, only tetracycline based host modulating agent i.e. SDD (Doxycycline hyclate 20 mg; Periostat, CollaGenex, Pharmaceuticals Newton PA) has been approved by FDA to be used as an adjunct to periodontal treatment. [25]

Tetracycline Analogues as Host Modulating Agents

Tetracycline belongs to a class of broad-spectrum antibiotics with activity against gram-positive, gram-negative and anaerobic microbes that exert their antimicrobial action by interfering with the protein synthesis at the ribosomal level. Based on their antimicrobial efficacy against putative periodontopathogens, these have long been considered useful adjuncts in periodontal therapy. Tetracycline with antibiotic activity consists of a tetracyclic naphthacene carboxamide ring system having a dimethylamine group at carbon 4 (C4) in ring "A" which is responsible for its antibacterial property. [34] However, about 3 deacades ago, Golub, et al. discovered that tetracyclines and its analogues have the unexpected ability to inhibit matrix metalloproteinases (MMPs), by mechanisms unrelated to its antibacterial properties. [35, 36] Mitscher LA did an extensive research on the chemistry of tetracyclines and demonstrated that a number of tetracycline analogs can be synthesized by deleting side-chain(s) or, in some cases, adding moieties to the parent tetracycline molecule. [37]

Based on this knowledge Golub and McNamara et al. synthesized a CMT by removing the dimethylamino group from the carbon-4 position of the "A" ring, resulting in the 4-de-dimethylaminotetracycline (CMT), which eliminated the drug's antimicrobial efficacy, but did not reduce the ability of the drug to block the activity of collagenases. [38, 39]

Later five different analogs were investigated regarding their ability to inhibit mammalian collagenase activity and bone resorption. These include CMT-1 (4-dedimethylomino TC), CMT-2 (TC nitrile), CMT-3 (6-demethyl 6-deoxy 4-dedimethylomino TC), CMT-4(7-ch1oro 4-dedimethylamino TC) and 8 CMT-5 (pyrozole) [40, 41] Golub et al. 1991 concluded that the C-4 moiety was not required for the anticollagenase activity of the tetracycline molecule. [40]

Ryan ME and Golub LM in their paper have listed the pleiotropic mechanisms by which Tetracyclines inhibit connective tissue breakdown. These have been grouped as those

a *Mediated by extracellular mechanisms:* Direct inhibition of active matrix metalloproteinases based on its Ca and Zn ions chelating properties, inhibition of oxidative activation of pro-matrix metalloproteinases, excessive proteolysis of pro-matrix metalloproteinases into enzymatically-inactive fragments, protection of α1-proteinase inhibitor, thus indirectly inhibits serine proteinase activity
b *Mediated by cellular regulation:* Tetracyclines decrease the level of cytokines, inducible nitric oxide synthase, phospholipase A2, prostaglandin synthase as well as affects protein kinase C, calmodulin
c *Mediated by pro-anabolic effects:* Increase collagen production, osteoblast activity and bone formation. [28]

More recently, the non-antibiotic properties of tetracycline i.e. biologic actions of tetracycline affecting inflammation, proteolysis, angiogenesis, apoptosis, metal chelation, ionophoresis, and bone metabolism have been discussed by Sapadin et al. [34]

Currently, 3 groups of tetracyclines are available: natural tetracycline, semisynthetic tetracycline (Doxycycline and minocycline), and chemically modified tetracyclines (CMTs). [34] Doxycycline, a semi-synthetic antibiotic, with a superior half-life in the circulation and fewer side-effects (e.g., less photosensitivity) compared to other tetracyclines has been preferred over other tetracyclines as an adjunctive antibiotic to scaling and root planning (SRP) in the non-surgical treatment of the periodontal patient. It has also been revealed that though tetracyclines inhibit tissue-destructive MMPs, it is the doxycycline (a semisynthetic tetracycline) which is the most potent MMP inhibitor and exhibits MMP inhibition in vivo at plasma levels that are subantimicrobial. [42, 43]

Though Golub et al. in 1990 introduced the Low dose doxycycline (later termed SDD), when they suggested that a regimen of low-dose doxycycline capsules might provide a safe and effective adjunct to non-surgical periodontal therapy in the management of pathologic collagenolysis in the periodontal patient without inducing tetracycline resistance in the subgingival plaque; [43] it was only in 1997 that the anticollagenolytic effect of SDD was acknowledged for the first time in human studies by Golub LM et al. [44] A typical prescription for Periostat (20-mg doxycycline tablets) is for at least 3 months (180 tablets, 1 tablet twice a day until complete), and refills may be provided for longer courses of therapy. [20] Till date various clinical trials performed to evaluate the efficacy of SDD as an adjunct to SRP have revealed statistically significant better results than SRP + placebo. [45-49]

Yet, in one of the study a rebound effect was seen in the subantimicrobial doxycycline group after cessation of doxycycline resulting in an increase in mean probing depths and attachment levels at the 6 month follow-up i.e. 3 months after completion of 3 months of drug therapy. [50]

Preshaw PM supports that the prolonged dosing of SDD for 9 months might lead to the achievement of maximum benefit with less chance of relapse upon stopping the medication. [4] Which is also demonstrated by a study done by Caton et al. in 2001 where no relapse was seen 3 months after patients finished a 9-month course of subantimicrobial dose doxycycline. [51]

Most recently, bisphosphonates, which are generally bone-sparing agents have been found to inhibit MMPs. [52, 53] Bisphosphonates will be discussed later in this chapter.

Host Modulating Agents Acting against Arachidonic Acid Metabolites

Free arachidonic acid (AA) is produced in the hosts when phospholipase A2 acts on the phospholipids present in plasma membranes of the cells, wherein the phospholipids have been made available to the phospholipase A2activity, due to the damage initiated by the bacterial as well as host factors. This AA can then be metabolized to produce prostaglandins, prostacyclin, and thromboxane via the cyclooxygenase (CO) pathway as well as leukotrienes and other hydroxyeicosatetraenoic acids via the lipoxygenase (LO) pathway. Furthermore, there are 2 isoforms of Cyclooxygenase (COX): COX-1which is important for physiologic functions including gastric cytoprotection; and COX-2 which is thought to be involved in inflammation as it is inducible and upregulated by proinflammatory cytokines. [54, 55]

Several authors over decades have demonstrated the role of arachidonic acid metabolites in the onset, progression as well as regulation of the magnitude of the tissue-destructive response in progressive periodontitis. [57, 58] Recently, Dybvig MW also validated that prostaglandins are an important mediator of bone loss in periodontitis. [59] Hence, one proposed approach to modulate the host response is inhibition of enzymes responsible for the release of these destructive products. [54] Nonsteroidal anti-inflammatory (NSAIDs) drugs block the activity of both cyclooxygenase isozymes (COX- 1 and -2), which mediate the production of arachidonic acid metabolites that are proinflammatory mediators implicated in a variety of bone resorptive and tissue degrading processes.

These anti-inflammatory drugs including analgesics such as ibuprofen and aspirin with multiple levels of anti-inflammatory effects also block platelet activity through thromboxane inhibition. [15]

Many authors have demonstrated the role of NSAIDs like flurbiprofen, [60] indomethacin, [61] and naproxen, [62] in inhibiting gingivitis and progression of periodontitis. Though after reviewing various studies it has been demonstrated that systemic daily administration of NSAIDs for periods upto three years results in a significant reduction in the rate of bone loss, yet, it has a major disadvantage of rebound effect following the cessation of the drug use. [63] Additionally, NSAIDs like ketorolac tromethamine rinse and S-ketoprofen dentifrice have also been evaluated for topical administration. [64] While inhibition of periodontal disease progression via the modulation of arachidonic acid metabolites with NSAIDs is evident from a number of studies, efforts are being taken to formulate specifically COX-2 inhibitors (In contrast to standard NSAIDs that inhibit both COX 1 and 2 and secondarily produce unwanted side effects related to the gastrointestinal tract, kidney and platelets) and lipoxins, as potential second and third-generation therapeutics. [65]

Lipoxins (LX) are generated endogenously late in inflammation via cell-cell interaction when a second lipoxygenase (eg. 5-LO) interacts with a lipoxygenase product (eg. hydroxyeicosatetraenoic acid) generated earlier from archidonic acid. [66]

Lipoxins possess both antiinflammatory and proresolving potential. Two lipoxin derivatives: lipoxin A4 and B4 have been identified which have been described as oxygenated arachidonic acid derivatives and termed "lipoxygenase interaction products" by Serhan et al. [67, 68, 65] of interest is the aspirin-triggered lipoxin (ATL) or 15-epi-lipoxins which are produced when, in the presence of aspirin, acetylated COX-2 loses its activity required to produce prostaglandin (PG)H2 but retains oxygenase activity to synthesize 15R-HETE from arachidonate which in turn is transformed to ATL. [69]

The pro-resolving actions of lipoxins have been summarized by Serhan et al. as reduction of neutrophil infiltration and recruitment, blocking cytokines and reactive oxygen species generation, thereby preventing connective tissue and bone loss. [70]

Serhan et al. in 2003 examined the response of transgenic rabbits overexpressing 15-LO (15-LO products can interact with 5-LO to generate lipoxins via transcellular biosynthesis) to inflammatory challenge and demonstrated that overexpression of 15-LO and lipoxins is associated with dampened neutrophil-mediated tissue degradation and bone loss, suggesting that enhanced anti-inflammation status is an active process. [71] This shows that LXs can be targets for host modulatory therapy against periodontitis.

Lipid-Inflammatory Mediators as Target for HMT

Among the other endogenous chemical mediators resolvins, protectins, and newly identified maresins, have emerged as a novel genus of potent and stereoselective players that mediate resolution and counter-regulate excessive acute inflammation [72] which are biosynthesized from precursors like omega-3 polyunsaturated fatty acids (PUFAs), eicosapentaenoic acid (EPA) and docosahexaenoic acid (DHA) via sequential steps involving lipoxygenases (LOX), and cyclooxygenases (COX). [70, 73, 74] Resolvins further can be categorized as the E-series and D-series of resolvins, derived from EPA and DHA, respectively. [73] The role of these endogenous chemical mediators is similar to that of lipoxins i.e. inhibition of neutrophil recruitment etc. [73, 72] Thus, designing pharmacological mimetics of naturally occurring pro-resolving mediators offers exciting new targets for drug design, [75] especially for host modulation therapy.

Host Modulating Agents Acting against Cytokines

Role of cytokines in the pathogenesis of periodontitis is well known. An intermediate mechanism that lies between bacterial stimulation and tissue destruction is the production of cytokines, which stimulates inflammatory events that activate effector mechanisms. [8] The detection of pro-inflammatory as well as anti-inflammatory cytokines have demonstrated a dual nature for host inflammatory immune responses in periodontal diseases, where the control of periodontal infection and the destruction of periodontal tissues seem to share similar cellular and molecular pathways. Where on one hand Pro-inflammatory cytokines (eg. IL-1α, IL-1β, IL-6, TNF-α, IFN-γ etc.) seem to play active roles in the control of periodontal infection through the chemoattraction and activation of phagocytes being considerably harmful from the tissue destruction viewpoint, triggering periodontal tissue destruction; on the other hand the anti-inflammatory cytokines (IL-4, IL-10 etc.) are associated with the attenuation of periodontal issue destruction with no compromise to the control of periodontopathogens. [76, 77] Thus, these molecules hold a great potential for controlling the adverse effects of the host immune response and/or augmenting the regenerative potential of cytokines and HMT against cytokines (cytokine therapy) may prove to be an effective strategy for treating periodontal diseases. [78]

These therapies aim at

a Antagonizing the pro-inflammatory cytokines via
   - *Cytokine receptor antagonist:* that binds to the receptor present on the target cell and prevents the cytokine from binding to the target cell. E.g. interleukin-1 receptor antagonist (IL-1ra) which is commercially available as Kineret - a recombinant, nonglycosylated form of the human IL-1ra (Anakinra, Amgen). [24, 79]
   - *Anti-cytokine antibodies*: eg. Antibodies against TNF-α, IL-6, IL-12, IL-15, IL-23, IL-17. Some of the anticytokine antibodies currently available are:
     - Anti TNF-α antibody: Adalimumab (Humira, manufacturered by Abbott Laboratories), Cetrolizumab pegol (Cimzea, manufacturered by Union chimique belge), Golimumab (Simponi, manufacturered by Centocor) etc.
     - Anti IL-6 antibody: Tocilizumab (RoActemra, manufacturered by Roche)
     - Anti IL-15 antibody: AMG714 (AMG714, manufacturerd by Novartis)
     - Anti IL-12 and IL-23 antibody: Ustekinumab (Stelara, manufacturered by Centacor)
     - Anti IL-17 antibody: AIN457 (AIN457, manufacturered by Novartis) [24]
   - *Soluble cytokine receptors:* that binds to the cytokines in solution and prevents signaling. eg. sIL-1R, sTNF-R, sIL-6R are the soluble receptors against IL-1β, TNF-α and IL-6 respectively. [79] Assuma et al. explored the role of soluble receptors of IL-1 and TNF in inhibiting periodontal destruction and reported that the soluble receptors inhibited roughly 80% of the inflammatory cell numbers, osteoclasts and bone resorption as well. [80] Promising results for host modulation have also been achieved through gene delivery of soluble proteins, such as tumor necrosis factor receptor-1, which have shown reduction in tumor necrosis factor activity and inhibition of alveolar bone loss. [81]

b Disrupting inflammatory cell-signalling pathways to inhibit the production of pro-inflammatory cytokines and/or stimulate anti-inflammatory cytokine production:

Cell-signalling pathways like MAPK, NFκB, JAK/STAT and Rank/ Rankl-OPG pathways as described earlier in this chapter are dependent on a number of signaling-intermediate molecules for its uninterrupted functioning. Targeting these pathways or the intermediate signaling molecules for their blockade with HMT may be more effective than targeting specific cytokines. [6] It has also been seen that the activity of cytokines is also controlled by the suppressors of cytokine signaling (SOCS - SOCS-1, -2 and -3 mRNA), which when expressed down-regulate the signal transduction and inflammatory cytokine production as part of an inhibitory feedback loop. [82, 83] The exploration of these molecules further open up many new possibilities for modulating host response.

Based on the clinical data Souza et al. have listed some of the inhibitors targeting these signalling pathways that have been developed and have demonstrated anti-inflammatory activity. These are: SD-282, SC-409, SB (SmithKline Beecham) -242235, AW-814141, BIRB-796 (Boehringer Ingelheim Pharmaceuticals Inc., Ridgefield, CT, US) and VX-702 that act as p38 inhibitors; SP600125 (Celgene Corporation, San Diego, California, US) as JNK inhibitor; FR180204 as ERK inhibitor; BMS (Bristol-Myers Squibb)-345541 as NFκB inhibitor; CP-690550 (Pfizer) as JK3 inhibitor. [6]

Lima et al. 2004 further demonstrated protective role of Pentoxifylline (PTX), a methylxanthine derivative, in experimental periodontitis as inhibitor of cytokine synthesis, mainly tumor necrosis factor. [84]

Likewise, a number of intracellular signaling pathways involved in osteoclastogenesis, activated upon RANK-RANKL binding are blocked by osteoprotegerin (a natural inhibitor of RANKL), which acts as a decoy and blocks the binding of RANKL to RANK. Moreover, increase in RANKL/osteoprotegerin ratio at periodontally inflamed sites has been associated with disease severity. [85]

Thus modulation of the RANKL/RANK/osteoprotegerin axis via pharmacotherapeutic agents, may lead to an increase in osteoprotegerin and a decrease in RANKL to a level consistent with an equilibrium state between bone formation and bone destruction. [24]

Jin et al. 2007 demonstrated that systemic delivery of OPG-Fc fusion protein inhibits alveolar bone resorption in experimental periodontitis, supporting the fact that RANKL inhibition may represent an important therapeutic strategy for the prevention of progressive alveolar bone loss. [86] Studies to date have indicated that RANKL inhibitors, such as a fully human monoclonal antibody that specifically targets RANKL currently available as denosumab (Denosumab, Amgen) can lead to increased bone mineral density and decreased bone resorption. [24]

Recombinant anti-inflammatory cytokine administration

Martuscelli et al. demonstrated that subcutaneous injections of rh IL-11 (anti-inflammatory cytokine) were able to slow the progression of attachment and radiographic alveolar bone loss in a ligature-induced beagle dog model. [87]

Host Modulating Agents Acting against Bone Resorption

Bisphosphonates (BPs) are pyrophosphate analogs that can suppress osteoclastic bone resorption. [88]

They all have a P-C-P backbone i.e. two phosphonate groups that share a common carbon atom, to which two side chains (R1 and R2) responsible for the large range of activity observed among the BPs are attached. The P-C-P group required both for binding to bone mineral and for cell-mediated antiresorptive activity is resistant to hydrolysis and hence excreted unaltered by the body. BPs are absorbed by the bones and then released locally during acidification associated with osteoclastic activity. [89] The chemistry and structure of R2 substituents determine the antiresorptive potency of the bisphosphonates. [90] Etidronate, Clodronate and Tiludronate are first generation BPs having a short R2 side chain as $-CH_3$, -Cl and chlorophenylthiomethylene respectively. Their potency is 10-1000 folds less than second-generation bisphosphonates such as in Pamidronate and Alendronate, which have a primary amino group at the R2 side chain.

Furthermore, the third-generation bisphosphonate Ibandronate is an analog of pamidronate that contains a tertiary amino group and is 10,000-fold more potent than the first-generation compounds. [91, 92] Bisphosphonates are known to bind to hydroxyapatite crystals and prevent their dissolution in addition to increasing osteoblast differentiation and inhibiting osteoclast activation. [4]

William V Giannobile has summarized and categorized the bone-specific actions of bisphosphonates at *the tissue level* (decrease bone turnover due to inhibition of bone resorption, decrease the number of new bone multicellular units resulting in a net positive whole body bone balance), *cellular level* (decrease osteoclast recruitment, osteoclast adhesion, depth of resorption site and release of cytokines by macrophages along with an increase in osteoclast apoptosis and osteoblast differentiation and number) and *at the molecular level* (inhibit mevalonate pathway resulting in perturbated cell activity and induction of apoptosis as well as decreasing post-translational prenylation of GTP binding proteins). [5, 93] Therefore, they have been used extensively in the management of osteoporosis and other bone resorptive conditions such as multiple myeloma and metastatic cancer to the bones and have resulted in statistically significant reduction in skeletal complications like compression of spinal cord, pathologic fractures and the need for subsequent radiotherapy or surgery to bone. [4, 94-96]

FDA has approved the use of these drugs orally or intravenously in the management of Paget's disease, osteoporosis and bone metastases. [97] Based on its bone-sparing properties there exists a possible use for bisphosphonates in the management of periodontal diseases as well also provision for an interesting management strategy to stimulate osteogenesis in conjunction with regenerative materials around osseous defects and may result in the promotion of bone formation around endosseous implants. [15]

Shoji et al. in 1995 demonstrated that systemic administration of a bisphosphonate, risedronate, could prevent alveolar bone resorption in rats with experimental periodontitis. [98] In 2003 Shinnawi et al. in a human clinical trial examined the effect of alendronate sodium on alveolar bone loss in periodontitis and observed a statistically significant difference in bone density ($P < 0.001$) between the two goups (one receiving the BP drug and other group receiving no drug as an adjunct to periodontal therapy) with increased bone density favouring the alendronate group. [99]

Yet, the use of BPs especially intravenous administration has been associated with a serious adverse effect of osteonecrosis of the jaws (ONJ) as documented in several publications. [100, 101] Nonetheless, bisphosphonates may still offer a promising therapeutic option for periodontal bone loss, if these drugs can be administrated locally without affecting the microvascular systems present in the alveolar bones. [102]

Similarly, Chemically modified tetracyclines (CMT) are also known to diminish bone resorption by a direct effect on osteoclast structure and function as well as inhibition of the activity of MMPs and inhibition of the secretion of other collagenolytic enzymes (i.e. lysosomal cathepsins). [15]

Furthermore, anti-integrins can also block the initial osteoclast adhesion to the matrix and prevent bone resorption. [3] Based on the well demonstrated role of estrogen on excessive bone resorption as well as its lack in the post-menopausal osteoporosis affecting the remodeling of the bone tissue in such a way that, in most patients with periodontitis the amount of bone resorbed exceeds that being formed, resulting in net bone loss, Inagaki et al. has also suggested the use of selective estrogen receptor modulators (SERM) and hormone replacement therapy (HRT) to improve the clinical outcome of periodontal disease as an adjunctive treatment to preserve periodontal bone mass. [103]

Shu et al. in 2008 also demonstrated in human periodontal cells that estrogen may play a significant role in modulating periodontal tissue responses to lipo-polysaccharide, and may exert its bone-sparing effects on periodontal tissues via altering the expression of inflammatory cytokines. [104] Yet, given the potentially large number of significant side-effects associated with hormone replacement therapy, it is difficult to see this being recommended as a management strategy for periodontitis. [24]

Modulation of NOS

Nitric oxide is a free radical with important physiological functions of maintaining homeostasis. While homeostasis requires low nitric oxide tissue levels, pro-inflammatory stimuli such as endotoxins leads to increased expression of the inducible nitric oxide synthase enzyme (iNOS) that produces a large amount of nitric oxide (NO) and peroxynitrite, which act as a cytotoxic molecule against the invading microorganism and may be related to beneficial effects, yet, it may also cause deleterious effects to host such as DNA damage, lipid peroxidation, protein damage and stimulation of inflammatory cytokine release. [105-107]

Lohinai et al. 1998 demonstrated the protective effects of mercaptoethylguanidine (MEG), a selective inhibitor of iNOS and a peroxynitrite scavenger against the enhanced concentration of NO and the associated extravasation and bone destruction in ligature-induced periodontitis in the rat. [108] Recently, Leitao et al. 2005 also proved that Nitric oxide synthase inhibitors prevents alveolar bone resorption in experimental periodontitis. [109]

Other Host Modulatory Therapies

Probiotic

Probiotics have demonstrated significant potential as therapeutic options for a variety of disease as they have been known to modulate cytokine secretion profiles, influence T lymphocyte populations, protect against physiologic stress, and enhance intestinal epithelial cell function and antibody secretion. [110] Recently, Teughels et al. 2011 explored whether the use of probiotics can influence the periodontal microbiota and periodontal health and concluded that probiotics might offer opportunities to manipulate the oral microbiota and, periodontal health by either direct microbiological interactions or by immunomodulatory interactions. [111]

Periodontal Vaccine

George Hajishengallis reported that Toll Like Receptors (TLRs) may offer novel targets for host-modulation therapy in periodontitis since manipulation of TLR signalling may contribute to control of infection or regulation of inflammation and, moreover, synthetic or natural TLR agonists could serve as novel periodontal vaccine adjuvants. [112]

Yokoyama et al. in 2007 also demonstrated that egg yolk antibody against Porphyromonas gingivalis (IgY-GP) proved to be an effective immunotherapeutic agent in the treatment of periodontitis. [113] Similarly, Choi et al. reported that prior immunization of mice to Fusobacterium nucleatum modulated the host immune responses to P. gingivalis at the humoral, cellular and molecular level. [114]

Nutrients

Nutrients, which include major extracellular antioxidants, include vitamin C, vitamin E, carotenoids, reduced glutathione and omega 3 fatty acids can also act as modulators of inflammation by scavenging free radicals as they are formed, sequestering transition metal ions and catalyzing formation of other molecules. [63] Studies have also demonstrated that cranberry juice contains molecules (A-type cranberry proanthocyanidins: AC-PACs) that inhibit MMPs, interleukin-6, interleukin-8, and prostaglandin E production by lipopolysaccharide-activated gingival fibroblasts and hence show potential for the development of novel host-modulating strategies to inhibit tissue destruction during periodontitis. [115, 116]

Locally Administered HMT

In addition, a number of local host modulatory agents have been investigated in clinical trials for their potential use as adjuncts to surgical procedures not only to improve on wound healing but also to stimulate regeneration of lost bone, periodontal ligament, and cementum, restoring the complete periodontal attachment apparatus. [20]

These agents include enamel matrix protcins (Emdogain), bone morphogenetic proteins 2 and 7, growth factors (platelet-derived growth factor and insulin-like growth factor), tetracyclines, NSAIDs, Bisphosphonates, Cimetidine, Hypochlorous Acid and Taurine-N-Monochloramine. [20, 64, 117-119]

Enamel Matrix Proteins (EMD)

It is believed that during development of root and attachment apparatus, there is a secretory phase in which Hertwig's epithelial root sheaths (HERS- the apical extension of the enamel organ), secretes enamel-related matrix proteins. [120]

The major fraction of the enamel matrix proteins is composed of the amelogenins, a family of hydrophobic proteins that constitute for more than 90% of the organic constituent of the enamel matrix while the remaining 10% includes proline-rich non-amelogenins, tuftelin, tuft protein, serum proteins and at least one salivary protein [121] Enamel matrix derivative is now commercially available for the treatment of periodontal defects as Emdogain® (Biora AB, Malmö, Sweden) which has received FDA approval. The other component of Emdogain is the vehicle, propylene glycol alginate, which facilitates its application. [122]

The enamel proteins are extracted from tooth buds derived from six-month-old piglets and the basic rationale behind using Emdogain is that it will act as a tissue-healing modulator that would mimic the events that occur during root development and help stimulate periodontal regeneration. [122-124] EMD initiates periodontal regeneration through recruitment of cementoblasts to the root-surface and stimulates these to form root-cementum, which will thereafter secondarily lead to regeneration of periodontal fibers and alveolar bone, [125] by enhancing proliferation rate, metabolism and protein synthesis, cellular attachment rate, and mineral nodule formation of PDL cells, cementoblasts and mature osteoblasts in addition to enhancement of PDL cell attachment. [120]

It has also been shown that EMD increases intracellular cAMP signalling and autocrine production of transforming growth factor (TGF-β), IL-6 and platelet-derived growth factors (PDGF AB), which contributes to periodontal healing and regeneration in a process mimicking natural root development. [126] Similarly, it has also been shown that amelogenin induces expression of nuclear protein that stimulates bone sialoprotein (BSP) gene transcription in osteoblasts, which is an early phenotypic marker of osteoblast and cementoblast differentiation and has been implicated in the nucleation of hydroxyapatite during bone formation. [127]

Local application of amelogenins also stimulates angiogenesis by inducing secretion of VEGF, PDGF, and matrix metalloproteinase-2 which aid in wound healing. [125] The above mentioned actions of EMD justify its role as a host modulating agent.

Bone Morphogenetic Protein (BMP)

BMPs are the members of transforming growth factor-β (TGF-β) superfamily, which play a crucial role in cell growth and differentiation. BMP guides modulation and differentiation of mesenchymal cells into bone and bone marrow cells. [128] Absorbable collagen sponge (ACS) containing recombinant human BMP-2 has been approved for clinical use in certain oral surgery procedures, including sinus augmentation and localized alveolar ridge augmentation, under the name INFUSE® Bone Graft (Medtronic, Minneapolis, MN, US) and InductOS™ (Wyeth, Maidenhead, UK). These ACS release the protein over time in the location where it is implanted and provides a scaffold on which new bone can grow. As the graft site heals, the ACS is absorbed and replaced by bone. [27] Studies have demonstrated the unparalleled osteoinductive potential of rhBMP to augment alveolar bone, support implant osseointegration, periodontal regeneration and wound healing. [129-131]

Platelet Derived Growth Factor (PGDF)

FDA approved Growth-factor Enhanced Matrix, GEM 21S® (Osteohealth, Shirley, NY) which is a combination of a bioactive highly purified recombinant human PDGF-BB with an osteoconductive bone matrix (β-tricalcium phosphate, β-TCP), and is the only product for dental therapy that contains PDGF, one of the main growth factors often referred to as "nature's wound healing agent". [27]

PDGF, as a host modulating agent can increase chemotaxis of neutrophils and monocytes, increase autocrine expression and generation of additional cytokines like TNF-alpha, IL-1beta, PDGF and chemokines, stimulate fibroblasts proliferation and extracellular matrix synthesis, increase chemotaxis, proliferation and differentiation of endothelial cells, stimulates proliferation of mesenchymal progenitor cells and differentiation of fibroblasts into myofibroblasts. [132]

Nebins et al. 2005 demonstrated that the purified rhPDGF-BB mixed with bone allograft results in robust periodontal regeneration in both Class II furcations and interproximal intrabony defects. [133]

Furthermore, high concentrations of the growth factors PDGF, TGF-B1, TGF-B2, and IGF (insulin-like growth factor) are also found in Platelet-rich plasma/ fibrin, which is an autologous product derived from whole blood and has been proved beneficial for periodontal regenerative therapy. [134, 135]

Bisphosphonate

Role and action of BPs has already being discussed above. Due to serious side-effects of systemically administered BPs leading to osteonecrosis of the jaws (ONJ) additional studies using topically administered bisphosphonates have been carried out which have reported a significant increase in the postoperative percentage of bone-defect fill, prevention of bone resorption as well as the boosting effect of BPs on the osteoconductive and regenerative potential of bone grafts used in periodontal therapy. [117, 136, 137]

NSAIDs

Role of NSAIDs as a host-modulating agent has been discussed above. Because NSAIDs are lipophilic and are well absorbed into gingival tissues its topical application is possible. NSAIDs that have been evaluated for topical administration include ketorolac tromethamine rinse and S-ketoprofen dentifrice. [64] Piroxicam [11] and meclofenamic acid [138] in inhibiting gingivitis and progression of periodontitis.

Hypochlorous Acid and Taurine-N-Monochloramine

It has been reported that Hypochlorous acid (HOCl) and taurine-N-monochloramine (TauCl) which are the end-products of the neutrophilic polymorphonuclear leukocyte (PMN) respiratory burst, modulate the host inflammatory response by inhibiting the production of interleukin-6, prostaglandins, nitric oxide and other proinflammatory substances, as well as increasing the capacity of α2-macroglobulin to bind Tumor Necrosis Factor-alpha, IL-2, and IL-6, as well as activating tyrosine kinase signaling cascades and facilitating the release of various growth factors.

Thus, HOCl and TauCl, playing a crucial role in the periodontal inflammatory process offer opportunities for the development of novel host-modulating therapies for the treatment of periodontitis. [118]

Recently, Lorenz et al. 2009 assessed the influence of 2% and 3% N-chlorotaurine mouth rinse on dental plaque and demonstrated that rinsing with 10 mL of the test solution two times daily for 4 days reduced the plaque vitality. [139]

Cimetidine

Cimetidine, a powerful H2-(Histamine) receptor antagonist and hence, eliminates histamine's inhibitory effects on immune response, thereby acting as a modulator of inflammation and immunity by inhibiting neutrophil chemotaxis and superoxide production, increasing cAMP levels and downregulating both TH1 and TH2 cytokines. Hasturk et al. 2006 provided morphological and histological evidence to prove that topically active cimetidine is a potent inhibitor of P. gingivalis-elicited periodontal inflammation and can arrest and/or prevent tissue destruction and influence cell populations present in the inflammatory cell infiltrate. [119]

Conclusion

The improved understanding of the host-bacterial interactions and the host immuno-inflammatory response leading to periodontal tissue destruction has led to the development of host modulatory therapy. The current chapter emphasizes the promising potential of various host-modulating agents in the management of periodontal diseases as well as explores various host responses that can serve as targets for host modulatory agents.

References

[1] Haffajee, A. D., Socransky, S. S. Microbial etiologic agents of destructive periodontal diseases. *Periodontol*. 2000. 1994;5:78-111

[2] (Carranza chapter 16)

[3] Kirkwood, K. L., Cirelli, J. A., Rogers, J. E., and Giannobile, W. V. Novel host response therapeutic approaches to treat periodontal diseases. *Periodontology* 2000. 2007;47:294-315

[4] Preshaw, P. M. Host response modulation in periodontics. *Periodontology* 2000. 2008; 48:92-110

[5] Giannobile, W. V. Host-Response Therapeutics for Periodontal Diseases. *J. Periodontol*. 2008;79:1592-1600.

[6] Souza, J. A., Rossa, C. Jr, Garlet, G. P., Nogueira, A. V., Cirelli, J. A. Modulation of host cell signaling pathways as a therapeutic approach in periodontal disease. *J. Appl. Oral Sci*. 2012;20(2):128-38.

[7] Ambili, R., Santhi, W. S., Janam, P., Nandakumar, K., Pillai, M. R. Expression of activated transcription factor nuclear factor-kappaB in periodontally diseased tissues. *J. Periodontol.* 2005;76:1148-53
[8] Graves, D. Cytokines that promote periodontal tissue destruction. *J. Periodontol.* 2008; 79:1585-91.
[9] Socransky, S. S., Haffajee, A. D. The bacterial etiology of destructive periodontal disease: current concepts. *J. Periodontol.* 1992;63(4 Suppl.): 322-31.
[10] Carranza chapter 53
[11] Howell, T. H., Fiorellini, J., Weber, H. P., Williams, R. C. Effect of the NSAID piroxicam, topically administered, on the development of gingivitis in beagle dogs. *J. Periodont. Res.* 1991;26:180-183.
[12] Page, R. C., Kornman, K. S. The pathogenesis of human periodontitis: An introduction. *Periodontol.* 2000. 1997;14:9-11.
[13] Lamster, I., Novak, M. J. Host mediators in gingival crevicular fluid: Implications for the pathogenesis of periodontal disease. *Crit. Rev. Oral Biol. Med.* 1992;3:31-60.
[14] Kinane, D. F. Causation and pathogenesis of periodontal disease. *Periodontol.* 2000. 2001;25:8-20.
[15] Kantarci, A., Hasturk, H., Van Dyke, T. E. Host-mediated resolution of inflammation in periodontal diseases. *Periodontol.* 2000. 2006;40:144-63
[16] Williams, R. C. Periodontal disease. *N Engl. J. Med.* 1990;322:373-382.
[17] Golub, L. M., Suomalainen, K., Sorsa, T. Host modulation with tetracyclines and their chemically modified analogues. *Curr. Opin. Dent.* 1992;2:80-90
[18] Information Paper. The pathogenesis of periodontal diseases. *J. Periodontol.* 1999; 70:457-470
[19] Thomson, R. G. Modulating the host response as an adjunctive treatment for periodontitis. *Periodontol.* 2000. 2001; 22(1):26-34
[20] Ryan, M. E. Nonsurgical Approaches for the treatment of periodontal diseases. *Dent. Clin. N Am.* 2005;49:611-636
[21] Preshaw, P. M., Hefti, A. F., Jepsen, S., Etienne, D., Walker, C., Bradshaw, M. H. Subantimicrobial dose doxycycline as adjunctive treatment for periodontitis. A review. *J. Clin. Periodontol.* 2004;31:697-707
[22] Lawrence, T., Willoughby, D. A., Gilroy, D. W. Anti-inflammatory lipid mediators and insights into the resolution of inflammation. *Nat. Rev. Immunol.* 2002;2:787-795
[23] Serhan, C. N. A search for endogenous mechanisms of anti-inflammation uncovers novel chemical mediators: missing links to resolution. *Histochem. Cell Biol.* 2004;122: 305-321.
[24] Bartold, P. M., Cantley, M. D. and Haynes, D. R. Mechanisms and control of pathologic bone loss in periodontitis. *Periodontology* 2000. 2010;53:55-69
[25] Caton, J., Ciancio, S., Crout, R., Hefti, A., Polson, A. Adjunctive use of subantimicrobial doxycycline therapy for periodontitis. *J. Dent. Res.* 1998;77:29-57 (abstr.)
[26] Ying Gu, Maria E. Ryan. Chapter 2: Overview of Periodontal Disease: Causes, Pathogenesis, and Characteristics. In: Genco, R. J., Williams, R. C. *Periodontal Disease and Overall Health: A Clinician's Guide.* US, Professional Audience Communications, Inc. 2005, pg 5-24

[27] Chen, F. M., An, Y., Zhang, R., Zhang, M. New insights into and novel applications of release technology for periodontal reconstructive therapies. *J. Control. Release*. 2011; 149(2):92-110.

[28] Ryan, M. E. and Golub, L. M. Modulation of matrix metalloproteinase activities in periodontitis as a treatment strategy. *Periodontol*. 2000. 2000;24:226-238

[29] Oyarzún, A., Arancibia, R., Hidalgo, R., Peñafiel, C., Cáceres, M., González, M. J., Martínez, J., Smith, P. C. Involvement of MT1-MMP and TIMP-2 in human periodontal disease. *Oral Dis*. 2010;16(4):388-95.

[30] Visse, R., Nagase, H. Matrix metalloproteinases and tissue inhibitors of metalloproteinases: structure, function, and biochemistry. *Circ. Res*. 2003. 2;92(8):827-39.

[31] McIntush, E. W., Smith, M. F. Matrix metalloproteinases and tissue inhibitors of metalloproteinases in ovarian function. *Rev. Reprod*. 1998; 3(1):23-30.

[32] Fisher, J. F., Mobashery, S. Recent advances in MMP inhibitor design. *Cancer Metastasis Rev*. 2006;25(1):115-36.

[33] Evrosimovska, B., Velickovski, B., Dimova, C., and Daniela,V. S. Matrix metalloproteinases (with accent to collagenases). *Journal of Cell and Animal Biology*. 2011;5(7):113-120

[34] Sapadin, A. N. and Fleischmajer, R. Tetracyclines: Nonantibiotic properties and their clinical implications. *J. Am. Acad. Dermatol*. 2006; 54(2):258-265

[35] Golub, L. M., Lee, H. M., Lehrer, G., Nemiroff, A., McNamara, T. F., Kaplan, R., and Ramamurthy, N. S. Minocycline reduces gingival collagenolytic activity during diabetes: preliminary observations and a proposed new mechanism of action. *J. Periodontal Res*.1983;18:516-526.

[36] Golub, L. M., Wolff, M., Lee, H. M., McNamara, T. F., Ramamurthy, N. S., Zambon, J., Ciancio, S. Further evidence that tetracyclines inhibit collagenase activity in human crevicular fluid and from other mammalian sources. *J. Periodontal Res*. 1985;20:12-23.

[37] L. A. Mitscher (1978) *The Chemistry of the Tetracycline Antibiotics*. Medicinal Research Series, Vol. 9. Marcel Dekker, New York. 172

[38] Golub, L. M., McNamara, T. F., D'Angelo, G., Greenwald, R. A., and Ramamurthy, N. S. A non-antibacterial chemically modified tetracycline inhibits mammalian collagenase activity. *J. Dent. Res*. 1987;66:1310

[39] McNamara, T. F., Golub, L. M., D'Angelo, G., and Ramamurthy, N. S. The synthesis and characterization of a non-antibacterial chemically-modified tetracycline (CMT). *J. Dent. Res*. 1986;65(Spec. Iss.):IADR Abstr. no. 515.

[40] Golub, L. M., Ramamurthy, N. S., McNamara, T. F., Greenwald, R. A., and Rifkin, B. R. Tetracyclines inhibit connective tissue breakdown: new therapeutic implications for an old family of drugs. *Crit. Rev. Oral Biol. Med*. 1991;2(3):297-321.

[41] Golub, L. M., Riflkin, B. R., Ramamurthy, N. S., Vernilo, A., Sanavi, F., and McNamara, T. F. Chemically-modified tetracyclines as probes of collagenase in bone resorption, In: *8th Int. Conf. on Periodontal Res.,* San Antonio, Texas, Nov. 15-18, 1990, Abstract.

[42] Golub, L. M., Lee, H. M., Ryan, M. E., Giannobile, W. V., Payne, J., Sorsa, T. Tetracyclines inhibit connective tissue breakdown by multiple non-antimicrobial mechanisms. *Adv. Dent. Res*. 1998;12(2):12-26.

[43] Golub, L. M., Ciancio, S., Ramamamurthy, N. S., Leung, M., McNamara, T. F. Low-dose doxycycline therapy: effect on gingival and crevicular fluid collagenase activity in humans. *J. Periodontal Res.* 1990; 25(6):321-330.

[44] Golub, L. M., Lee, H. M., Greenwald, R. A., Ryan, M. E., Sorsa, T., Salo, T., Giannobile, W. V. A matrix metalloproteinase inhibitor reduces bone-type collagen degradation fragments and specific collagenases in gingival crevicular fluid during adult periodontitis. *Inflamm. Res.* 1997; 46:310-319.

[45] Preshaw, P. M., Hefti, A. F., Novak, M. J., Michalowicz, B. S., Pihlstrom, B. L., Schoor, R., Trummel, C. L., Dean, J., Van Dyke, T. E., Walker, C. B., Bradshaw, M. H. Subantimicrobial dose doxycycline enhances the efficacy of scaling and root planning in chronic periodontitis: a multicenter trial. *J. Periodontol.* 2004;75:1068-1076.

[46] Lee, J. Y., Lee, Y. M., Shin, S. Y., Seol, Y. J., Ku, Y., Rhyu, I. C., Chung, C. P., Han, S. B. Effect of subantimicrobial dose doxycycline as an effective adjunct to scaling and root planing. *J. Periodontol.* 2004; 75: 1500-1508.

[47] Caton, J. G., Ciancio, S. G., Blieden, T. M., Bradshaw, M., Crout, R. J., Hefti, A. F., Massaro, J. M., Polson, A. M., Thomas, J., Walker, C. Treatment with subantimicrobial dose doxycycline improves the efficacy of scaling and root planing in patients with adult periodontitis. *J. Periodontol.* 2000;71:521-532.

[48] Mohammad, A. R., Preshaw, P. M., Bradshaw, M. H., Hefti, A. F., Powala, C. V., Romanowicz, M. Adjunctive subantimicrobial dose doxycycline in the management of institutionalized geriatric patients with chronic periodontitis. *Gerodontology.* 2005; 22:37-43.

[49] Preshaw, P. M., Hefti, A. F., Bradshaw, M. H. Adjunctive subantimicrobial dose doxycycline in smokers and non-smokers with chronic periodontitis. *J. Clin. Periodontol.* 2005;32:610-616.

[50] Haffajee, A. D., Torresyap, G., Socransky, S. S. Clinical changes following four different periodontal therapies for the treatment of chronic periodontitis: 1-year results. *J. Clin. Periodontol.* 2007;34:243-253.

[51] Caton, J. G., Ciancio, S. G., Blieden, T. M., Bradshaw, M., Crout, R. J., Hefti, A. F., et al. Subantimicrobial dose doxycycline as an adjunct to scaling and root planing: post-treatment effects. *J. Clin. Periodontol.* 2001;28:782-789.

[52] Teronen, O., Konttinen, Y., Lindqvist, C., Salo, T., Ingman, T., Lauhio, A., Ding, Y., et al. Human neutrophil collagenase MMP-8 in peri-implant sulcus fluid and its inhibition by clodronate. *J. Dent. Res.* 1997; 76:1529-1537.

[53] Teronen, O., Konttinen, Y., Lindqvist, C., Salo, T., Ingman, T., Lauhio, A., et al. Inhibition of matrix metalloproteinase-1 by dichloromethylene bisphosphonate (clodronate). *Calcif. Tissue Int.* 1997;61:59-61.

[54] Informational Paper. Modulation of the Host Response in Periodontal Therapy. *J. Periodontol.* 2002;73:460-470.

[55] DeWitt, D. L., Meade, E. A., Smith, W. L. PGH synthase isoenzyme selectivity: The potential safer anti-inflammatory drugs. *Am. J. Med.* 1993;95:40S-44S

[56] Smith, M. A., Braswell, L. D., Collins, J. G., Boyd, D. L., Jeffcoat, M. K., Reddy, M., et al. Changes in inflammatory mediators in experimental periodontitis in the rhesus monkey. *Infect. Immun.* 1993;61(4):1453-1459.

[57] Saffar, J. L. Arachidonic acid derivatives in periodontitis. *J. Parodontol.* 1990 May;9 (2):163-7.

[58] Eberhard, J., Jepsen, S., Albers, H. K., Açil, Y. Quantitation of arachidonic acid metabolites in small tissue biopsies by reversed-phase high-performance liquid chromatography. *Analytical Biochemistry*. 2000;280(2):258-263

[59] Weaks-Dybvig, M., Sanavi, F., Zander, H., and Rifkin, B. R. The effect of indomethacin on alveolar bone loss in experimental periodontitis. *J. Periodontal Res.* 1982;17(1):90-100.

[60] Heasman, P. A., Offenbacher, S., Collins, J. G., Edwards, G., Seymour, R. A. Flurbiprofen in the prevention and treatment of experimental gingivitis. *J. Clin. Periodontol.* 1993; 20:732-738.

[61] Nyman, S., Schroeder, H. E., Lindhe, J. Suppression of inflammation and bone resorption by indomethacin during experimental periodontitis in dogs. *J. Periodontol.* 1979;50:450-461

[62] Howell, T. H., Jeffcoat, M. K., Goldhaber, P., Reddy, M. S., Kaplan, M. L., Johnson, H. G., Hall, C. M., Williams, R. C. Inhibition of alveolar bone loss in beagles with the NSAID naproxen. *J. Periodontal Res.* 1991;26:498-501.

[63] Reddy, S., Kaul, S., Asutkar, H., Bhowmik, N., Amudha. Host modulation in periodontics. *e-Journal of Dentistry*. 2011;1(3):51-62

[64] Zeshmukh, J., Jawali, M. A., Kulkarni, V. K. Host modulation therapy – a promising new concept in treating periodontal diseases. *International Journal of Dental Clinics*. 2011:3(2):48-53

[65] Paquette, D. W. and Williams, R. C. Modulation of host inflammatory mediators as a treatment strategy for periodontal diseases. *Periodontol.* 2000. 2000;24:239–252

[66] Van Dyke, T. E. Control of inflammation and periodontitis. *Periodontology* 2000. 2007;45:158-166

[67] Serhan, C. N., Takano, T., Maddox, J. F. Aspirin-triggered 15- epi-lipoxin A4 and stable analogs on lipoxin A4 are potent inhibitors of acute inflammation. Receptors and pathways. *Adv. Exp. Med. Biol.* 1999;447:133-149.

[68] Serhan, C. N. Lipoxins and novel aspirin-triggered 15-epilipoxins (ATL): a jungle of cell-cell interactions or a therapeutic opportunity? *Prostaglandins*. 1997;53:107-137

[69] Claria, J., Serhan, C. N. Aspirin triggers previously undescribed bioactive eicosanoids by human endothelial cell-leukocyte interactions. *Proc. Natl. Acad. Sci. US*. 1995;92: 9475-9479.

[70] Serhan, C. N., Chiang, N. and Van Dyke, T. E. Resolving inflammation: dual anti-inflammatory and pro-resolution lipid mediators. *Nat. Rev. Immunol.* 2008;8(5):349-361.

[71] Serhan, C. N., Jain, A., Marleau, S., Clish, C., Kantarci, A., Behbehani, B., et al. Reduced inflammation and tissue damage in transgenic rabbits overexpressing 15-lipoxygenase and endogenous anti-inflammatory lipid mediators. *J. Immunol.* 2003; 171:6856-6865

[72] Spite, M., Serhan, C. N. Novel lipid mediators promote resolution of acute inflammation: impact of aspirin and statins. *Circ. Res.* 2010; 107 (10):1170-84

[73] Janakiram, N. B., Rao, C. V. Role of lipoxins and resolvins as anti-inflammatory and proresolving mediators in colon cancer. *Curr. Mol. Med.* 2009;9(5):565-79.

[74] Fredman, G., Oh, S. F., Ayilavarapu, S., Hasturk, H., Serhan, C. N., Van Dyke, T. E. Impaired Phagocytosis in Localized Aggressive Periodontitis: Rescue by Resolvin E1. *PLoS One*. 2011;6(9):e24422.

[75] Kohli, P. and Levy, B. D. Resolvins and protectins: mediating solutions to inflammation. *Br. J. Pharmacol.* 2009;158(4):960-971.
[76] Garlet, G. P. Destructive and protective roles of cytokines in periodontitis: a re-appraisal from host defense and tissue destruction viewpoints. *J. Dent. Res.* 2010;89 (12):1349-63.
[77] Loo, W. T., Fan, C. B., Bai, L. J., Yue, Y., Dou, Y. D., Wang, M., Liang, H., Cheung, M. N., Chow, L. W., Li, J. L., Tian, Y., Qing, L. Gene polymorphism and protein of human pro and anti-inflammatory cytokines in Chinese healthy subjects and chronic periodontitis patients. *J. Transl. Med.* 2012;19(10 Suppl.):1-S8.
[78] Riccelli, A. E., Agarwal, S., Piesco, N. P., Hoffman, R. D., Suzuki, J. B. Role of cytokines in periodontal diseases. *J. Calif. Dent. Assoc.* 1995;23 (8):48-51.
[79] Waykole, Y. P., Doiphode, S. S., Rakhewar, P. S., Mhaske, M. Anticytokine therapy for periodontal diseases: Where are we now? *J. Indian Soc. Periodontol.* 2009;13:64-8.
[80] Assuma, R., Oates, T., Cochran, D., Amar, S., Graves, D. T. IL-1 and TNF antagonists inhibit the inflammatory response and bone loss in experimental periodontitis. *J. Immunol.* 1998:1;160(1):403-9.
[81] Taba, M., Abramson, Z., Sugai, J., Huffer, H., Kreider, J., Goldstein, S., Ramseier, C., Lustig, K., Burstein, H., Giannobile, W. Gene delivery of TNFR:Fc by adeno-associated virus vector blocks progression of periodontitis [abstract 677]. *Programs and abstracts of the American Society of Gene Therapy's Eighth Annual Meeting*; American Society of Gene Therapy; Saint Louis (MO). 2005. p. 262.
[82] Garlet, G. P., Cardoso, C. R., Campanelli, A. P., Martins, W. Jr, Silva, J. S. Expression of suppressors of cytokine signaling in diseased periodontal tissues: a stop signal for disease progression? *J. Periodontal Res.* 2006;41(6):580-4
[83] De Souza, J. A., Nogueira, A. V., de Souza, P. P., Cirelli, J. A., Garlet, G. P., Rossa, C. Jr. Expression of suppressor of cytokine signaling 1 and 3 in ligature-induced periodontitis in rats. *Arch. Oral Biol.* 2011;56 (10): 1120-8
[84] Lima, V., Vidal, F. D., Rocha, F. A., Brito, G. A., Ribeiro, R. A. Effects of tumor necrosis factor-alpha inhibitors pentoxifylline and thalidomide on alveolar bone loss in short-term experimental periodontal disease in rats. *J. Periodontol.* 2004;75(1):162-8.
[85] Cochran, D. L. Inflammation and bone loss in periodontal disease. *J. Periodontol.* 2008;79(8 suppl.):1569-1576.
[86] Jin, Q., Cirelli, J. A., Park, C. H., Sugai, J. V., Taba, M. Jr, Kostenuik, P. J., et al. RANKL Inhibition Through Osteoprotegerin Blocks Bone Loss in Experimental Periodontitis. *J. Periodontol.* 2007;78(7):1300–1308.
[87] Martuscelli, G., Fiorellini, J. P., Crohin, C. C., Howell, T. H. The effect of interleukin-11 on the progression of ligature-induced periodontal disease in the beagle dog. *J. Periodontol.* 2000;71:573-578
[88] Shinoda, H., Takeyama, S., Suzuki, K., Murakami, S., Yamada, S. Pharmacological topics of bone metabolism: a novel bisphosphonate for the treatment of periodontitis. *J. Pharmacol. Sci.* 2008;106(4):555-8.
[89] Reddy, M. S., Geurs, N. C., Gunsolley, J. C. Periodontal host modulation with antiproteinase, anti-inflammatory, and bone-sparing agents. A systematic review. *Ann. Periodontol.* 2003;8(1):12-37.
[90] Ebetino, F. H., Francis, M. D., Rogers, M. J., Russell, R. G. G. Mechanisms of action of etidronate and other bisphosphonates. *Rev. Contemp. Pharmacother.* 1998;9:233-243.

[91] Geddes, A. D., D'Souza, S. M., Ebetino, F. H., Ibbotson, K. J. Bisphosphonates: Structure-activity relationships and therapeutic implications. *In: Bone and Mineral Research.* 1994;8:265-306.

[92] Benford, H. L., Frith, J. C., Auriola, S., Mönkkönen, J., Rogers, M. J. Farnesol and geranylgeraniol prevent activation of caspases by aminobisphosphonates: biochemical evidence for two distinct pharmacological classes of bisphosphonate drugs. *Mol. Pharmacol.* 1999;56(1):131-40.

[93] Tenenbaum, H. C., Shelemay, A., Girard, B., Zohar, R., Fritz, P. C. Bisphosphonates and periodontics: Potential applications for regulation of bone mass in the periodontium and other therapeutic/ diagnostic uses. *J. Periodontol.* 2002;73:813-822.

[94] Lipton, A., Theriault, R. L., Hortobagyi, G. N., Simeone, J., Knight, R. D., Mellars, K., Reitsma, D. J., Heffernan, M., Seaman, J. J. Pamidronate prevents skeletal complications and is effective palliative treatment in women with breast carcinoma and osteolytic bone metastases: long term follow-up of two randomized, placebo-controlled trials. *Cancer.* 2000;88:1082-90.

[95] Berenson, J. R., Rosen, L. S., Howell, A., Porter, L., Coleman, R. E., Morley, W., Dreicer, R., Kuross, S. A., Lipton, A., Seaman, J. J. Zoledronic acid reduces skeletal-related events in patients with osteolytic metastases. *Cancer.* 2001;91:1191-200.

[96] Saad, F. Clinical benefit of zoledronic acid for the prevention of skeletal complications in advanced prostate cancer. *Clin. Prostate Cancer.* 2005; 4:31-7.

[97] Ronald Man-Lung Yip. Bisphosphonates and Osteonecrosis of the Jaw. *Hong Kong Bull. Rheum. Dis.* 2008;8:19-25.

[98] Shoji, K., Horiuchi, H., Shinoda, H. Inhibitory effects of acbisphosphonate (risedronate) on experimental periodontitis in rats. *J. Periodontal. Res.* 1995;30:277-284.

[99] El-Shinnawi, U. M., El-Tantawy, S. I. The effect of alendronate sodium on alveolar bone loss in periodontitis (clinical trial). *J. Int. Acad. Periodontol.* 2003;5:5-10.

[100] Ficarra, G., Beninati, F., Rubino, I., Vannucchi, A., Longo, G., Tonelli, P., Pini Prato, G. Osteonecrosis of the jaws in periodontal patients with a history of bis-phosphonates treatment. *J. Clin. Periodontol.* 2005;32: 1123-1128.

[101] Khosla, S., Burr, D., Cauley, J., Dempster, D. W., Ebeling, P. R., Felsenberg, D., et al. American Society for Bone and Mineral Research. Bisphosphonate-associated osteonecrosis of the jaw: Report of a task force of the American Society for Bone and Mineral Research. *J. Bone Miner Res.* 2007;22:1479-1491.

[102] Han, X., Kawai, T., Taubman, M. A. Interference with immune cell-mediated bone resorption in periodontal disease. *Periodontol.* 2000. 2007;45:76-94

[103] Inagaki, K., Kurosu, Y., Sakano, M., Yamamoto, G., Kikuchi, T., Noguchi, T., et al. Oral osteoporosis: a review and its dental implications. *Clin. Calcium.* 2007;17(2):157-63

[104] Shu, L., Guan, S. M., Fu, S. M., Guo, T., Cao, M., Ding, Y. Estrogen modulates cytokine expression in human periodontal ligament cells. *J. Dent. Res.* 2008;87(2):142-7.

[105] Southan, G. J., Szabo, C. Selective pharmacological inhibition of distinct nitric oxide synthase isoforms. *Biochem. Pharmacol.* 1996;51:383-394.

[106] Chapple, I. L. Reactive oxygen species and antioxidants in inflammatory diseases. *J. Clin. Periodontol.* 1997;24:287-296.

[107] Batista, A.C., Silva, T. A., Chun, J. H., Lara, V. S. Nitric oxide synthesis and severity of human periodontal disease. *Oral Dis*. 2002;8(5):254-60.

[108] Lohinai, Z., Benedek, P., Feher, E., Gyorfi, A., Rosivall, L., Fazekas, A., et al. Protective effects of mercaptoethylguanidine, a selective inhibitor of inducible nitric oxide synthase, in ligature-induced periodontitis in the rat. *Br. J. Pharmacol*. 1998;123: 353-360.

[109] Leitao, R. F., Ribeiro, R. A., Chaves, H. V., Rocha, F. A., Lima, V., Brito, G. A. Nitric oxide synthase inhibition prevents alveolar bone resorption in experimental periodontitis in rats. *J. Periodontol*. 2005; 76: 956-963.

[110] Thomas, C. M., Versalovic, J. Probiotics-host communication: Modulation of signaling pathways in the intestine. *Gut. Microbes*. 2010; 1(3):148-63.

[111] Teughels, W., Loozen, G., Quirynen, M.: Do probiotics offer opportunities to manipulate the periodontal oral microbiota? *J. Clin. Periodontol.* 2011;38(Suppl. 11): 159-177.

[112] Hajishengallis, G. Toll gates to periodontal host modulation and vaccine therapy. *Periodontol*. 2000. 2009;51:181-207.

[113] Kyosuke Yokoyama, Naoyuki Sugano, Teruko Shimada, Rahman AKM Shofiqur, El-Sayed M Ibrahim et al. Effects of egg yolk antibody against Porphyromonas gingivalis gingipains in periodontitis patients. *Journal of Oral Science*. 2007; 49(3):201-6.

[114] Choi, J., Borrello, M. A., Smith, E., Cutler, C. W., Sojar, H., Zauderer, M. Prior exposure of mice to Fusobacterium nucleatum modulates host response to Porphyromonas gingivalis. *Oral Microbiol. Immunol*. 2001; 16 (6):338-44.

[115] La, V. D., Howell, A. B., Grenier, D. Cranberry proanthocyanidins inhibit MMP production and activity. *J. Dent. Res*. 2009;88(7):627-32.

[116] Bodet, C., Chandad, F., Grenier, D. Cranberry components inhibit interleukin-6, interleukin-8, and prostaglandin E production by lipopolysaccharide-activated gingival fibroblasts. *Eur. J. Oral Sci*. 2007; 115 (1):64-70.

[117] Mitsuta, T., Horiuchi, H., Shinoda, H. Effects of topical administration of clodronate on alveolar bone resorption in rats with experimental periodontitis. *J. Periodontol*. 2002; 73(5):479-86.

[118] Mainnemare, A., Mégarbane, B., Soueidan, A., Daniel, A., Chapple, I. L. C. Hypochlorous Acid and Taurine-N-Monochloramine in Periodontal Diseases. *JDR* 2004;83(11):823-831

[119] Hasturk, H., Kantarci, A., Ebrahimi, N., Andry, C., Holick, M., Jones, V. L., Van Dyke, T. E. Topical H2 antagonist prevents periodontitis in a rabbit model. *Infect. Immun*. 2006;74(4):2402-14.

[120] Venezia, E., Goldstein, M., Boyan, B. D., Schwartz, Z. The use of enamel matrix derivative in the treatment of periodontal defects: A literature review and meta-analysis. *Crit. Rev. Oral Biol. Med*. 2004; 15 (6):371-391

[121] Brookes, S. J., Robinson, C., Kirkham, J., Bonass, W. A. Biochemistry and molecular biology of amelogenin proteins of developing dental enamel. *Archives of Oral Biology*. 1995;40:1-14

[122] Hammarström, L., Heijl, L., Gestrelius, S. Periodontal regeneration in a buccal dehiscence model in monkeys after application of enamel matrix proteins. *J. Clin. Periodontol*. 1997;24:669-677

[123] Hammarström, L. Enamel matrix, cementum development and regeneration. *J. Clin. Periodontol.* 1997;24:658-668

[124] Heijl, L., Heden, G., Svardström, G., Ostgren, A. Enamel matrix derivative (Emdogain) in the treatment of intrabony periodontal defects. *J. Clin. Periodontol.* 1997;24:705-714.

[125] Lyngstadaas, S. P., Wohlfahrt, J. C., Brookes, S. J., Paine, M. L., Snead, M. L., Reseland, J. E. Enamel matrix proteins; old molecules for new applications. *Orthod. Craniofac. Res.* 2009; 12(3):243-253

[126] Lyngstadaas, S. P., Lundberg, E., Ekdahl, H., Andersson, C., Gestrelius, S. Autocrine growth factors in human periodontal ligament cells cultured on enamel matrix derivative. *J. Clin. Periodontol.* 2001;28(2):181-8.

[127] Shimizu, E., Saito, R., Nakayama, Y., Nakajima, Y., Kato, N., Takai, H., et al. Amelogenin stimulates bone sialoprotein (BSP) expression through fibroblast growth factor 2 response element and transforming growth factor-β1 activation element in the promoter of the BSP Gene. *J. Periodontol.* 2005;76:1482-9.

[128] Urist, M. R., Strates, B. S. The Classic: Bone Morphogenetic Protein. *Clin. Orthop. Relat. Res.* 2009;467(12):3051-3062.

[129] Wikesjö, U. M., Qahash, M., Huang, Y. H., Xiropaidis, A., Polimeni, G., Susin, C. Bone morphogenetic proteins for periodontal and alveolar indications; biological observations - clinical implications. *Orthod. Craniofac. Res.* 2009;12(3):263-70.

[130] Levine, J. P., Bradley, J., Turk, A. E., Ricci, J. L., Benedict, J. J., Steiner, G. ,et al. Bone morphogenetic protein promotes vascularization and osteoinduction in preformed hydroxyapatite in the rabbit. *Ann. Plast. Surg.* 1997;39(2):158-68.

[131] Takahashi, Y., Yamamoto, M., Tabata, Y. Enhanced osteoinduction by controlled release of bone morphogenetic protein-2 from biodegradable sponge composed of gelatin and beta-tricalcium phosphate. *Biomaterials.* 2005;26(23):4856-65.

[132] Sood, S., Gupta, S., Mahendra, A. Gene therapy with growth factors for periodontal tissue engineering–A review. *Med. Oral Patol. Oral Cir. Bucal.* 2012;17(2):e301-10

[133] Nevins, M., Giannobile, W. V., McGuire, M. K., Kao, R. T., Mellonig, J. T., Hinrichs, J. E., et al. Platelet derived growth factor (rhPDGF-BB) stimulates bone fill and rate of attachment level gain, results of a large, multicenter randomized controlled trial, *J. Periodontol.* 2005;76:2205-2215.

[134] Okuda, K., Kawase, T., Momose, M., Murata, M., Saito, Y., Suzuki, H., et al. Platelet-rich plasma contains high levels of platelet-derived growth factor and transforming growth factor-beta and modulates the proliferation of periodontally related cells in vitro. *J. Periodontol.* 2003; 74(6):849-57.

[135] Kawase, T., Okuda, K., Wolff, L. F., Yoshie, H. Platelet-rich plasma-derived fibrin clot formation stimulates collagen synthesis in periodontal ligament and osteoblastic cells in vitro. *J. Periodontol.* 2003 Jun.;74 (6):858-64.

[136] Houshmand, B., Rahimi, H., Ghanavati, F., Alisadr, A., Eslami, B. Boosting effect of bisphosphonates on osteoconductive materials: a histologic in vivo evaluation. *J. Periodontal Res.* 2007;42:119-123

[137] Veena, H. R., Prasad, D. Evaluation of an aminobisphosphonate (alendronate) in the management of periodontal osseous defects. *J. Indian Soc. Periodontol.* 2010;14:40-5

[138] Kornman, K. S., Blodgett, R. F., Brunsvold, M., Holt, S. C. Effects of topical applications of meclofenamic acid and ibuprofen on bone loss, subgingival microbiota

and gingival PMN response in the primate Macaca fascicularis. *J. Periodont. Res.* 1990; 25:300-307.

[139] Lorenz, K., Mayer, D., Bruhn, G., Noack, B., Brecx, M., Heumann, C., et al. Effect of N-chlorotaurine mouth rinses on plaque regrowth and plaque vitality. *Clin. Oral Investig.* 2009;13(1):9-14.

In: Current Trends in Periodontics and Implant Dentistry ISBN: 978-1-62618-819-8
Editors: Vishal Anand and Minkle Gulati

Chapter VII

Recurrence, Progression of Periodontitis and Tooth Loss Associated with Surgical or Non-Surgical Procedures in Periodontal Maintenance Therapy: An Overview

Fernando Oliveira Costa,[1] Alcione Maria Soares Dutra Oliveira,[2] José Roberto Cortelli,[3] Luís Otávio Miranda Cota[1] and Peterson Antonio Dutra Oliveira

[1]Departament of Periodontology, Dentistry School,
Federal University of Minas Gerais, Belo Horizonte, Brazil
[2]Department of Periodontology, Faculty of Dentistry,
Pontific Catholic University of Minas Gerais, Brazil
[3]Departament of Dentistry, Periodontics Research Division,
University of Taubaté, Taubaté, São Paulo, Brazil

Abstract

The benefits of periodontal maintenance therapy (PMT) in maintaining the homeostasis of periodontal tissues obtained after active periodontal therapy, which includes surgical and non-surgical procedures, has been extensively documented in numerous studies. A classic problem in PMT programs is difficulty in maintaining the patient's cooperation and in scheduling regular maintenance visits. However, without establishing a regular program of clinical re-evaluation, adequate biofilm control, and reinforcement of oral hygiene instructions, the benefits of PMT cannot be maintained.

Several indicators or risk factors and biological, behavioral, and social conditions can influence the periodontal status of individuals undergoing PMT. Moreover, neglecting a regular PMT program has been associated with a higher risk of recurrence and with the progression of periodontitis. In this chapter, smoking, diabetes, and poor oral hygiene were strongly associated with recurrence, progression of periodontitis and tooth loss in individuals under PMT. The efficiency of surgical and non-surgical periodontal procedures in the context of periodontal therapy has been widely reported.

Review studies on surgical or nonsurgical periodontal therapy have concluded that: (a) the comparison of the efficacy of surgical and nonsurgical procedures revealed that scaling and root planing alone or in combination with flap procedures are effective methods for the treatment of chronic periodontitis; (b) the consistent message is that in treating deep pockets, open-flap debridement results in greater probing pocket depth reduction and clinical attachment gain than nonsurgical modalities; (c) Nonsurgical modalities in shallower pockets consistently involve less post-therapy recession and are clearly recognized as being more conservative.

Additionally, recurrence of periodontitis and tooth loss has been reported in studies in the absence of periodontal treatment, as well as in many PMT retrospective and prospective studies. However, these results have been very controversial, primarily related to the type of surgical or non-surgical procedures performed during PMT.

In this sense, several issues related to the recurrence, progression of periodontitis and tooth loss during periodontal maintenance therapy require clarification. The aim of this chapter is to review the periodontal literature and summarize the main findings of different study designs, in attempt to a greater understanding of the influence of risk factors associated with surgical or non-surgical procedures performed during periodontal maintenance therapy on the occurrence of these adverse outcomes.

Keywords: Periodontitis, periodontal maintenance therapy, surgical and non-surgical procedures, risk factors, progression and recurrence, tooth loss

Conceptual Issues in Periodontal Maintenance Therapy

The aim of effective treatment of periodontal diseases is to arrest the inflammatory disease process by removal of the supragingival and subgingival biofilm compatible with periodontal health. Reduction of probing depths, maintenance or improvement of clinical attachment levels and reduction in bleeding on probing are the most common outcome measures used to determine whether treatment is successful. The treatment offered to the periodontal disease patients by the dentist during active periodontal therapy may be nonsurgical or surgical mechanical procedures. After re-evaluation of all clinical periodontal parameters and once established periodontal health, individuals should be included in an effective program - the periodontal maintenance therapy (PMT).

PMT is an integral part of periodontal therapy. It is performed by a dentist, although components of PMT can be performed by a dental hygienist under the supervision of the dentist. PMT should include an update of medical and dental histories, radiographic review, extraoral and intraoral soft tissue examination, dental examination, periodontal evaluation, removal of dental biofilm from the supragingival and subgingival sites, scaling and root planing where indicated, polishing of the teeth and a review of the patient's plaque control efficacy and other appropriate behavior modification.[1]

The American Academy of Periodontology (2005) [2] stressed that the therapeutic goals of PMT are: to minimize the recurrence of periodontal disease in individuals who have been previously treated for gingivitis and periodontitis; to reduce the incidence of tooth loss (TL)

by monitoring the dentition and any prosthetic replacements of natural teeth when necessary; and to increase the probability of locating and treating, in a timely manner, other diseases or conditions found within the oral cavity. It is highlighted that the main aims of the PMT are shown in Figure 1.

The benefits of PMT in maintaining the homeostasis of periodontal tissues obtained after active periodontal therapy, which includes surgical and non-surgical procedures, has been extensively documented in numerous studies. [3-10]

However, without establishing a regular program of clinical re-evaluation, adequate biofilm control, and reinforcement of oral hygiene instructions, the benefits of PMT cannot be maintained. [11,6,7] Several indicators or risk factors and biological, behavioral, and social conditions can influence the periodontal status of individuals undergoing PMT. [3,12,9]

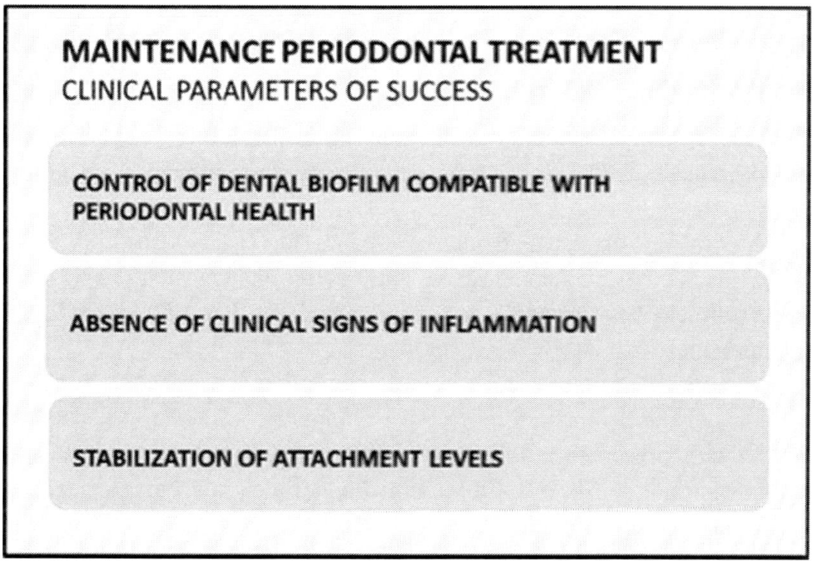

Figure 1. Main aims of periodontal maintenance therapy.

PMT visits can be considered a critical factor for success in controlling periodontal disease. Moreover, neglecting a regular PMT program has been associated with a higher risk of recurrence and with the progression of periodontitis. [13,3,14]

The efficiency of surgical and non-surgical periodontal procedures in the context of periodontal therapy has been widely reported. [15-19] Furthermore, recurrence and progression of periodontitis has been reported in studies in the absence of periodontal treatment, [19-21] as well as in many PMT retrospective studies [11,13,22-26] and in relatively few prospective studies. [6,7,27,28]

In addition, no prospective studies to date on PMT have reported a direct influence of the performance of surgical and non-surgical procedures on the recurrence and progression of periodontitis associated with the degree of compliance of individuals.

The aim of this chapter is to review the periodontal literature and summarize the main findings of different study designs, in attempt to a greater understanding of the influence of risk factors associated with surgical or non-surgical procedures performed during periodontal maintenance therapy on the occurrence of these adverse outcomes, i.e, recurrence and progression of periodontitis and tooth loss.

2. Frequency, Efficacy and Compliance

Several studies have shown that minor clinical attachment loss occurs, and fewer teeth are lost when patients maintain regular PMT intervals compared with patients seen less often or not at all. [29] A counterpoint to the efficacy of frequent PMT visits has been offered in a limited number of studies that found no difference in recurrence and progression of periodontitis in individuals seen less frequently compared with those who received more frequent PMT. Most of the individuals in this last group of studies maintained relatively high levels of oral hygiene.

Despite this knowledge, a classic problem in PMT programs is difficulty in maintaining the patient's cooperation and in scheduling regular maintenance visits.[1] The frequency of visits in the literature conflicts greatly, with the intervals between visits considered as regularly as 3-4, [11,3,2] 6 months, [13,30] or a maximum of 12 months when considering the risk profile of the individual. [31,16,4,3,12,7,8]

However, there is more consensus in the literature that the majority of individuals with a history of chronic periodontitis should be seen at least three times a year, because that interval will result in a decreased likelihood of progressive disease as compared with individuals seen less frequently.[7-10,32]

Compliance with suggested PMT intervals can affect the success of treatment. [33] Individuals treated for periodontal disease who comply suggested PMT intervals will experience less clinical attachment loss and tooth loss than individuals who do not demonstrate compliance with the PMT schedule.

Costa et al. demonstrated that regular complier individuals presented lower oral impacts on daily performance when compared to irregular compliers. [8] Moreover, personality traits, especially neuroticism, presented a significant influence on these indicators of impact. In this manner, personality traits can be used to estimate adherence and compliance, especially in PMT that demands monitoring and constant control during life, independently of the performance of surgical or non-surgical during PMT.

A recent publication [34] indicated that, non-compliance with periodontal maintenance cannot be solely explained by one determinant but rather might involve an individual's health beliefs, emotional intelligence, psychological stressors, and personality traits.[7] Thus, it provides, for the health professional, a holistic view of the periodontally susceptible individual.

3. Re-evaluation

Follow-up periodic assessment must be performed to determine whether treatment of periodontal disease is successful. This reassessment guides future therapy. These re-examinations are performed during therapy and at PMT visits. Since most periodontal diseases are chronic, the perspective gained by comparing current data with the last baseline is invaluable. Retreatment is seldom discussed.

The reasons are varied, but include the complexity of the individuals, limited knowledge of the disease process, reluctance to discuss apparent failure with colleagues and inaccuracy in measuring disease progression. The good way to decide when to re-treat would be to use a method that accurately predicts future clinical attachment loss. Two measurements are used: changes in clinical attachment loss or probing depth and tissue signs, especially bleeding upon probing and suppuration.[29]

4. Adverse Outcomes in Periodontal Maintenance Therapy

The main adverse outcomes that may occur during PMT are recurrence, progression of periodontitis and tooth loss, with tooth loss being considered a full and indisputable failure during monitoring of individuals in PMT.

4.1. Recurrence and Progression of Periodontitis

The definitions of recurrence and progression of periodontitis has been the target of much discussion for many years. What magnitude of alterations in clinical attachment loss and/or probing depth measures as occurring in a given period can be considered relevant? Currently it is consensual: (a) *Progression of periodontitis*: was defined as interproximal clinical attachment loss ≥ 3 mm in at least 2 teeth between 2 different observation points, according to the 5th European Workshop on Periodontology; [14] *(b) Recurrence of periodontitis:* Sites showing probing depth ≥4mm and clinical attachment loss ≥3 mm, together with the presence of bleeding on probing and/or suppuration, during any of the PMT visits.[14,6,7,8]

During PMT, individuals diagnosed with recurrence or having sites with residual probing depth increases can be re-treated with mechanical subgingival debridement (nonsurgical treatment) or surgical procedures as necessary (preferably Widman modified flap surgery).

4.2. Tooth Loss

The tooth mortality is a generic term used to define the dental loss without, however, specifying the cause. Periodontics defines that the progression of periodontal disease can lead to clinical attachment loss resulting in loss of functionality due to tooth mortality.

Due to it multifactorial etiology, the diagnostic decision and/or prognosis for teeth affected by periodontal disease is often a decision with a high degree of clinical difficulty.

The determination to retain teeth involved is very complex and depends on the treatment philosophy of the professional and the quality of treatment offered. High success rates with dental implants therapy and reports of probable association of periodontal infection on systemic condition of individuals have influenced the planning of dental treatment. [35]

Several reported studies have examined the factors at systemic and / or local levels as predictors of tooth loss during phase of PMT after non-surgical and surgical treatment demonstrating that tooth loss was more prevalent in molars [36-38] while the mandibular teeth [37] and the canines seem to be less committed. [36] Factors associated with patient [37] as age and gender were analyzed by several authors, [39-44] who reported a positive association of tooth loss with age ≥60 years, whereas the association with gender has been demonstrated in studies by Fardal et al. (2004) [39] and Eickholz et al. (2008).[42] The smokers had a positive association with tooth loss in most studies: [37,39-42,45-47] while only Pretzl et al. 2008 did not find an association with smoking.[43]

Periodontal parameters such as bone loss and initial furcation involvement have been shown to be positive predictors of tooth loss in the studies of Mc Guire and Nunn 1996,[37] Muzzi et al. 2006 [38] and Pretzl et al. 2008. [43] The probing depth ≥ 6 mm and bleeding on probing ≥ 30% represented a risk factor for tooth loss in the study by Matuliene et al. (2008). [46] The influence of variables such as high plaque index and irregular participation of patients during periodontal maintenance was analyzed and showed statistically significant association with tooth loss. [41-43,47]

The results of studies that analyzed the causes of tooth loss in patients undergoing active periodontal therapy (non-surgical and / or surgical treatment) followed by periodontal maintenance, demonstrated that long-term follow-up resulted in a low rate of tooth loss associated with periodontal disease. Hirschfeled and Wasserman (1978) [48] found that 1312 teeth (2.2 teeth / patient) were lost in 600 patients diagnosed with advanced periodontal disease, under a maintenance interval of 4-6 months between visits. A retrospective study of McFall (1982) [49] enrolling a group of 100 patients in periodontal maintenance, with an average of 19 years follow-up, showed a rate of 2.6 teeth loss per patient during the study. Becker et al. (1984) [50] investigating 95 patients on periodontal maintenance, found a tooth loss rate of 1.6 teeth per patient. Lindhe and Nyman (1984),[51] in a longitudinal study of 14 years, reported a loss of 2.3% of teeth with attachment loss >50% in 61 patients, with a mean number of tooth loss being 0.49 per patient.

Nabers et al. (1988)52 evaluated 1535 individuals that were recalled during 12.9 years (average) from the completion of non-surgical and surgical periodontal treatment. Of the 1535 patients, 73.5% required resective or regenerative surgical procedures in selected areas and only 26.5% were subjected to non-surgical treatment. It was found that 1371 patients had not lost any teeth by periodontal disease and that the total number of loss occurred in only 164 patients.

Wood et al. (1989) [36] reported that after completion of periodontal therapy out of 1607 teeth present 115 (7.1%) were lost during the maintenance period and of these 88 (5.0%) were lost due to periodontal reasons. McGuire and Nunn (1996) [37] evaluated 100 patients diagnosed with moderate or advanced chronic periodontitis at visits of 2-3 months. After the active periodontal therapy the number of teeth lost during the periodontal maintenance phase was 131 (1.3 teeth / patient). 51 patients (51%) did not lose any teeth and 1.7% lost teeth for exclusively periodontal reasons. Tonetti et al. (2000) [53] conducted a study with 273 patients and the results indicated that 574 out of a total of 6503 teeth were extracted; 311 teeth were extracted during active periodontal therapy and 263 during the supportive periodontal care. 46% of patients received the tooth extractions as part of their active treatment and 41% during their participation in the secondary prevention program.

Chambrone and Chambrone (2006) [40] reported that among the 2927 teeth present only 53 (1.8%) were lost due to periodontal disease, 16 (0.5%) due to root fracture, 6 (0.2%) due to caries, 5 (0.2%) for endodontic reasons and 31 (1%) due to extraction of 3rd molars. Matuliene et al. (2008) [46] examined 172 patients after surgical and non-surgical treatment. Compared with PPD ≤3 mm, PPD ≥5 mm represented a risk factor for tooth loss, demonstrating that the increase of the probing depth was a risk factor for tooth loss. Chambrone et al. (2010) [54] systematically reviewed 13 retrospective studies in which subjects after undergoing periodontal therapy were followed for a minimum period of 5 years, and reported that the percentage of teeth lost due to periodontal reasons ranged from 1.5% to 9.8%. Matuliene et al. (2010) [12] analyzed the association of the periodontal risk assessment model categories with tooth loss during supportive periodontal therapy and also explored the role of patient compliance. Patients with high risk profile lost significantly more teeth (2.59 ± 3.9) than patients with moderate profile (1.02 ± 1.8) or low risk (1.18 ± 1.9). Patient with erratic compliance lost significantly more teeth (11.3 ± 4.5) than patients compliant with maintenance therapy (1.7 ± 1.6). Martin et al. (2010) [55] evaluated the loss of teeth of treated periodontal patients categorized by severity and risk. The stepwise regression analysis showed that disease ($p = 0.0000478$) and risk ($p = 0.00129$) scores predicted the mean tooth loss rate.

The main studies reporting tooth loss in patients who underwent non-surgical and surgical treatment with periodontal maintenance are summarized in table 1.

There are limited numbers of studies that have evaluated the tooth loss in patients who received active periodontal therapy but were not followed up after completion of treatment. Becker et al. (1984) [56] reported data on a sample of 44 patients 5.25 years after the completion of basic therapy who elected not to accept maintenance therapy and found a tooth loss of 33.5%, in addition to bone loss >75%, probing depth 8 to 10 mm, Class III furcation involvement, tooth mobility and history of repeated periodontal abscess formation. The mean tooth loss was 0.22 teeth / patient / year.

Checchi et al. (2002) [23] conducted a study that included 92 patients who were divided into two groups: those who complied with the recommended maintenance schedule and those whose compliance was erratic. Patients complying erratically with PMT were at 5.6 times greater risk for tooth loss following active periodontal therapy than regularly compliant patients. Leung et al. (2006) [41] re-called 97 individuals who responded favorably to periodontal treatment performed 5-12 years previously and were advised to seek regular supportive periodontal care on discharge. It was found that 256 teeth had been lost of which 195 were lost due to periodontal reasons as reported by the patient.

Ng et al. (2011) [44] compared retrospective data collected from 273 patients (all compliers) and cross-sectional data from 39 patients after discontinuation of periodontal maintenance (non-compliers).

All compliers lost 1.3 teeth / patient during active periodontal therapy and 0.9 teeth / patient during the maintenance phase, i.e. tooth loss due to periodontitis was 0.03 teeth / patient / year. Whereas non-complier individuals lost 1.1 teeth/patient during active periodontal therapy and 2.7 teeth / patient during discontinuation i.e. tooth loss due to periodontitis was 0.22 teeth / patient / year, a sevenfold increase ($p < 0.05$) compared with compliers.

The data also suggests that tooth loss is not evenly distributed and that only a small group of patients may exhibit the highest tooth mortality rates after completion of therapy. The low rates of mortality in the patients who underwent treatment and were followed up with maintenance care was in sharp contrast to the tooth loss occurring in patients treated but not provided continued maintenance care. This highlights the importance of care after active periodontal therapy in maintaining periodontal health and, consequently, the tooth mortality.

The main studies reporting tooth loss in patients who underwent non-surgical and surgical treatment without periodontal maintenance are summarized in table 2.

Table 1. Characteristics of the Included Studies on the Tooth Loss in Individuals with Periodontal Maintenance Therapy

Author / year	Study design/ location	Sample	Mean duration study	Mean tooth loss during maintenance / Main findings
Becker et al. (1984)	Retrospective (USA)	95 patients	6.58 years	(1.6teeth /patients)
Chambrone and Chambrone (2006)	Retrospective Practice-based Brazil	120 patients	17.4 (range 10-36 years)	Total number of teeth lost=111 (0.9 teeth / patients / years)
Chambrone et al. (2010)	Systematic review of 13 Retrospective studiesBrazil	2.147 patients	≥ 5 years	Total number of teeth lost=3919 – range 1.5 a 9.8%
Checchi et al. (2002)	Retrospective Practice-based Italy	92 patients	6.7 (range 3-12 years)	Total number of teeth lost=44 (0.07teeth / patients / years)
Hirschfeled and Wasserman (1978)	Retrospective Practice-based (USA)	600 patients	22.0 (range 15-53 years)	Total number of teeth lost=1312 (2.2teeth / patients)
Lindhe and Nyman (1984)	Longitudinal	61 patients	14 years	Total number of teeth lost=30 (0.49teeth / patients)
Martin et al. (2010)	Retrospective Practice-based (USA)	776 patients	13.2±7 (range 3-32.5 years)	Total number of teeth lost=980 1,26±2.53 teeth / patients
Matuliene et al. (2008)	Cohort retrospective Universiy-based Switzerland	172 patients	11.3 (range 3-27 years)	Probing Depth ≥ 6mm and bleeding on probing ≥30% representaram fator de risco para perda dental. Total number of teeth lost=597 /4138 Total number of teeth lost during PMT=294 (49.2%)
Matuliene et al. (2010)	Cohort retrospective Universiy-based Switzerland	172 patients	9.5±4.5years	Total number of teeth lost=1.61±2.8teeth /patients
McFall (1982)	Retrospective Universiy-based (USA)	100 patients	19 (range 15-29 years)	Total number of teeth lost=299 (3.0 teeth / patients)
McGuire and Nunn (1996)	Retrospective	100 patients	9.9 (range 5-16 years)	Total number of teeth lost=131 (1.3 teeth / patients)
Muzzi et al. (2006)	Retrospective Practice-based Italy	60 patients	10 (range 12.7±2.2 years)	Total number of teeth lost=52 (3.3%)
Nabers et al. (1988)	Retrospective	1.535 patients	12.9 years	Total number of teeth lost=444 (0.29 teeth / patients)
Ng et al. (2011)	Retrospective National DentalCentre Singapura	273 patients	10.7 (range 7-20.4 years)	0.9 teeth / patients / years tooth loss due periodontitis (0.03 teeth / patients/years)
Tonetti et al. (1998)	Retrospective Universiy-based Switzerland	273 patients	67±46 months (range 5 months – 23 years)	Total number of teeth lost=297 (0.23±0.49teeth / patients/years)
Tonetti et al. (2000)	Retrospective Universiy-based Switzerland	273 patients	67±46 months (range 5 – 278 months)	Total number of teeth lost during PMT=263 (0.4±0.37teeth / patients/years)
Wood et al. (1989)	Retrospective Universiy-based (USA)	63 patients	13.6 (range 10-34 years)	Total number of teeth lost=115 (1.8teeth / patients)

Table 2. Characteristics of the Included Studies on the Tooth Loss Individuals without Periodontal Maintenance Therapy

Author / year	Study design / location	Sample	Mean duration study	Mean tooth loss during maintenance
Becker et al. (1984)	Retrospective (USA)	44 patients	5.0 years	(0.22 teeth / patients / years)
Checchi et al. (2002)	Retrospective Practice-based Italy	92 patients	6.7 (range 3-12 years)	Patients complying erratically with suportive periodontal therapy were at a 5.6 times greater risk for tooth loss following active therapy than regularly compliant patients.
Leung et al. (2006)	Retrospective Universiy-based – China	97 patients	5-12 years	Total number of teeth lost= 256
Ng et al. (2011)	Cross-sectional National Dental Centre Singapura	39 patients	9.6 years	(2.7teeth /patients/years) sevenfold increase ($p<0.05$) compared with compliers (0.22teeth / patients/years) tooth loss due periodontitis

5. Risk Factors in PMT

Several indicators or risk factors, including biological, behavioral and social variables, can influence the periodontal status of individuals under PMT. Evidence in the literature demonstrates a direct and significant link between several risk factors and periodontal disease.

Among these risk factors, periodontal literature unanimously highlights the association of poor biofilm control, diabetes mellitus, and smoking with recurrence, progression of periodontitis and dental loss.

5.1. The Control of Biofilm

According to "The American Academy of Periodontology" (2000) [57] periodontal maintenance is an integral part of periodontal therapy for patients with a history of inflammatory periodontal diseases and part of this therapy includes assessment of personal oral hygiene status, removal of subgingival and supragingival plaque and calculus and oral hygiene reinstructions if needful.

Nowadays, over 700 species of bacteria have been found to reside in the human oral cavity. Of these, over 400 species have been found in the periodontal pocket, whereas the remaining 300 species have been localized to other sites within the oral cavity, such as the tongue, oral mucous membranes, carious lesions and root canals (Paster et al. 2006).[58] Although many of these species could be considered commensal, only a few of them are associated with different oral infections, such as periodontal diseases. [59,60]

Periodontitis differ from many other types of infections in the human body, as they are not caused by a single bacterium but rather by a group of bacteria. [61,62] Most bacteria colonizing higher-order organisms grow into populations by adhering to solid surfaces, ultimately forming mixed culture biofilms. The early colonizers of dental plaque are of great importance in the successive stages of biofilm formation and its overall effect on the oral health of the host. [63] Hence, biofilm induced periodontitis, and together with caries, is considered the most important cause of tooth extraction among adults. [64,65]

Since a long time, good oral hygiene habits associated with scaling and root planning therapies have been considered effective in maintaining periodontal attachment and reducing periodontal pocket depths. [66] However, the presence of high quantity of biofilm on the surfaces of the teeth for a long period of time can provoke more periodontal destruction. [67]

Hellström et al (1996) [68] investigated if carefully practiced supragingival plaque control influenced the subgingival microbiota at periodontal sites with suprabony, infrabony, or furcation pockets. They found that professionally delivered and frequently repeated supragingival tooth cleaning, combined with careful self-performed plaque control had a marked effect on the subgingival microbiota of moderate to deep periodontal pockets. Thus, at sites with suprabony and infrabony pockets, as well as at furcation sites, the meticulous and prolonged supragingival plaque removal reduced the total number of microorganisms that could be harvested, as well as the % of sites with *P. gingivalis*.

As pointed out by Petersilka et al. (2002) [69] personal oral hygiene coupled with regular professional supragingival debridement may further improve the level of plaque control but still fails to achieve a completely plaque-free dentition. These remaining bacteria were considered the primary source for the subgingival recolonization. These authors stressed that as a basis for the restoration and maintenance of periodontal health, repeated subgingival debridement, as performed in supportive periodontal therapy, can reduce the number and proportions of periodontopathogenic bacteria in subgingival plaque. However, intensive subgingival scaling and root planing should be avoided in sites that probe less than 3 mm, as this is likely to traumatize the periodontium and cause attachment loss.

There is an interesting fact about the presence of *P. gingivalis* and failure of periodontal maintenance therapy. *P. gingivalis,* a gram-negative anaerobe that colonizes distinct niches in the human oral cavity, is described as one of the major pathogens associated with periodontal breakdown. [70] After the profound effects of active periodontal treatment on *P. gingivalis* elimination were previously demonstrated, Fujise et al (2006) [71] revealed that the subsequent *P. gingivalis* free or suppressed status seems to be maintained during early periodontal maintenance, therefore, severe periodontitis sites before active periodontal treatment seemed to place them at risk of *P. gingivalis* recolonization in the early periodontal maintenance period, and this microbial restoration could be a cause of recurrent periodontitis.

In sum, specific microorganisms are associated with periodontitis. The subgingival population of these bacteria is suppressed following scaling and root planning used during PMT but may return to baseline levels days to months later. [72] The average time for return can vary dramatically in different individuals.[73]

5.2. Diabetes Mellitus

Periodontitis and Diabetes Mellitus (DM) are two chronic diseases that have long been considered to be biologically linked. [74,75,76] The epidemiological associations between periodontitis and diabetes mellitus could be the result of at least two similar, but distinct, pathogenic pathways: a direct causal relationship in which the consequences of diabetes act as modifiers of periodontitis expression or, alternatively, a common pathological defect that results in a host susceptible to either, or both, diseases. [77,78,32]

An increase in the prevalence and severity of periodontitis in individuals with diabetes mellitus is due to reduced polymorphonuclear leukocytes chemotaxis, phagocytic defects, and depressed humoral response. In addition to a hyperglycemic environment, numerous proteins undergo glycosylation to form advanced glycation end products (AGEs). AGEs-mediated events are of primary importance in the pathogenesis of diabetes mellitus complications and may also contribute to tissue changes within the periodontium. [79]

Current evidence regarding the biologic link between diabetes mellitus and periodontitis supports persistent hyperglycemia leading to an exaggerated immuno-inflammatory response to the periodontal pathogenic bacterial challenge, resulting in a more rapid and severe destruction of periodontal tissues.[76]

A large amount of case reports, cross-sectional and longitudinal studies, as well as literature reviews, reported the adverse effects of diabetes mellitus on the onset, progression, and severity of periodontitis. [80,81] Additionally, several studies reported a two- to five-fold higher risk for periodontitis among individuals with diabetes mellitus. Moreover, several retrospective and prospective studies in PMT have shown that the number of maintenance visits, smoking, and diabetic individuals with poor glycemic control have a strong influence on periodontal status.

Bandyopadhyayet al. (2010) [81] conducted a study to evaluate associations between glycemic control and the progression of periodontitis among Gullah African Americans with type-2 DM, who had received no recent periodontal therapy. Authors showed that tooth sites from Gullah with poor glycaemic control had significantly increased odds for PPD progression compared with tooth sites from subjects with well-controlled type-2 DM and this association was significantly modified by PPD at baseline for the particular tooth site. A recent case-control study [82] was conducted to evaluate the relationship between blood glucose levels and clinical parameters of periodontal disease in 65 diabetic and 81 non-diabetic individuals. Authors concluded that periodontal clinical attachment loss were increased by hyperglycemia in diabetic individuals (odds ratio=2.24).

A widely discussed matter these days is the effect of periodontal treatment on glycemic control among diabetic individuals. In a recent systematic review and meta-analysis, it was concluded that periodontal treatment leads to an improvement of glycemic control in type-2 diabetic individuals for at least 3 months. The author's emphasized the need for follow-up periods greater than 6 months and larger samples to allow separate analysis of individuals with moderate to advanced periodontitis. [83]

Costa et al. (2012) [32] in a prospective study investigating an association between glycemic control and periodontitis in 92 individuals under PMT revealed that progression of periodontitis and tooth loss was significantly higher among diabetic individuals with poor glycemic control when compared to diabetics with good glycemic control and non-diabetic individuals. This result highlights the influence of the glycemic control in maintaining a good periodontal status.

5.3. Smoking

Smoking has been reported as the strongest modifiable risk factor for periodontitis, secondary to dental biofilm. A great number of epidemiological studies have also reported a higher prevalence and severity of periodontitis among current-smokers and former-smokers. [84,85,9,86] It is important to highlight that smoking is recognized as an important risk factor for recurrence and progression of periodontitis and the adverse effects on periodontal tissues have been extensively reported, particularly in heavy smokers under PMT. [9,10,32] A great number of studies have demonstrated that smoking is associated with an increased risk for attachment loss, bone loss, and tooth loss. In addition, it has also been demonstrated that smokers respond less propitiously to all forms of periodontal treatment and present less improvement in probing depth and clinical attachment loss.

Scientific evidence suggests that cumulative smoking exposure and duration of smoking cessation are directly associated with periodontitis. [86] Different studies showed that smoking cessation has beneficial effects on periodontal status and that the risk for periodontitis significantly decreases with an increase in the duration of smoking cessation. [87,84,86] However, only a few studies have reported the time interval of smoking cessation which will determine these beneficial effects and hence, indicates the need for additional studies.

Costa et al. in a sequence of studies of individuals in PMT revealed that smoking was associated with a 3-5 times greater chance for recurrence, progression of periodontitis and tooth loss.[7, 8]

This chapter shows that inadequate biofilm control, smoking and diabetes are strong risk factors for progression and recurrence of periodontitis. Thus, the identification of these risk factors, and severity of disease, underscores the need for individual risk assessment of individuals in setting the frequency of visits for PMT.

6. Surgical and Non-Surgical Periodontal Procedures in the PMT

Review studies on surgical or non-surgical periodontal therapy have concluded that: (a) comparisons of the efficacy of surgical and non-surgical procedures have revealed that scaling and root planing alone or in combination with flap procedures are effective methods for the treatment of chronic periodontitis; (b) the consistent message is that, in treating deep pockets, open-flap debridement results in greater probing pocket depth reduction and clinical attachment gain than non-surgical modalities; and (c) non-surgical modalities in shallower pockets consistently involve less post-therapy recession and are clearly recognized as being more conservative. [88,89,5,90] In contrast, studies on the influence of surgical or non-surgical modalities after active therapy in PMT programs are scarce and, when available, were performed with retrospective designs, [3] small samples, and short periods of observation. [30,91] Still, numerous authors point out the limitations of gaining access to difficult areas including depth pockets and furcations using non-surgical techniques. Non-surgical techniques may be operator-dependent and require multiple appointments over prolonged treatment times. [92, 93] They further suggest that debridement with surgical access may in many cases be more effective and efficient than in a closed environment. Wylam et al. 1993 , [94] however, do not support the idea that surgical access may be more efficient use of time, since their results show no difference between time spent in root surface instrumentation for the closed approach (15.2 minutes on average, range 9.5 to 21.8) versus open flap approach (13.6 minutes on average, range 9.5 to 20.5 minutes). Harrel et al., (2001) [19] in a retrospective study with the objective of evaluating the effect of no periodontal treatment, non-surgical treatment only, and a combination of non-surgical and surgical treatment on the progression of periodontitis, showed that surgical treatment yielded much more favorable results than non-surgical treatment alone. The authors concluded that compliance with periodontal maintenance recommendations could be a major contributor to this finding. In addition, the authors also recognized that non-surgical procedures were more common in non-cooperative individuals with future recommendations for PMT. Hung and Douglas (2002) [95] in a meta-analysis of the effect of scaling and root planning, surgical treatment and antibiotic therapies on periodontal probing depth and attachment loss concluded that: (a) surgical treatment is better for reduction of periodontal probing depth and these benefits become greater with the increase of initial probing depth; (b) differences in the gain of attachment level indicates an advantage for nonsurgical treatment in shallow and medium initial periodontal probing depths; (c) for deep initial periodontal probing depths, surgical therapy showed similar attachment gains when compared with scaling and root planning. Several studies reported surgical treatment was performed significantly more frequently in irregular compliers. [96,30,91,5] The literature consistently reports that non-surgical periodontal therapy is more often performed in non-molar teeth compared to the molars. Clearly these findings reflect a greater difficulty in correct root instrumentation only with non-surgical procedures in molar teeth, compared to non-molars. [97,17,18,5] The main factors for these findings are the morphology of the posterior teeth, especially when associated with furcation lesions. [17,96] With regard to the accumulation of plaque after treatment, there is insufficient evidence showing differences between surgical and non-surgical treatments or between various surgical procedures. [98,5] Furthermore, studies have shown that the degree of cooperation could be inversely correlated with plaque index values. [91,6] A systematic review conducted by Heitz-Mayfield et al. 2005 [5] concluded: (a) a substantial reduction in the percentage of sites with BOP following both treatment modalities, reflecting the systematic approach to plaque control incorporated in the studies; (b) When sites with an initial probing pocket depth of 1-3 mm were treated by open flap debridement there was more clinical attachment level loss than after scaling and root planning (weighted mean differences -0.51 mm); (c) When sites with an initial probing depth of 4-6 mm were treated by open flap debridement there was less clinical attachment level gain than after scaling and root planning (weighted mean differences – 0.37 mm); (d) Though there was a greater reduction in probing pocket depth reduction after the open flap debridement procedure (weighted mean difference 0.35 mm); (e) When sites with an initial probing pocket depth of > 6mm were treated by open flap debridement, there was a greater increase in the clinical attachment level than after scaling and root planning (weighted mean difference 0.19 mm); (f) Open flap debridement resulted in a greater reduction in probing depth than scaling and root planning in these deep pockets (weighted mean difference 0.58 mm); (g) There is limited evidence (no meta-analysis) suggesting differences between open flap debridement and scaling and root planning when treating furcations or angular bony defects; (h)There are no data available to address the important issue of patient-centered treatment outcomes and the evaluation of adverse effects. A meta-analysis conducted by Heitz-Mayfield (2005) including 5 studies also corroborates these findings, showing that sites with an initial probing pocket depth of 1-3 mm presented significant clinical attachment loss after open flap debridement when compared to scaling and root planning. However, several authors [88,27,3,5,90] have pointed out that most studies comparing surgical versus non-surgical therapy are heterogeneous because they have been conducted comparing different techniques and populations, with too many different designs and follow-up times and no intended treatment; thus, they have reported different results.

7. Final Considerations

The literature showed that patients who comply with periodontal maintenance in the long-term after the completion of non-surgical and surgical active periodontal therapy had a low level of recurrence, progression of periodontitis, and tooth loss. Smokers and individuals with poor glycemic control are at increased risk for adverse effects on periodontal status even in a regular periodontal maintenance therapy. The modality of surgical or non-surgical treatment during PMT does not exercise influence on periodontal condition in the presence of a good control of biofilm and maintenance at regular intervals determined by an individual risk assessment.

8. Implications for Future Research

This chapter identified a number of important issues which need to be addressed in future research, including the evaluation of adverse effects, and individual-based outcomes, such as aesthetics and aspects related to quality of life of individuals. The choice of nonsurgical or surgical periodontal procedures in the PMT should be based on a careful consideration and discussion of the benefits and harm for those particular individuals and sites.

References

[1] Wilson Jr TG. Supportive periodontal treatment introduction- definition, extent of need, therapeutic objectives, frequency and efficacy. *Periodontology* 2000. 1996;12:11-15.

[2] American Academy of Periodontology. Position Paper. Epidemiology of periodontal diseases. *Journal of Periodontology*. 2005;76:1406-1419.

[3] Renvert S, Persson GR. Supportive periodontal therapy. *Periodontology* 2000. 2004;36:179-195.

[4] Axelsson P, Nystrom B, Lindhe J. The long-term effect of a plaque control program on tooth mortality, caries and periodontal disease in adults: Results after 30 years of maintenance. *Journal of Clinical Periodontology*. 2004;31:749-757.

[5] Heitz-Mayfield LJA. How effective is surgical therapy compared with non-surgical debridement? *Periodontology* 2000. 2005;37:72-87.

[6] Lorentz TCM, Cota LOM, Cortelli JR, Vargas AMD, Costa FO. Prospective study of complier individuals under periodontal maintenance therapy: analysis of clinical periodontal parameters, risk predictors and the progression of periodontitis. *Journal of Clinical Periodontology*. 2009;36:58-67.

[7] Costa FO, Cota LOM, Lages EJP et al. Progression of periodontitis in a sample of regular and irregular compliers under maintenance therapy: a 3-year follow-up study. *Journal of Periodontology*. 2011a;82:1279-1287.

[8] Costa FO LOM, Lages EJP, Câmara GCV, Cortelli SC, Cortelli JR, Costa JE et al. Oral Impact on Daily Performance, Personality Traits, and Compliance in Periodontal Maintenance Therapy. *Journal of Periodontology*. 2011b;82:1146-1154.

[9] Costa FO, Cota LOM, Lages EJP, Oliveira APL, Cortelli SC, Cortelli JR et al. Periodontal Risk Assessment Model in a Sample of Regular and Irregular Compliers Under Maintenance Therapy: A 3-Year Prospective Study. *Journal of Periodontology*. 2012a;83:292-300.

[10] Costa FO, Santuchi CC, Lages EJP et al. Prospective Study in Periodontal Maintenance Therapy: Comparative Analysis Between Academic and Private Practices. *Journal of Periodontology*. 2012b;83:301-311.

[11] Cattabriga M, Rotundo R, Muzzi L, Nieri M, Verrocchi G, Cairo F et al. Retrospective evaluation of the influence of the interleukin-1 genotype on radiographic bone levels in treated periodontal patients over 10 years. *Journal of Periodontology*. 2001;72:767-773.

[12] Matuliene G, Studer R, Lang NP, Schmidlin K, Pjetursson BE, Salvi GE et al. Significance of periodontal risk assessment in the recurrence of periodontitis and tooth loss. *Journal of Clinical Periodontology*. 2010:37:191-199.

[13] Koning J, Plagmann HC, Langenfeld N, Kocher T. Retrospective comparison of clinical variables between compliant and non-compliant patients. *Journal of Clinical Periodontology*. 2001;28:227-232.

[14] Tonetti MS, Claffey N. European Workshop in Periodontology Group C. Advances in the progression of periodontitis and proposal of definitions of a periodontitis case and disease progression for use in risk factor research. Group C consensus report of the 5th European Workshop in Periodontology. *Journal of Clinical Periodontology*. 2005;32(Suppl.6):210-213.

[15] Badersten A, Nilvéus R, Egelberg J. Scores of plaque, bleeding, suppuration and probing depth to predict probing attachment loss: 5 years of observation following nonsurgical periodontal therapy. *Journal of Clinical Periodontology*. 1990;17:102-107.

[16] Kaldahl WB, Kalkwarf KL, Patil KD, Molvar MP, Dyer JK. Long term evaluation of periodontal therapy: I. Response to 4 therapeutic modalities. *Journal of Periodontology*. 1996;67:93-102.

[17] Claffey N, Polyzois I, Ziaka P. An overview of non-surgical and surgical therapy. *Periodontology* 2000. 2000;36:35-44.

[18] Becker W, Becker BE, Caffesse R, Kerry G, Ochsenbein C, Morrison E et al. A longitudinal study comparing scaling, osseous surgery, and modified Widman procedures: results after 5 years. *Journal of Periodontology*. 2001;72:1675-1684.

[19] Harrel SK, Nunn ME. Longitudinal comparison of the periodontal satus of patients with moderate and severe periodontal disease receiving no treatment, non-surgical treatment, and surgical treatment utilizing individual sites for analysis. *Journal of Periodontology*. 2001;72:1509-1519.

[20] Becker W, Berg L, Becker BE. Untreated periodontal disease: a longitudinal study. *Journal of Periodontology*. 1979;50:234-244.

[21] Oliveira Costa F, Cota LOM, Costa JE, Pordeus IA. Periodontal disease progression among young subjects with no preventive dental care: a 52-month follow-up study. *Journal of Periodontology*. 2007;78:198-203.

[22] Macleod DE, Lainson PA, Spivey JD. The predictability of periodontal treatment as measured by tooth loss: a retrospective study. *Quintessence International*. 1989;29:631-635.

[23] Checchi L, Montevecchi M, Gatto MRA, Trombelli L. Retrospective study of tooth loss in 92 treated periodontal patients. *Journal of Clinical Periodontology*. 2002;29:651-656.

[24] Miyamoto T, Kumagai T, Lang MS, Nunn ME. Compliance as a Prognostic Indicator. II. Impact of Patient's Compliance to the Individual Tooth Survival, *Journal of Periodontology*. 2010;81:1280-1288.

[25] Famili P, Short E. Compliance with periodontal maintenance at the University of Pittsburgh: Retrospective analysis of 315 cases. *General Dentistry*. 2010;58:e42-e47.

[26] Leininger M, Tenenbaum H, Davideau JL. Modified periodontal risk assessment score: long-term predictive value of treatment outcomes. A retrospective study. *Journal of Clinical Periodontology*. 2010;37:427-435.

[27] Papantopoulos GH. Effect of periodontal therapy in smokers and non-smokers with advanced periodontal disease: results after maintenance therapy for a minimum of 5 years. *Journal of Periodontology*. 2004;75:838-843.

[28] Fisher S, Kells L, Picard JP, Gelskey SC, Singer DL, Lix L et al. Progression of Periodontal Disease in a Maintenance Population of Smokers and Non-Smokers: A 3-Year Longitudinal Study. *Journal of Periodontology*. 2008;79:461-468.

[29] Wilson Jr TG, Kornman KS. Retreatment for patients with inflammatory periodontal disease. *Periodontology* 2000. 1996;12:119-121.

[30] Rosling B, Serino G, Hellstrom MK, Socransky SS, Lindhe J. Longitudinal periodontal tissue alterations during supportive therapy. Findings from individuals with normal and high susceptibility of periodontitis. *Journal of Clinical Periodontology*. 2001;28:241-249.

[31] Renvert S, Nilveus R, Dahlén G, Slots J, Egelberg J. 5 year follow up of periodontal intraosseous defects treated by root planning or flap surgery. *Journal of Clinical Periodontology*. 1990;17:356-363.

[32] Costa FO, Cota LOM, Lages EJP et al. Progression of periodontitis and tooth loss associated with glycemic control individuals under periodontal maintenance therapy: a 5-year follow-up study. *Journal of Periodontology*. 2012c Doi::10.1902/jop.2012.120255.

[33] Mendoza AR, Newcomb GM, Nixon KC. Compliance with supportive periodontal therapy. *Journal of Periodontology*. 1991;62:731-736.

[34] Umaki TM, Umaki MR, Cobb CM. The Psychology of Patient Compliance: A Focused Review of the Literature. *Journal of Periodontology*. 2012;83:395-400.

[35] Kwok V, Caton JG. Prognosis revisited: A system for assigning periodontal prognosis. *Journal of Periodontology*. 2007;78:2063-2071.

[36] Wood WR, Greco GW, McFall WT Jr. Tooth loss in patients with periodontitis after treatment and long-term maintenance care. *Journal of Periodontology*. 1989;60:516-520.

[37] McGuire MK, Nunn ME. Prognosis versus actual outcome. III. The effectiveness of clinical parameters in accurately predicting tooth survival. *Journal of Periodontology*. 1996;67:666-674.

[38] Muzzi L, Nieri M, Cattabriga M, Rotundo R, Cairo F, Pini Prato GP. The potential prognostic value of some periodontal factors for tooth loss: A retrospective multilevel analysis on periodontal patients treated and maintained over 10 years. *Journal of Periodontology*. 2006;77:2084-2089.

[39] Fardal O, Johannessen AC, Linden GJ. Tooth loss during maintenance following periodontal treatment in a periodontal practice in Norway. *Journal of Clinical Periodontology*. 2004;31:550-555.

[40] Chambrone LA, Chambrone L. Tooth loss in well maintained patients with chronic periodontitis during long-term supportive therapy in Brazil. *Journal of Clinical Periodontology*. 2006;33:759-764.

[41] Leung WK, Ng DKC, Jin L, Corbet EF. Tooth loss in treated periodontitis patients responsible for their supportive care arrangements. *Journal of Clinical Periodontology*. 2006;33:265-275.

[42] Eickholz P, Kaltschmitt J, Berbig J, Reitmeir P, Pretzl B. Tooth loss after active periodontal therapy. 1: patient-related factors for risk, prognosis, and quality of outcome. *Journal of Clinical Periodontology*. 2008;35:165-174.

[43] Pretzl B, Kaltschmitt J, Kim TS, Reitmeir P, Eickholz P. Tooth loss after active periodontal therapy 2: tooth-related factors. *Journal of Clinical Periodontology*. 2008;35:175-182.

[44] Ng MCH, Ong MMa, Lim LP, Koh CG, Chan YT. Tooth loss in compliant and non compliant periodontally treated patients: 7 years after active periodontal therapy. *Journal of Clinical Periodontology*. 2011;38:499-508.

[45] Jansson L, Lagervall M. Periodontitis progression in patients subjected to supportive maintenance care. *Swed Dental Journal*. 2008;32:105-114.

[46] Matuliene G, Pjetursson BE, Salvi GE, Schmidlin K, Brägger U, Zwahlen M et al. Influence of residual pockets on progression of periodontitis and tooth: Results after 11 years of maintenance. *Journal of Clinical Periodontology*. 2008;35:685-695.

[47] Tsami A, Pepelassi E, Kodovazenitis G, Komboli M. Parameters affecting tooth loss during periodontal maintenance in a Greek population. *Journal of American Dental Association*. 2009;140:1100-1107.

[48] Hirschfeld L, Wasserman B. A long-term survey of tooth loss in 600 treated periodontal patients. *Journal of Periodontology*. 1978;49:225-237.

[49] McFall WT Jr. Tooth loss in 100 treated patients with periodontal disease. A long-term study. *Journal of Periodontology*. 1982;53:539-548.

[50] Becker W, Becker BE, Berg L. Periodontal treatment without maintenance. A retrospective study in 44 patients, *Journal of Periodontology*. 1984a;55:505-509.

[51] Lindhe J, Nyman S. Long-term maintenance of patients treated for advanced periodontal disease. *Journal of Clinical Periodontology*. 1984;11:504-514.

[52] Nabers CL, Stalker WH, Esparza D, Naylor B, Canales S. Tooth loss in 1535 treated periodontal patients. *Journal of Periodontology*. 1998;59:297-300.

[53] Tonetti MS, Steffen P, Muller-Campanile V, Suvan J, Lang NP. Initial extractions and tooth loss during supportive care in a periodontal population seeking comprehensive care. *Journal of Clinical Periodontology*. 2000;27:824-831.
[54] Chambrone L, Chambrone D, Lima LA, Chambrone LA. Predictors of tooth loss during long-term periodontal maintenance: a systematic review of observational studies. *Journal of Clinical Periodontology*. 2010;37:675-684.
[55] Martin JA, Page RC, Loeb CF, Levi PA Jr. Tooth loss in 776 treated periodontal patients. *Journal of Periodontology*. 2010;81:244-250.
[56] Becker W, Berg L, Becker BE. The long-term evaluation of periodontal treatment and maintenance in 95 patients. *International Journal of Periodontics Restorative Dentistry*. 1984b;4:54-71.
[57] American Academy of Periodontology. Parameter on Periodontal Maintenance. *Journal of Periodontology*. 2000;71(Supplement):849-850.
[58] Paster BJ, Olsen I, Aas JA, Dewhirst F. The breadth of bacterial diversity in the human periodontal pocket and other oral sites. *Periodontology* 2000. 2006;42:80–87.
[59] Jenkinson HF, Lamont RJ. Oral microbial communities in sickness and in health. *Trends in Microbiology*. 2005;13:589–595.
[60] Socransky SS, Haffajee AD. Periodontal microbial ecology. *Periodontology* 2000. 2005;38:135–187.
[61] Nonnenmacher C, Dalpke A, Mutters R, Heeg K. Quantitative detection of periodontopathogens by real-time PCR. *Journal of Microbiological Methods*. 2004;59:117–125.
[62] Haffajee AD, Socransky SS, Patel MR, Song X. Microbial complexes in supragingival plaque. *Oral Microbiology and Immunology*. 2008;23:196–205.
[63] Li J, Helmerhorst EJ, Leone CW, Troxler RF, Yaskell T, Haffajee AD et al. Identification of early microbial colonizers in human dental biofilm. *Journal of Applied Microbiology*. 2004;97:1311–1318.
[64] Caldas AF Jr. Reasons for tooth extraction in a Brazilian population. *International Dental Journal*. 2000;50:267–273.
[65] Aida J, Ando Y, Akhter R, Aoyama H, Masui M, Morita M. Reasons for permanent tooth extractions in Japan. *Journal of Epidemiology*. 2006;16:214–219.
[66] Suomi JD, Greene JC, Vermillion JR, Chang JJ, Leatherwood EC. The effect of controlled oral hygiene procedures on the progression of periodontal disease in adults: results after two years. *Journal of Periodontology*. 1969;40:416-420.
[67] Ramfjord SP, Knowles JW, Nissle RR, Shick RA, Burgett FG. Longitudinal study of periodontal therapy. *Journal of Periodontology*. 1973;44:66-77.
[68] Hellström MK, Ramberg P, Krok L, Lindhe J. The effect of supragingival plaque control on the subgingival microflora in human periodontitis. *Journal of Clinical Periodontology*. 1996;23:934-40.
[69] Petersilka GJ, Ehmke B, Flemmig TF. Antimicrobial effects of mechanical debridement. *Periodontology* 2000. 2002;28:56-71.
[70] Zambon JJ. Periodontal diseases: microbial factors. *Annals of Periodontology*. 1996;1:879-925.
[71] Fujise O, Miura M, Hamachi T, Maeda K. Risk of Porphyromonas gingivalis recolonization during the early period of periodontal maintenance in initially severe periodontitis sites. *Journal of Periodontology*. 2006;77:1333-9.

[72] Sbordone L, Ramaglia l, Guletta E, Iacomo V. Recolonization of the subgingival microflora after scaling and root planing in human periodontitis. *Journal of Periodontology*. 1990;61:579-584.
[73] Greenstein G. Periodontal response to mechanical non-surgical therapy: a review. *Journal of Periodontology*. 1992;63.118-130.
[74] Fernandes JK, Wiegand RE, Salinas CF et al. Periodontal disease status in Gullah African Americans with type 2 diabetes living in South Carolina. *Journal of Periodontology*. 2009;80:1062-1068.
[75] Sotherland JH, Taylor GW, Moss K, Beck JD, Offenbacher S. Commonality in chronic inflammatory diseases: Periodontitis, diabetes, and coronary artery disease. *Periodontol 2000*. 2006;40:130-143.
[76] Marlow NM, Slate EH, Bandyopadhyay D, Fernandes JK, Leite RS. Health insurance status is associated with periodontal disease progression among Gullah African-Americans with type 2 diabetes mellitus. *Journal of Public Health Dentistry*. 2011;7:143-151.
[77] Loe H. Periodontal disease: The sixth complication of diabetes mellitus. *Diabetes Care*. 1993;16:329-334.
[78] Ylostalo PV, Knuuttila ML. Confounding and effect modification: possible explanation for variation in the results on the association between oral and systemic diseases. *Journal of Clinical Periodontology*. 2006;33:104-108.
[79] Campus G, Salem A, Uzzau S, Baldoni E, Tonolo G. Diabetes and Periodontal disease: a case-control study. *Journal of Periodontology*. 2005;76:418-425.
[80] Taylor GW, Borgnakke WS. Periodontal disease: associations with diabetes, glycemic control and complications. *Oral Disease*. 2008;14:191-203.
[81] Bandyopadhyay D, Marlow NM, Fernandes JK, Leite RS. Periodontal disease progression and glycaemic control among Gullah African Americans with type-2 diabetes. *Journal of Clinical Periodontology*. 2010;37:501-509.
[82] Botero JE, Yepes FL, Roldán N et al. Tooth and periodontal clinical attachment loss are associated with hyperglycemia in diabetic patients. *Journal of Periodontology*. 2012 doi:10.1902/jop.2012.110681.
[83] Teeuw JW, Gerdes VEA, Loss B. Effect of periodontal treatment on glycemic control of diabetic patients. A systematic review and meta-analysis. *Diabetes Care*. 2010;33:421-427.
[84] Torrungruang K, Tamsailom S, Rojanasomsith K, Sutdhibhisal S, Nisapakulton K, Vanichjakvong O et al. Risk indicators of periodontal disease in older Thai adults. *Journal of Periodontology*. 2005;76:558–65.
[85] Thomson MW, Broadbent JM, Welch D, Beck JD, Poulton R. Cigarette smoking and periodontal disease among 32-year-olds, a prospective study of a representative birth cohort. *Journal Clinical of Periodontology*. 2007;34:828–834.
[86] Patel RA, Wilson RF, Palme RM. The Effect of Smoking on Periodontal Bone Regeneration, A Systematic Review and Meta-Analysis. *Journal of Periodontology*. 2012;83:143-155.
[87] Labriola A, Needleman I, Moles DR. Systematic review of the effect of smoking on nonsurgical periodontal therapy. *Periodontology* 2000. 2005;37:124-137.
[88] Kaldhal WB, Kalkwarf KL, Patil KD. A review of longitudinal studies that compared periodontal therapies. *Journal of Periodontology*. 1993;64:243-253.

[89] Ishikawa I, Baehini P. Non-surgical periodontal therapy-where do we stand now? *Periodontology* 2000. 2004;36:9-13.

[90] Apatzidou DA, Kinane DF. Non-surgical mechanical treatment strategies for periodontal disease. *Dental Clinical North American*. 2010;54:1-12.

[91] Serino G, Rosling B, Ramberg P, Hellstrom MK, Socransky SS, Lindhe J. The long-term effect of systemic tetracycline used as an adjunt to non-surgical treatment of advanced periodontitis. *Journal of Clinical Periodontology*. 2001;28:446-452.

[92] Lang NP. Indications and rationale for non-surgical periodontal therapy. *International Dental Journal*. 1983;33:127-136.

[93] Grossi SG, Skrepcinski FB, Decaro T, Robertson DC Ho AW, Dunford RG, Genco RJ. Treatment of periodontal disease reduces glycated hemoglobin. *Journal of Periodontology*. 1997;68:713-719.

[94] Wylam JM, Mealey BL, Mills MP, Waldrop TC, Moskowicz DC. The clinical effectiveness of open versus closed scaling and root planing on multi-rooted teeth. *Journal of Periodontology*. 1993;64:1023-1028.

[95] Hung HC, Douglas CW. Meta-analysis of the effect of scaling and root planning, surgical treatment and antibiotic therapies on periodontal probing depth and attachment loss. *Journal of Clinical Periodontology*. 2002;29: 975-986.

[96] Svärdström G, Wennström JL. Periodontal treatment decisions for molars: an analysis of influencing factors and long-term outcome. *Journal of Periodontology*. 2000;1:579-85.

[97] Nordland P, Garret S, Kiger R, Vanooteghem R, Hutchens LH, Egelberg J. The effect of plaque control and root debridement in molar teeth. *Journal of Clinical Periodontology*. 1987;14:231-236.

[98] Isidor F, Karring T. Long-term effect or surgical and non-surgical periodontal treatment. A 5-year clinical study. *Journal of Periodontal Research*. 1986;21:462-472.

In: Current Trends in Periodontics and Implant Dentistry ISBN: 978-1-62618-819-8
Editors: Vishal Anand and Minkle Gulati

Chapter VIII

Supportive Periodontal Therapy

Minkle Gulati[1] and Vishal Anand[2]
[1]Department of Periodontics, BBDCODS, Uttar Pradesh, India
[2]Department of Periodontics, Faculty of Dental Sciences, KGMU, Uttar Pradesh, India

Abstract

Chronic periodontitis is an infection disease caused by an opportunistic microflora. The infection triggers host inflammatory responses resulting in the destruction of the tooth supporting tissues. Periodontal maintenance measures implicate the elimination of plaque and calculus, and an assessment geared toward categorizing aspects that may impede with oral health. Scientific exploration has established that with meticulous day-to-day plaque removal and periodontal maintenance procedures, the reappearance and progression of periodontal disease can be minimized.

Introduction

The initial intraoral deposit formed on a polished hydroxyapatite surface is a condensate of salivary proteins termed pellicle. Since this coating forms so rapidly, it has been hypothesized that the bacterial colonization would be unlikely to begin on any surface without the initial formation of pellicle [1]. The initial colonizers of the tooth surface have been reported to be members of the primary colonizer's species and attachment of these microorganisms is mediated through proteoglycans as well as proteins in fimbriae and pilli. The earliest accumulations of these deposits occur at protected sites, such as the gingival margin and interdental areas. Once the initial adherence has occurred, the plaque undergoes a process of maturation including a succession of dominant microorganisms and an increase of plaque thickness, which occurs primarily by the growth of the microorganisms rather than through the adhesion of additional microorganisms [2, 3]. Plaque development and maturation have been described as a process of orderly succession of microbial populations from predominantly gram-positive, facultative cocci to that represented by a gram negative, anaerobic microbiota [1]. Once supragingival microbial deposits have established an ecological niche, subgingival deposits begin to form. The composition of the subgingival microflora has been studied intensively, as it is these deposits that are thought to be involved in causing the destructive periodontal diseases. Changing in the supragingival microflora have been reported to cause changes in the subgingival composition [1, 4].

Plaque has been implicated as the primary etiologic agent in most forms of periodontal diseases and from this brief overview, it becomes apparent that there can be several potential means of developing preventive strategies to control dental plaque formation (and consequently preventing and managing periodontal diseases) through inhibition of microbial attachment, through alteration of the structure of the deposits or through interfering with the pattern of plaque development [5, 6]. Primary prevention can also be accomplished once the microbial plaque deposit have been formed, through reducing existing plaque, selectively inhibiting these particular microbes associated with disease or inhibiting the expression of virulence determinants [7].

With all these strategies, primary prevention and supportive periodontal treatment are inexorably interwined. Prevention is related to making the occurrence or progression of a disease process unlikely or impossible [8]. The application of preventive measures has been divided into three categories depending upon when during the disease process they are to be applied [9]. Strategies designed to ensure that the disease process fails to become clinically evident are termed as primary prevention. Primary prevention is, arguably, the most cost effective health care measure, as it eliminates the need for further treatment and the pain and suffering associated with diseases. Once a disease has become clinically evident, the focus of prevention shifts from prevention of inception to prevention of disease progression.

This second stage of prevention is entitled secondary stage of prevention and is also highly cost-effective. In this the debilitating or disfiguring effects of the disease can be minimized. For secondary prevention to become most effective, early recognition and treatment of the disease processes are therefore essential. Diagnosis and early treatment of the inflammatory periodontal diseases and their role in prevention requires some notation of current concepts and advances in this area. It should also be noted that the distinction between primary and secondary prevention is not a sharp separation, as many preventive strategies may be equally applied both before and following inception of the disease process.

As a disease progresses, defects in the host begin to become evident and require correction. Prevention as a part of corrective therapy is termed tertiary prevention and encompasses the dual goals of disability limitation as well as rehabilitation. Supportive periodontal treatment could be considered a part of tertiary prevention as it deals with some aspects of rehabilitation; but it also has a strong foothold in both primary and secondary prevention, as prevention of disease progression also falls within the definition of this entity.

According to the American Academy of Periodontology, "supportive periodontal treatment is an integral part of periodontal therapy". It is performed by a dentist, although components of supportive periodontal treatment can be performed by a dental hygienist under the supervision of a dentist. Supportive periodontal treatment should include an update of medical and dental histories, radiographic review, extraoral and intraoral soft tissue examination, dental examination, periodontal evaluation, removal of bacterial plaque from the supragingival and subgingival regimes, scaling and root planning where indicated, polishing of the teeth and a review of the patients plaque control efficacy and other appropriate behaviour modification [10].

There procedures are performed at selected intervals to assist the periodontal patient in maintaining oral health. Supportive periodontal treatment is usually started after the completion of active periodontal therapy and continues at varying intervals for the entire life of the dentition or its implant replacements. The patient may move back into active care if the disease undergoes a period of exacerbation.

Rationale for Supportive Periodontal Therapy

Preservation of the periodontal health of the treated patient requires as positive a program as that required for the elimination of periodontal disease. After phase I therapy is completed, patients are placed on a schedule of periodic recall visit for maintenance care to prevent recurrence of the disease.

Transfer of the patient from active treatment status to a maintenance program is a definitive step in total patient care that requires time and effort on the part of the dentist and staff as well. Patients must understand the purpose of the maintenance program, and the dentists must focus on maintenance therapy. Patients who are not maintained on a supervised recall program subsequent to active treatment show obvious signs of recurrent periodontitis (e.g., increased pocket depth, bone loss, tooth loss) [11, 12]. The more often the patients present for recommended supportive periodontal treatment (SPT), the less likely they are to loose teeth [13].

Studies have shown that even with appropriate periodontal therapy, some progression of disease is possible [14, 15]. One likely explanation for the recurrence of periodontal disease is incomplete subgingival plaque removal [16]. If subgingival plaque is left behind during scaling; it regrows within the pocket. The regrowth of subgingival plaque is a slow process compared with that of supragingival plaque. During this period (perhaps months), the subgingival plaque may not induce inflammatory reactions that can be discerned at the gingival margin.

The clinical diagnosis may be further confused by the introduction of adequate supragingival plaque control, because the inflammatory reactions caused by the plaque in the soft tissue wall of the pocket are not likely to be manifested clinically as gingivitis. Thus, inadequate subgingival plaque control can lead to continued loss of attachment, even without the presence of clinical gingival inflammation.

Bacteria are present in the gingival tissues in chronic and aggressive periodontitis case [17, 18]. Eradication of intragingival microorganisms may be necessary for a stable periodontal result. Scaling, root planning, and even flap surgery may not eliminate intragingival bacteria in some areas [19]. These bacteria may recolonize the pocket and cause recurrent disease.

Bacteria associated with periodontitis can be transmitted between spouses and other family members [20, 21]. Patients who appear to be successfully treated can become infected or reinfected with potential pathogens. This is especially likely in patients with remaining pockets.

Another possible explanation for the recurrence of periodontal disease is the microscopic nature of the dentogingival unit healing after periodontal treatment. Histologic studies have shown that after periodontal procedures, tissues usually do not heal by formation of new connective tissue attachment to root surfaces [22, 23]. but reunite in a long junctional epithelium. It has been speculated that this type of dentogingival unit may be weaker and that inflammation may rapidly separate the long junctional epithelium from the tooth. Thus, treated periodontal patients may be predisposed to recurrent pocket formation if maintenance care is not optimal. Subgingival scaling alters the microflora of periodontal pockets [24, 25]. Although pocket debridement suppresses components of the subgingival microflora associated with periodontitis, periodontal pathogens may return to baseline levels within days or months [26, 27]. The return of pathogens to pretreatment levels generally occurs in approximately 9 to 11 weeks but can vary dramatically among patients [26]. Both the mechanical debridement performed by the therapist and the motivational environment provided by the recall appointments seem to be necessary for good maintenance results. Patients tend to reduce their oral hygiene efforts between appointments [11, 28]. Knowing that their hygiene will be evaluated motivates them to perform better oral hygiene in anticipation of the appointment.

Salutary Goals of Supportive Periodontlogy Therapy

Gingivitis left untreated may lead to periodontitis [29]. This progression can be prevented or limited by either optimal personal oral hygiene [30, 31] and / or periodic maintenance care under the supervision of a dentist [32]. Since patients are rarely completely effective in removing plaque accumulation, supportive periodontal treatment can reduce the possibility of future attachment loss. Although the prevalence of gingivitis has not been completely determined, this disease affects millions of people [33, 34]. The fact that gingivitis may lead to periodontitis [29] and the fact that it cannot yet be accurately predicted when, or even whether, gingivitis will progress to periodontitis dictates the need for monitoring and professional removal of plaque and its related products for patients treated for this periodontal disease [7, 31] This monitoring and professional therapy are provided during supportive periodontal treatment. Patients with a history of periodontitis usually require periodic supportive periodontal treatment since personal supragingival oral hygiene alone has not been shown to control attachment loss in these patients [35, 36]. It can therefore be concluded that a large percentage of the population would benefit from regular supportive periodontal treatment. The therapeutic objectives of supportive periodontal therapy are:

- To prevent the progression and recurrence of periodontal disease in patients who have previously been treated for gingivitis and periodontitis.
- To prevent the loss of dental implants after clinical stability has been achieved.
- To reduce tooth loss by monitoring the dentition and any prosthetic replacements of the natural teeth; and
- To diagnose and manage in a timely manner, other diseases or conditions found within or related to the oral cavity.

Numerous studies have shown that less attachment loss occurs and fewer teeth are lost when patients maintain regular supportive periodontal treatment intervals [37, 38] compared with patients seen less often [39, 40] or not at all [41, 42]. Occasionally despite the best efforts of clinicians and patients, some individuals may lose teeth despite maintaining a regular supportive periodontal treatment schedule [43, 44]. This last group of individuals often benefits from additional diagnostic procedures such as microbial analysis and therapy that includes antimicrobial agents [45, 46]. A counterpoint to the efficacy of frequent supportive periodontal treatment visits has been offered in a limited number of studies that found no difference in the progression of periodontal diseases in patients receiving less frequent supportive periodontal treatment as compared with those who received more frequent supportive periodontal treatment [47, 48]. Most of the patients in this last group of studies maintained relatively high levels of oral hygiene.

For most patients with gingivitis but no previous attachment loss, supportive treatment twice a year will suffice [49]. For patients with a previous history of periodontitis, the results from a number of clinical trials suggest that the frequency of supportive periodontal should be less than 6 months. Intervals of 2 weeks [50, 51], 2-3 months [11], 3 months [52, 53], 3-4 months [31, 54], 3-6 months [55, 56], and 4-6 months [43] have been proposed for patients with a history of chronic periodontitis and these patients should be seen at least four times a year, because that interval will result in a decrease in disease progression or recurrence as compared with patients seen less frequently [37, 38].

Specific microorganisms are associated with periodontitis [57, 58]. The subgingival population of these bacteria is suppressed following root planning used during supportive periodontal treatment but may return to baseline levels days to months later [59, 60]. If the clinician wishes to prevent re-establishment of suspected pathogens, supportive periodontal treatment intervals of 3 months or less appear to be required.

Compliance with suggested supportive periodontal treatment intervals can affect the success of treatment. Patients treated for periodontitis who comply with suggested supportive periodontal treatment intervals will experience less attachment loss and tooth than patients who do not demonstrate compliance with the supportive periodontal treatment schedule [61, 62].

This body of data supports the concept that it is advantageous if supportive periodontal treatment visits are performed every 3 months. This interval should be individualized. Supportive periodontal treatment intervals can be tailored to the individual's need of each patient and further modified based on the ongoing clinical studies. Supportive periodontal treatment patients often need to be returned to active care. Sites that have experienced previous attachment loss are most likely to need active therapy in the future and may involve nonsurgical or surgical treatment.

Supportive Periodontal Appointments for Patients with Periodontal Disease

Supportive periodontal treatment varies greatly from office to office, therapist to therapist, patient to patient, and for the same patient over time. However, all supportive periodontal treatment visits have a common thread: moving from cleaning teeth towards diagnosing and treating disease found during these visits. As disease prediction becomes more accurate, therapy for most patients will become increasingly localized.

This section covers the specific procedures performed at a typical supportive periodontal treatment visit for a patient with an inflammatory periodontal disease. These suggestions should be tailored (and improved upon) for each specific situation, office and patient.

Chart Appraisal

The therapist and the patient will benefit from a professional review of the patient's health history and record of the previous supportive periodontal treatment visits before any current treatment. Any medicines needed before supportive periodontal treatment (such as antibiotic prophylaxis to reduce the chance of subacute bacterial endocarditis in a patient with a heart murmur) or any special needs (such as local anaesthesia) can thus be determined before the patient is seen.

Operatory and Instrument Infection Control

Providing a safe, clean environment for patient care has always been important. However, the recent rise in highly infectious viral diseases and antibiotic-resistant tuberculosis bacterial strains have heightened the need for these procedures. On the positive side, when infection control procedures are used, less cross-contamination occurs. On the negative side, a great deal of time and material must be expended towards infection control, which impacts the economics of the delivery of care.

Health History Update

Patients can undergo significant medical and dental health changes in the few weeks or months between supportive periodontal treatment visits. The questions that follow often uncover important new information for the health history. Any changes should be recorded in the patient's chart:

- Has there been any change in your health or medicines, or have you been hospitalized since your last visit?
- Is there anything about your mouth or jaw that is of concern to you?
- Have you had any dental work since your last visit?
- What do you routinely do to clean your teeth?

Conversation with the Patient

The fact that most periodontal diseases are chronic in nature runs counter to the fact that health care trends are forcing many dental practitioners to spend less and less time with individual patients. Professionals sometimes then fall into the trap of seeing patients as "mouths to be repaired", not people who have long-term dental problems. Taking a few moments during each visit to get to know one another will benefit both the therapist and the patient. Such interchanges can lead to better care and compliance for the patient and increased job satisfaction for the professional.

Extraoral Examination

The extraoral (facial) and intraoral soft tissues are examined visually for any abnormalities, and alternative findings are noted.

Clinical Examination

One of the critical issues in supportive periodontal treatment is how to best use the allotted time. In the past it was assumed that each surface of each tooth should be thoroughly scaled and root planed. At present, areas of previous attachment loss or sites of current signs of inflammation should be identified and treated appropriately. In the future it may be possible to predict areas of future attachment loss or patients more at risk for loss, and provide appropriate local or systemic therapy to intervene. In the meantime emphasis should begin to shift from "cleaning teeth" to diagnosing and treating disease.

Dental Examination

Tooth Loss

Any teeth lost since the last charting should be recorded.

Caries and Prosthetic Examination

The natural teeth are examined for overt signs of dental caries and any prosthetic replacements of the natural dentition checked.

Fremitus

Movement of the teeth during function (fremitus) is simple to measure and has been associated with advancing disease. Therefore, it should be checked, noted, and eliminated (when possible) if it is found on a tooth that has clinical signs of inflammation.

Periodontal Examination

Probing depth has been defined as the distance from the gingival margin to the apical depth of periodontal probe tip penetration. Probing depth measurements should be taken and recorded at six points around each tooth. The readings are best obtained by moving a periodontal probe through the sulcus (pocket), with the long axis of the probe parallel to the long axis of the tooth.

Records are made at the midfacial and midlingual depths as well as at the mesiolingual and distolingual and mesiobuccal and distobuccal (facial) aspects of the tooth. Interproximal readings are best made not at the line angles of the tooth, but by placing the probe tip in the deepest part of the pocket (usually under the contact area) while keeping it as parallel as possible to the tooth's long axis. Patients with aggressive periodontitis should be completely checked at each supportive periodontal treatment visit and any changes from baseline should be recorded.

Individuals with chronic periodontitis may be checked every 6 months and those with gingivitis each year. Patients with chronic diseases featuring localized severe loss of attachment should have those areas checked at each supportive periodontal treatment visit. The accuracy and reproducibility of this measurement depend on the diameter of the probe, how forcefully the probe tip is introduced into the pocket, the relative health of the tissue and the skill and experience of the operator. Recent advances in the mechanical probes can make these devices very desirable when they become more cost effective for the dentist and more comfortable for the patient.

Gingival Recession

As long as the clinician measures probing depth and not the attachment levels, gingival recession should be included in routine measurements at supportive periodontal treatment visits. This is important not only to document any continued recession but also to provide a perspective for probing depth measurements. A 3-mm probing depth associated with 7 mm of recession is of more concern than the same depth where no recession is found.

Inflammation

In the foreseeable future a number of more accurate tests to predict disease activity should be available. At present it is helpful to assess bleeding upon probing and suppuration. Bleeding on probing is found by dragging a probe through the sulcus. A force of 25 N has been suggested as optimal to measure bleeding. Suppuration can also be detected by applying coronal finger pressure on the gingival tissues. These data are important because they may provide information about whether the gingival tissues are inflamed and therefore should be measured and recorded at each supportive periodontal treatment visit where probing depths are recorded.

Radiographic Examination

Conventional parallel or right-angle radiographs, although limited to showing only gross amounts of bone loss, still provide important information, especially when several sets exposed over a number of years are available for comparison. The number of radiographs should be limited for safety reasons, but in cases of apparently active disease, a full-mouth series every 3-5 years with seven vertical bite-wing radiographs every year is helpful in making an accurate assessment of the bone stability. As advancements continue in digital and subtraction radiography, and as the economic factor decreases, these methods will supplement or replace conventional radiographs.

Microbiological Monitoring

For patients who have an aggressive form of periodontitis, microbiological monitoring and antibiotic sensitivity testing can be useful. When used in these cases and combined with traditional approaches to therapy, including subgingival scaling and root planing, the appropriate antibiotic and antimicrobial therapy often yields results superior to scaling and root planing alone. When the possible causal organisms remain after this therapy or if generalized attachment loss or inflammation continues or recurs, periodic microbial monitoring is suggested.

Personal Oral Hygiene Review

Patients who clean their teeth well tend to keep their teeth longer than those who do not clean optimally. Therefore, personal oral hygiene is of great importance. Unfortunately, a large percentage of patients do not brush well and clean much less between their teeth. Newer electric toothbrushes offer improved results compared with manual brushes and have been well accepted by many patients. Most of the periodontal diseases start interproximally and in areas usually unreached by the toothbrush, and when no interproximal gingival recession exists, patients must use dental floss. The problem remains that the average patient does not floss at all or does it incorrectly.

Most dentists are looking for a single problem-free method to rid patients of dental plaque, but this method does not exist. However, in a very small group of patients who will not or cannot comply with suggested oral hygiene, chlorhexidine rinses have been shown to be useful on a short-term basis.

Removal of Subgingival Accretions

After assessment of attachment loss and inflammation along with monitoring and reinforcing personal oral hygiene, removal of subgingival accretions is the next most important step. This is technically one of the most difficult procedures performed by the dental professional. Inadequate removal of deposits by subgingival scaling and root planing often produces a positive gingival response that may lead the inexperienced clinician to believe that the disease process has been arrested, when in fact only gingival health has been improved and bone loss continues. Several studies have shown that, with long and diligent efforts, the clinician can successfully remove subgingival tooth-borne plaque and calculus from teeth that have 3-mm probing depths using closed subgingival scaling and root planing.

These same studies have also shown that with probing depths greater than 5 mm, the probability of removing all subgingival accretions diminishes in spite of spending up to 45 minutes per tooth for cleaning. In deeper probing depths, surgery is often needed to provide easier access to the dental accretions and to reduce the probing depths so as to facilitate access by the patient and the professional.

If time for the scaling and root planing segment of the supportive periodontal treatment visit is short, then areas that have increased probing depths and / or clinical signs of inflammation (color changes, bleeding upon probing or suppuration) should be the first to receive closed subgingival scaling and root planing. The patient should then be reappointed for removal of the remaining accretions.

Removal of Supragingival Deposits

Unfortunately, a great deal of time that could be best spent on more important facets of supportive periodontal treatment is used for mechanical removal of supragingival accretions. For this reason the dental professional providing the care at the supportive periodontal treatment visit should complete the necessary disease assessment, oral hygiene procedures and subgingival scaling and root planing before beginning to remove materials that have accumulated supragingivally. This may require additional visits by the patient.

Behaviour Modification

Patient compliance with professional suggestions is critical to long-term success in the treatment of inflammatory periodontal diseases. However, the average patient does not completely comply with the recommendations concerning personal health. Most people understand that compliance with suggestions made by health care providers can lengthen and enrich their lives. Still, most people find it difficult to adhere to the myriad rules needed for positive change. Therefore, the professionals should be realistic when placing demands on patients.

It can also be assumed that the average patient will not make sweeping behavioural changes, especially in the long term. A noncomplier may occasionally be turned into a complete complier, but these victories will be few and far between. Since periodontics deal with chronic diseases for the most part, they must take these facts into consideration during all phases of dental therapy.

Expecting a patient with a past history of noncompliance with suggested oral hygiene and supportive periodontal treatment to respond well to procedures that require rigid compliance is illogical. Therapy should be based on facilitating compliance, not making it more difficult. It is possible to improve patient compliance to some degree in almost every case using accepted practices for behaviour modification.

Maintenance procedures are under the supervision of the dentist and include an update of the medical and dental histories, extraoral and intraoral soft tissue examination, dental examination, periodontal evaluation, radiographic review, removal of bacterial plaque from supragingival and subgingival regions, scaling and root planing where indicated, polishing of the teeth, and review of the patient's plaque control efficacy. An interval of 3 months between appointments appears to be an effective treatment schedule, but this can vary depending upon the clinical judgment of the dentist and the disease status of the patient. When new or recurring periodontal disease appears, additional diagnostic and treatment procedures must be considered. The successful long-term control of periodontal disease depends upon active maintenance care through supportive periodontal treatment.

Recent evidence suggests that the control and prevention of oral disease, especially periodontitis, is especially important for patients with various systemic conditions that can be impacted by oral infections. It is far better for patients and therapists to practice primary and even secondary prevention with effective plaque control and regular, consistent supportive periodontal therapy, than having to rely on tertiary prevention for disease that has progressed to a level that requires costly treatment, is time-consuming and carries a greater risk of morbidity.

Conclusion

Successful periodontal therapy with regular SPT can promote periodontal health and reduce tooth loss. Following active periodontal therapy, an interval is established for periodic ongoing care. Active periodontal therapy consists of non-surgical and/or surgical treatment.

Supportive periodontal treatment following active therapy is not synonymous with a prophylaxis.

References

[1] Adell R, Lekholm U, Rockler B, Brgnemark PI. A 15-year study of osseointegrated implants in the treatment of the edentulous jaw. *Int. J. Oral. Surg.,* 1981;10:387-416.

[2] Adriaens PA, DeBoever JA, Loesche WJ. Bacterial invasion in root cementum and radicular dentin of periodontally diseased teeth in humans-a reservoir of periodontopathic bacteria. *J. Periodontol.,* 1988;59:222-230.

[3] Adriaens E Edwards C, DeBoever J, Lesche W. Ultrastructural observations on bacterial invasion in cementum and radicular dentin of periodontally diseased human teeth. *J. Periodontol.,* 1988;59:493-503.

[4] Aguero A, Garnick JJ, Keagle J, Steflik DE, Thompson WO. Histological location of a standardized periodontal probe in man. *J. Periodontol.,* 19951;66:184-190.

[5] Albrektsson T, Dahl E, Enbom L, Engevall S, Engquist B, Erikksson AR et al. Osseointegrated oral implants-a Swedish multicenter study of 8139 consecutively inserted Nobel-pharma implants. *J. Periodontol.,* 1988;59:287-296.

[6] Aleo JJ, DeRenzis FA, Farber PA. In vitro attachment of human gingival fibroblasts to root surfaces. *J. Periodontol.,* 1976;46:639-645.

[7] Allison C, Simor AE, Mock D, Tenenbaum HC. Prosolchlorhexidine irrigation reduces the incidence of bacteremia during ultrasonic scaling with the Cavi-Med: a pilot investigation. *J. Can. Dent. Assoc.,* 1993;59:673-682.

[8] Al-Yahfoufi Z, Mombelli A, Wicki A, Lang NP. The effect of plaque control in subjects with shallow pockets and high prevalence of periodontal pathogens. *J. Clin. Periodontol.,* 1995;22:78-84.

[9] Alaluusua S, Asikaninen S, Lai CH. Intrafamilial transmission of Actinobacillus actinomycetemcomitans. *J. Periodontol.,* 1991;62:207.

[10] American Academy of Periodontology. Glossary of periodontal terms. Chicago: American Academy of Periodontology, 1992:39.

[11] American Academy of Periodontology: Position Paper: Periodontal maintenance. *J. Periodontol.,* 2003;74:1395.

[12] American Academy of Periodontology. Proceedings of the World Workshop in Clinical Periodontics. Chicago: American Academy of Periodontology: 1989.

[13] American Academy of Periodontology, Current terminology for periodontics and insurance reporting manual. 6th edn. Chicago: American Academy of Periodontology, 1991:22.

[14] The American Academy of Periodontology. Current Terminology for Periodontics and Insurance Reporting Manual, 7th ed. Chicago: The American Academy of Periodontology: 1995:49.

[15] Apse f Zarb GA, Schmitt A, Lewis DW. The longitudinal effectiveness of osseointegrated dental implants. The Toronto study: peri-implant mucosal response. *Int. J. Periodontics Restorative Dent.,* 1991;11:95-111.

[16] Armitage GC. Clinical evaluation of periodontal diseases. *Periodontogy,* 2000. 1995;7:39-53.

[17] Armitage GC, Jeffcoat MK, Chadwick DE, Taggert EJ, Numabe Y, Landis JR et al. Longitudinal evaluation of elastase as a marker for the progression of periodontitis. *J. Periodontol.,* 1994;5:120-128.

[18] Armitage GC, Svanberg GK, Loe H. Microscopic evaluation of clinical measurements of connective tissue attachment levels. *J. Clin. Periodontol.,* 1977;4:173-190.

[19] Atassi Newman HN, Bulman JS. Probe tine diameter and probing depth. *J. Clin. Periodontol.,* 1992;19:301-304.

[20] Axelsson P, Lindhe J. Effect of controlled oral hygiene procedures on caries and periodontal disease in adults. *J. Clin. Periodontol.,* 1978;5:133-151.

[21] Axelsson P, Lindhe J. Effect of controlled oral hygiene procedures on caries and periodontal disease in adults. *J. Clin. Periodontol.,* 1981;8:239-248.

[22] Axelsson P: Lindhe J. The significance of maintenance care in the treatment of periodontal disease. *J. Clin. Periodontol.,* 1981;8:281-294.

[23] Axelsson I: Lindhe J, Nystrom B. On the prevention of caries and periodontal disease: result of a 15 year longitudinal study in adults. *J. Clin. Periodontol.,* 1991;18:182-189.

[24] Baab D, Weinstein P. Oral hygiene instruction using a self inspection plaque index. *Commiinity Dent. Oral. Epidemiol.,* 1983;11:174-179.

[25] Baab DA, Weinstein P Longitudinal evaluation of a self inspection plaque index in periodontal recall patients. *J. Clin. Periodontol.,* 1986;13:313-318.

[26] Ball R. National health insurance: comments on selected issues. *Science,* 1978;200:864-866.

[27] Badersten A, Nilveus R, Egelberg J. Effect of nonsurgical periodontal therapy I. Moderately advanced periodontitis. *J. Clin. Periodontol.,* 1981; 8:57-72.

[28] Badersten A, Nilveus R, Egelberg J. Effect of nonsurgical periodontal therapy II. Severely advanced periodontitis. *J. Clin. Periodontol.,* 1984;11:63-76.

[29] Badersten A, Nilveus R, Egelberg J. Effect of nonsurgical periodontal therapy VII. Bleeding, suppuration and probing depth in sites with probing attachment loss. *J. Clin. Periodontol.,* 1985;12:432-440.

[30] Addy M, Hassan H, Wade W, Newcombe R. Use of antimicrobial containing acrylic strips in the treatment of chronic periodontal disease. A three month follow-up study. *J. Periodontol.,* 1988;59:577-564.

[31] Badersten A, Nilveus R, Egelberg J. Scores of plaque, bleeding, suppuration and probing depths to predict probing attachment loss. *J. Clin. Periodontol.,* 1990;17:102-107.

[32] Badersten A, Nilveus R, Egelberg J. Reproducibility of probing attachment level measurements. *J. Clin. Periodontol.,* 1984;11:475-485.

[33] Barnes JE, Schaffer EM. Subgingival root planing: a comparison using files, howes, and curets. *J. Periodontol.,* 1960;31:300-303.

[34] Barofsky 1. Compliance, adherence and the therapeutic alliance: steps in the development of self care. SOC Sci Med. 1978;12:369-376.

[35] Barrickman R, Penhall O. Graphing indexes reduces plaque. *J. Am. Dent. Assoc.,* 1973;87:1404-1408.

[36] Bauman GR, Mills M, Rapley JW et al. Plaque-induced inflammation around implants. *Int. J. Oral. Maxillofac Implants,* 1992;7:330.

[37] Bauman GR, Rapley JW, Hallmon WW et al. The periodontal sulcus. *Int. J. Oral. Maxillofac Implants,* 1993;8:273.

[38] Becker BE, Becker W, Caffesse RG, Kerry GJ, Ochsenbein C, Morrison EC. Three modalities of periodontal therapy: 5-year final results. *J. Dent. Res.,* 1990;69:219 (abstr 882).

[39] Becker W, Berg L, Becker BE. Untreated periodontal disease: a longitudinal study. *J. Periodontol.,* 1979;50:234-244.

[40] Becker W, Becker BE, Berg LE. Periodontal treatment without maintenance. A retrospective study in 44 patients. *J. Periodontol.,* 1984;55:505-509.

[41] Bowers JE, Hawley CE, Romberg E. A clinical test for proteolytic enzymes in gingival crevicular fluid: comparison with periodontal probing depth and bleeding on probing. *Int. J. Periodontics Restorative Dent.,* 1991;11:411422.

[42] Bowers JE, Zahradnik RT. Evaluation of a chairside gingival protease test for use in periodontal diagnosis. *J. Clin. Dent.,* 1989;1:106-109.

[43] Becker W, Becker BE, Ochsenbein C, Kerry G, Caffesse R, Morrison EC et al. A longitudinal study comparing scaling, osseous surgery and modified Widman procedures-results after one year. *J. Periodontol.,* 1988;59:351-365.

[44] Becker W, Berg L, Becker BE. The long term evaluation of periodontal maintenance in 95 patients. *Int. J. Periodontics Restorative Dent.,* 1984;2:55-71.

[45] Becker B, Karp C, Becker W, Berg L. Personality differences and stressful life events. Differences between treated periodontal patients with and without maintenance. *J. Clin. Periodontol.,* 1988;15:49-52.

[46] Bellin H, Anernd A, Monstafa M. Disclosing wafers in an oral hygiene program. *Odontol. Revy.,* 1974;25:247-253.

[47] Benfenati MP, Montesani MT, Benfenati SF Nathanson D. Scanning electron microscope: an SEM study of periodontally instrumented root surfaces, comparing sharp, dull, and damaged curettes and ultrasonic instruments. *Int. J. Periodontics Restorative Dent.,* 1987;7:50-67.

[48] Bakdash B. Oral hygiene and compliance as risk factors in periodontitis. *J. Periodontol.,* 1994;65:539-544.

[49] Buchanan SA, Robertson PB. Calculus removal by scaling/ root planing with and without surgical access. *J. Periodontol.,* 1987;58:159-163.

[50] Berglundh T, Lindhe J, Marinello C, Ericsson I, Liljenberg B. Soft tissue reaction to de novo plaque formation on implants and teeth. An experimental study in the dog. *Clin. Oral. Impl. Res.,* 1992;3:1-8.

[51] Berndsen M, Eijkman M, Hoogstraten J. Compliance perceived by Dutch periodontists and hygienists. *J. Clin. Periodontol.,* 1993;20:668-72.

[52] Bernstein D. Modification of smoking behavior: an evaluative review. *Psychol. Bull.,* 1969;71:418-422.

[53] Beube FE. Periodontology. *New York Macmillan.* 1953;376-378.

[54] Biagini G, Checchi L, Miccoli MC, Vasi V, Castaldini C. Root curettage and gingival repair in periodontitis. *J. Periodontol.,* 1988;59:124-129

[55] Birek P, McCulloch CAG, Hardy V. Gingival attachment level measurements with an automated periodontal probe. *J. Clin. Periodontol.,* 1987;14:472-477.

[56] Biro P, Hewson N. A survey of patients' attitudes to their dentist. *Aust. Dent. J.,* 1976;21:388-394.

[57] Black GV. Special dental pathology. 1st edn. Chicago: Medico-Dental Publishing Co., 1915: 371.

[58] Blomlöf L, Lindskog S, Appelgren R, Jonsson B, Weintraub A, Hammarström L. New attachment in monkeys with experimental periodontitis with and without removal of the cementum. *J. Clin. Periodontol.,* 1987;14:136-143.

[59] Boretti G, Zappa IJ, Graf H, Case D. Short-term effects of phase I therapy on crevicular cell populations. *J. Periodontol.,* 1995;66:235-240.

[60] Borghetti A, Mattout P, Mattout C. How much root planning is necessary to remove the cementum from the root surface? *Int. J. Periodontics Restorative Dent.,* 1987;4:22-29.

[61] Bowers JE, Hawley CE, Romberg E. A clinical test for proteolytic enzymes in gingival crevicular fluid: comparison with periodontal probing depth and bleeding on probing. *Int. J. Periodontics Restorative Dent.,* 1991;11:411-422.

[62] Bowers JE, Zahradnik RT. Evaluation of a chairside gingival protease test for use in periodontal diagnosis. *J. Clin. Dent.,* 1989;1:106-109.

In: Current Trends in Periodontics and Implant Dentistry
Editors: Vishal Anand and Minkle Gulati
ISBN: 978-1-62618-819-8

Chapter IX

Implant Related Complications and their Management

***Rohit Bahuguna*[1] *and Bhargavi Anand*[2]**
[1]Department of Prosthodontics, Crown & Bridge, Oral Implantology and Dental Materials, Seema Dental College and Hospital, Rishikesh, Uttrakhand, India
[2]Department of Prosthodontics, Crown & Bridge, Oral Implantology and Dental Materials, Rama Dental College and Hospital, Kanpur, Uttar Pradesh, India

Abstract

With the introduction of endosseous dental implants for rehabilitating partial and completely edentulous patients, dental treatment has been revolutionized. The high survival rates of osseointegrated dental implants have validated these implant supported restorations as a predictable method for oral rehabilitation. It is becoming increasingly clear that successfully integrated implants are susceptible to disease conditions and complications that may eventually lead to the loss of the implant. Therefore, careful treatment planning based on accurate preoperative anatomic assessments and an understanding of all potential implant related complications is very important for the successful placement and functioning of an implant. It is also necessary to know the various types of biological, technical, surgical and esthetic failures and the management of these failures.

Keywords: Endosseous, osseointegrated dental implants, oral rehabilitation, complications

Introduction

Dental treatment has been revolutionized with the introduction of endosseous dental implants for rehabilitating partial and completely edentulous patients. Though the documented high survival rate of osseointegrated dental implants have validated these implant supported restorations as a predictable method for oral rehabilitation, it is becoming increasingly clear that successfully integrated implants are susceptible to disease conditions and complications that may eventually lead to the loss of the implant. [1]

Therefore, careful treatment planning based on accurate preoperative anatomic assessments and an understanding of all potential implant related complications is very important for the successful placement and functioning of an implant. Although various success criteria for implant have been proposed over decades, yet the difference between the "implant survival" and "implant success" has not been clearly defined. "Implant Success" is defined as any implant-retained restoration in which [2]

1. The original treatment plan is performed as intended without complications
2. All implants that were placed remain stable and functioning without problems
3. Peri implant hard and soft tissues are healthy
4. Both the patient and the treating clinicians) are pleased with the results

"Implant survival" on the other hand, is simply defined as any implant that remains in place at the time of evaluation, regardless of any untoward signs, symptoms or history of problems. These surviving implants may or may not be connected to any restoration i.e. they may not be functioning. These non-functioning implants are referred to as "*sleepers*" and should not be considered successful merely because they are present and remain osseointegrated.

Rather, these sleeper implants that are included under the category of "surviving" implants should be counted as "failures" because they failed to fulfill the originally intended treatment. [2]

In addition, three other implant conditions have been proposed i.e. AILING, FAILING and FAILED implants.

Thus, the surviving implants that do not fit in the category of successful implants, can also be categorized under one of these three conditions: with implants showing radiographical bone loss without inflammatory signs or mobility being considered as ailing implants; implants with progressive bone loss, signs of inflammation but no mobility being considered as failing implants; and those with progressive bone loss, clinical mobility and loss of function being considered as failed implants. [3]

Implant failures can be further classified as "Early implant failure" that occurs shortly after placement as osseointegration is never really achieved and "Late implant failure" that occurs in a successfully integrated implant some time after placement and subsequent restoration probably due to marginal infection/disease or biomechanical overload. [4] Implant complications that eventually may lead to implant failure can be due to a number of reasons including prosthesis instability, implant mobility, occlusal trauma, fractured components, pain, inflammation, infection and neuropathy etc. [5]

This chapter reviews implant related complications and various strategies to manage these complications. These complications can be categorized as biologic, technical, surgical and esthetic complications, some of which are relatively minor and easy to correct, but others may result in loss of implants and failure of prostheses. [2]

Biologic Complications and Failures

Those that involve the peri-implant supporting hard and soft tissues resulting in soft tissue inflammation and proliferation, along with progressive bone loss and ultimately may lead to biologic loss of implants due to lack of osseointegration in the early stages before restoration or by a loss of osseo-integration as a result of bone loss after the restoration is installed and functioning. These include: Peri-implant mucosistis, Peri-implantitis and Biologic failure of implants. [2, 6]

Peri-implantitis is an inflammatory process affecting the tissues around an osseointegrated implant in function, resulting in loss of supporting bone. The differential diagnosis of peri-implantitis needs discrimination from peri-implant mucositis, which is a reversible inflammation of the soft tissues with no loss of supporting bone. [7]

Main Diagnostic Differences between Peri-Implant Mucositis and Peri-Implantitis

Clinical parameter	Peri-implant mucositis	Peri-implantitis
Increased probing depth	+/-	+
BOP	+	+
Suppuration	+/-	+
Mobility	-	+/-
Radiographic bone loss	-	+

Mombelli et al have listed various signs and symptoms which are typical for peri-implantitis lesions: [7]

- Radiological evidence for vertical destruction of the crestal bone which may develop as a saucer-shaped or wedge-shaped defect along the implant and may proceed without any notable signs of implant mobility until osseointegration is completely lost
- Vertical bone destruction associated with the formation of a peri-implant pocket
- Bleeding on gentle probing with a blunt instrument
- Suppuration from the pocket
- Hyperplasia in cases where implants are located in an area with nonkeratinized mucosa or if the suprastructure is an overdenture
- Pain is not a typical feature of peri-implantitis [7]

Although various stages of peri-implantitis can be classified on the basis of the clinical status of the peri-implant bone, yet no clear cut demarcations exist between these stages. [8]

Jovanovic and Spiekermann's classification of peri-implantitis (1995)

1. Peri-implantitis class 1: Minimum horizontal bone destruction with slight peri-implant bone loss
2. Peri-implantitis class 2: Moderate bone destruction with solitary vertical loss

3. Peri-implantitis class 3: Moderate or intense horizontal bone destruction with extensive circumferential bone lysis
4. Peri-implantitis class 4: Intense horizontal bone destruction with extensive circumferential bone lysis and loss of lingual or vestibular bone wall [8, 9]

Continous and unchecked bone loss around implants eventually results in implant failure. Hence, it is critical to include sensitive parameters for the detection of early signs and symptoms of peri-implant mucositis and peri-implantitis so that early therapeutic intervention may be possible before a substantial portion of the supporting bone is lost.

Treatment of peri-implant mucositis is principally focused on controlling bacterial plaque, although other surgical treatments may be performed to eliminate the peri-implant soft tissue hyperplasia as well as to graft keratinised gingiva, if necessary. The treatment consists of professional as well as personal peri-implant hygiene achievement. Professional peri-implant hygiene phase includes mechanical elimination of bacterial plaque with carbon fibre curettes, irrigation of the sulcus-pocket with 0.12% chlorhexidine, buffing of exposed implant surface with gauze strips soaked in chlorhexidine (0.2%), removal and disinfection of the prosthesis and abutments, modification of unhygienic prosthesis designs, diode LASER treatment especially in refractory cases and sometimes a partial-thickness flap is reflected to irrigate with sterile physiological saline, followed by the application of a tetracycline cream. [10, 11] The personal peri-implant hygiene is maintained by regular mechanical (brushing, flossing etc) and chemical (chlorhexidine mouth wash) plaque control. [12, 13]

Peri-implantitis management and treatment can be divided into two phases:

- *Initial therapeutic phase*: which includes occlusal therapy, anti-infective therapy carried out with LASERs, manual-mechanical and chemical methods to control bacterial plaque (similar to mucositis). Further the chemical methods may be local (0.12% chlorhexidine, citric acid, local application of tetracycline) or systemic (antibiotic therapy) [11,14]
- *Surgical phase*: the surgical techniques that are presently advocated for the control of peri-implant lesions are modified from techniques used to treat bone defects around teeth. It mainly consists of *peri-implant regenerative or resective therapy*. Peri-implant resective therapy along with apically displaced flap techniques are used to degranulate osseous defect, correct horizontal bone loss and moderate vertical (< 3 mm) bone defects and prepare the implant surfaces with chemicals and air abrasives to reduce overall pocket depth. [14] Indications for peri-implant resective therapy is moderate to severe horizontal bone loss, one- and two – wall bone defects and implant position in unesthetic area. [2]

Peri-implant regenerative therapy on the other hand allows regeneration of lost bone tissue via guided bone regeneration (GBR) and bone graft techniques. [14] Guided bone regeneration therapy can be in the form of submerged or pergingival regenerative therapy depending on the type of implant in place allows reosseintegration. Reosseointegration can be defined as the growth of new bone in direct contact to the previously contaminated implant surface without an intervening band of organized connective tissue. [15]

Since, it is known that regeneration of bone is enhanced if the area is isolated from the oral environment, in case of two-piece implants, submerged regenerative therapy is performed wherein the implant prosthesis are removed 4 to 8 weeks prior to the regenerative surgical procedure with a newly attached cover screw in place to allow the soft tissue to collapse and heal over the implant site. A membrane is then trimmed to extend 3 to 4 mm beyond the margins of the bone defect and secured with fixation screws, which is then left undisturbed, submerged under the flap for at least 4 to 6 months.

Whereas in case of one-piece implants, a pergingival regenerative therapy is performed wherein the membrane is perforated with a 3-mm hole and slid over the implant to ensure complete coverage and isolation of the vertical bone defect with flap sutured closely to the implant neck. In this case membranes must be removed after 6 to 8 to overcome the potential risk of membrane and periimplant infection due to pergingival oral environment. Various bone graft materials can be used in conjunction with GBR therapies. [2]

Indications submerged regenerative therapy are: implant allowing complete closure with flaps, moderate to advanced circumferential vertical defects, two and three-wall bone defects and detoxification of implant surface. [2]

Indications pergingival regenerative therapy are: one-stage implant or non-retrievable prostheses, moderate to advanced circumferential vertical defects, three-wall bone defects and detoxification of implant surface. [2]

Treatment can also vary depending on the various stages of periimplantitis.

1. Class 1 peri-implantitis is initially targeted towards conservative elimination of etiologic factors. If no improvement is observed, surgical therapy is performed which includes cleaning the implant surface, revising the osseous topography, pocket elimination via apical repositioning of the soft tissue and adjunctive antibiotic treatment if indicated. [8]
2. Class 2 peri-implantitis initial therapy targeted toward elimination of causative factors is performed along with surgical therapy as in the case described above.
3. Class 3 peri-implantitis is managed by an initial cause-related therapy along with surgical therapy which involves cleaning of the implants surface, pocket elimination via apical repositioning of soft tissues, possibly pocket elimination via osseous regeneration techniques; adjunctive antibiotic treatment.
4. Class 4 peri-implantitis is also managed in a way similar to Class 3 peri-implantitis management and includes initial cause-related therapy along with surgical therapy comprising of cleaning of the implant surface, pocket elimination via bone regeneration techniques, possibly using autologous bone transplants; adjunctive antibiotic therapy. [10]

According to Norton, the following surgical protocol has proven reliable and predictable in the treatment of advanced peri-implantitis lesions:

1. Systemic antibiotics equivalent to Metronidazole 400mg TDS for three days pre-operatively.
2. Pre-operative 1 minute mouthwash with 0.2% chlorhexidine.
3. Full thickness flap elevation extending beyond the infected area to sound tissues
4. Comprehensive debridement and curettage down to fresh bone. Mechanical curettage of implant surface with carbon fibre curettes

5. Pack gauze strips soaked in 0.2% chlorhexidine around implant, into defect and under the mucoperiosteal flap. Leave in situ for 5 minutes.
6. Remove gauze and wash defect with tetracycline solution 1g in 20mL of sterile saline.
7. Graft defect with hydroxyapatite bone mineral of allogeneic or xenogenic derivation rehydrated in the tetracycline solution
8. Trim and overlay graft with double layer of resorbable collagen membrane, rehydrated in tetracycline solution.

However, in cases where osseointegration has been reduced severely and bone loss has extended into the apical half of the implant, or if the implant demonstrates mobility or the implants do not complement the overall treatment plan, implant removal should be recommended to the patient. After the implants are removed, the ridge defects can be reconstructed. This treatment will usually enable the clinician to place new implants in a previously compromised situation. [14]

Novel Approach for the Management of Peri-Implantitis

Since, conventional mechanical methods are apparently ineffective for complete debridement of the bone defect as well as of the contaminated microstructured implant surface, recently, a new type of noninvasive phototherapy, called photodynamic therapy, which uses low-level laser has been proposed as an adjunctive for bacterial elimination in the treatment of peri-implantitis, based on its successful application in the treatment of periodontitis. The liquid photosensitizer is placed directly in the peri-implant pocket, which easily gains access to the entire exposed implant surface before being activated by the laser light through placement of the optical fiber directly in the pocket. Using lasers in antimicrobial photodynamic therapy, not only results in highly efficient bactericidal effects, but also produces additional photo-biomodulatory effects, which are essential to achieve effective healing with regeneration of the lost bone around the affected implants. [16]

Technical Complications and Failures

It typically occurs in the form of material failure, such as abutment and prosthetic screw loosening or fractures. Though many of these mechanical problems are minor and manageable yet, some technical complications are not salvageable, such as implant fractures. [2]

These include:

a. Implant fracture
b. Screw loosening and fracture
c. Fracture of restorative materials

a. Implant Fracture

Implant fractures is an infrequent and late biomechanical complication with a serious clinical outcome. An early diagnosis of the signs alerting to implant fatigue, such as loosening, torsion or fracture of the post screws and prosthetic ceramic fracture, can help prevent an undesirable outcome. [17]

Etiopathogenesis

Classified into three groups: [18]

1. Failure in implant design or material
2. Non-passive fitting of the crown of the prosthetic super-structure
3. Overloading secondary to deleterious parafunctional habits

Clinical Manifestations

Patients may often report spontaneous bleeding and mobility. Exploration (manually or electronically) in turn confirms increased mobility, increased pocket depth and gingival indexes, and occasionally also plaque accumulation resulting from patient fear of the pain triggered by brushing. Radiologically, separation of the fragments and bone loss may be seen. [17]

Treatment

- Complete removal of the fractured implant using explantation trephines
- Removal of the coronal portion of the fractured implant with the purpose of placing a new prosthetic post
- Removal of the coronal portion of the fractured implant, leaving the remaining apical part integrated in the bone

Complete implant extraction is considered to be the treatment of choice. However, when percentage of contact with bone is high, and fracture is not located too far apical, restoration of the connection between post and implant may be a valid option and should be contemplated only if there are still sufficient remaining internal threads to guarantee adequate prosthetic post retention. [17, 18]

b. Screw Loosening

Abutment or prosthesis screw loosening is often corrected by retightening the screws. Over time, however screws become fatigued and eventually fracture. The biomechanical support (and resistance) for the restoration must be evaluated and, if possible, changed to prevent recurrence of the problem. [2]

Esthetic Complications

It arises when patient expectations are not met. Patient satisfaction with the esthetic outcome of the implant prosthesis will vary from patient to patient depending on several factors. The risk for esthetic complications is increased for patients with high esthetic expectations and less-than-optimal patient-related factors (e.g., bone quantity and quality). [2]

To provide a patient with an implant-supported restoration that is functional and aesthetic, an effective diagnosis and an appropriate sequencing of treatment is required which must be guided by a three-dimensional analysis of the implant site: mesiodistal, faciolingual and apicocoronal. [19]

Esthetic complications can be caused either by malpositioned implants, inappropriate number and/or size of utilized implants, or peri-implant infection progressively leading to the destruction of peri-implant bone, or by existing bone or soft-tissue deficiencies in the alveolar process. [20]

The configuration and tissue components of certain ridge deformities require a staged approach designed to compensate for all of the deficiencies. In these instances, orthodontic movement, guided tissue regeneration to increase the osseous volume, and soft tissue surgery may all or in different combinations be used. [19]

Esthetic complications due to implant malpositions can be managed either by reducing the diameter of the implant platform (esp. for tissue-level implant designs) or by soft-tissue grafting in cases where blunting or loss of the papillae (often involving the adjacent natural tooth), or recession of the facial marginal mucosa has occurred due to implant malposition. [21]

Soft-tissue grafting procedures to augment edentulous ridges should be accomplished 2-4 months before implant placement, whereas placement of a subepithelial connective tissue graft can also be done during stage I surgery or stage II surgery which will aid in creating the appropriate inter- and intratooth relationships as well as allow repositioning of the tissue for creating the appropriate dimension of keratinized tissue and align the mucogingival junction. [19]

Two approaches may be used to correct recession of the facial marginal mucosa with soft-tissue grafts. In the first approach, connective tissue is grafted to the facial surface of the implant with the crown in situ and in the second approach, grafting with soft tissue is performed after removing the crown and abutment, and then using the soft-tissue graft/flap advancement to submerge partially or completely the implant. However, in cases where the malposition cannot be corrected with soft tissue grafting, and the attainment of a good esthetic outcome is essential for the patient, there is usually no alternative but to remove the implant and reinsert the implant in a proper 3D position. [21]

Chen ST and Buser D have suggested certain guidelines to avoid esthetic complications due to implant placement. [21]

Carefully assessment of the hard- and soft-tissue dimensions of the planned implant site.

- Maintaining 2 mm of thickness of the facial bone, which may require ridge site augmentation to optimize the hard- and soft-tissue conditions before placing the implant.

- Selecting an implant with the correct restorative platform in relation to the dimensions of the tooth to be replaced.
- Ensure correct placement of implant according to the restoratively determined 3D position. The implant should be placed: in the mesiodistal plane, at least 1.5 mm away from the roots of adjacent teeth; in the apicocoronal plane, between 2 and 3 mm (depending on the design of the implant) apical to the anticipated mucosal margin of the implant restoration; in the orofacial plane, at about 1.5 mm orally to the facial curvature of the arch at the level of the gingival margin.
- In complicated cases especially in sites with multiple missing teeth, a surgical guide stent should be considered.
- Abort the procedure if there are any doubts about the position of the implant at the time of surgery instead of placing the implant into an incorrect position.

Surgical Complications

There are the risks involved in the surgical procedures used for implant site development, implant placement, and implant exposure.[2]

These include: [22, 23]

a. Hemorrhage during drilling that can occur due to injury to an artery but can be managed by applying pressure pack either intraorally or extraorally from the submental region against the body of mandible. Furthermore, implant placement will stop the bleeding.
b. Nerve injury that is possibly caused by stretching, compression, and partial or total transection of the nerve due to poor flap design, traumatic flap reflection, accidental intraneural injection, traction on the mental nerve in an elevated flap, penetration of the osteotomy preparation or compression of the implant body into the canal. [24-26] In such cases either the implant is removed or high dose anti-inflammatory drugs along with adjunct drugs such as clonazepam, carbamazepine, or vitamin B-complex are prescribed, which might alleviate neuritis via their known neuronal anti-inflammatory actions.
c. Fracture of mandible may occur in cases of atrophic mandible that calls for immediate implant retrieval and fracture management with bone graft and monocortical miniplates. [23] Penetration of nasal/sinus floor especially when the bone in the maxilla is type IV bone. Primary closure of the exposed site along with antibiotic, decongestant and chlorhexidine mouth wash prescription is the line of management. [23]
d. Lack of primary stability is encountered in cases of type IV bone, grafted bone, imprecise preparation and excessive countersinking. In such a situation either the implant has to be removed or replaced with larger diameter or longer implant. [23]
e. Maxillary sinus lift procedures are associated with complications like Schneiderian membrane perforation, loss of the implant or graft materials into the maxillary sinus, postoperative maxillary sinusitis and hemorrhage. Such complications can be avoided by pre-operative treatment planning with the aid of cone-beam CT scan.

Management strategies for such complications include sealing the exposed site by folding the excess membrane/collagen membrane, packing with bone graft and achieving primary closure along with antibiotics, decongestant and chlorhexidine mouth wash prescription. [26, 23]

f. Devitalization of adjacent teeth due to injury caused to the tooth during implant placement as a result of insufficient space between implant and the adjacent tooth. Use of a surgical guide, radiographic analysis and CT scan can help locate the implant placement, thereby avoiding damage to adjacent teeth. Endodontic treatment is the line of management to save the injured tooth. [26, 23]

Supportive Periodontal Therapy with Dental Implants

Because peri-implant complications are difficult to treat, it is also extremely important to provide good supportive therapy with implant patients. In general, procedures for maintenance of patients with implants are similar to those for patients with natural teeth with the following three differences:

1. Special instrumentation that will not scratch the implants is used for calculus removal on the implants. These include plastic instruments or specially designed gold-plated curettes for calculus removal which will not scratch or alter the implant titanium surfaces as seen with metal hand instruments and ultrasonic and sonic tips.
2. Acid fluoride prophylactic agents are avoided because they cause surface damage to titanium abutments
3. Nonabrasive prophy pastes are used.

During the phase after uncovering the implants, patients must use ultrasoft brushes, chemotherapeutic rinses, tartar control pastes, irrigation devices, and yarnlike materials to keep the implants and natural teeth clean. Patients often are reluctant to touch the implants but must be encouraged to keep the areas clean. [2]

Conclusion

Dental treatment has been revolutionized with the introduction of endosseous dental implants for rehabilitating partial and completely edentulous patients. It is becoming increasingly clear that successfully integrated implants are susceptible to disease conditions and complications that may eventually lead to the loss of the implant. Careful treatment planning based on accurate preoperative anatomic assessments and an understanding of all potential implant related complications is very important for the successful placement and functioning of an implant. It is also necessary to differentiate between the "implant survival" and "implant success and also ailing, failing and failed implants. The difference between "Early implant failure" and "Late implant failure" and peri-implant mucositis and periimplantitis must also be recognized. Various procedures such as lasers, manual-mechanical and chemical methods such as using chlorhexidine mouth wash and surgical procedures, as *peri-implant regenerative or resective therapy* performed to maintin the implant in its proper site.

References

[1] Tonetti M. Risk factors for osseodisintegration. *Periodontol* 2000 1998;17:55-62.

[2] Newman GM, Takei HH, Carranza A. *Carranza's Clinical periodontology.*W.B. Saunders company, ed. 9th. 2002.

[3] El Askary AS, Meffert RM, Griffin T. Why Do Dental Implants Fail part. *Implant Dent* 1999;173-185.

[4] Chen S, Darby I. Dental implants: maintenance, care and treatment of peri-implant infection. Aust Dent J. 2003;48(4):212-20; quiz 263.

[5] American Academy of Periodontology. Parameter on placement and management of the dental implant. *J Periodontol* 2000;71:870-872.

[6] Lang NP, Wilson TG, Corbet EF. Biological complications with dental implants: their prevention, diagnosis and treatment. *Clin Oral Implants Res* 2000:11 Suppl 1:146-155.

[7] Mombelli A, Lang NP. The diagnosis and treatment of periimplantitis. *Periodontol* 2000. 1998;17:63-76.

[8] Spiekerman H. Chapter- Periimplant Pathology. Rateitschak KH, Wolf HF. *Color atlas of dental medicine-Implantology.* Thieme Medical Publishers, New York. 1995. 317-328

[9] Jovanovic SA,Diagnosis and treatment of peri-implant disease. *Curr Opin Periodontol* 1994;2:194-204.

[10] The decontamination and treatment of peri-implant mucositis and peri-implantitis. Michael Norton, *Implant practice* May 2009 Volume 2 Number 2, pg 14-17

[11] Bowen-Antolín A, Pascua-García MT, Nasimi A. Infections in implantology: From prophylaxis to treatment. *Med Oral Patol Oral Cir Bucal* 2007;12:E323-30.

[12] Implant maintenance : *Dent Clin N Am* 50 (2006) 463-478. Sue Humphrey

[13] The Expanding Esthetic Practice: Implant Maintenance-Part 2. *Contemporary Esthetics and Restorative Practice*, May 2005. Ronald E. Goldstein

[14] Sascha A. Jovanovic. Peri-Implant Tissue Response To Pathological Insults. *Adv Dent Res.* 1999;13:82-86.

[15] Shantipriya Reddy, Chapter 47- dental implants: periodontal considerations. *Essentials of Clinical Periodontology and Periodontics.* Shantipriya Reddy. 2nd edition. Jaypee brothers medical publishers (P) ltd., India. 2008. Pg 381-388.

[16] Periodontol 2000. 2009;51:109-40. *Application of antimicrobial photodynamic therapy in periodontal and peri-implant diseases.* Takasaki AA, Aoki A, Mizutani K, Schwarz F, Sculean A, Wang CY, Koshy G, Romanos G, Ishikawa I, Izumi Y.

[17] Arturo Sánchez-Pérez, Ma José Moya Villaescusa, Alfonso Jornet García, Santiago Gomez. Etiology, risk factors and management of implant fractures. *Med Oral Patol Oral Cir Bucal.* 2010;15(3):e504-8.

[18] Balshi TJ. An analysis and management of fractured implants: a clinical report. *Int J Oral Maxillofac Implants.* 1996;11:660-6.

[19] Aesthetics and implant dentistry. Tarnow DP, Eskow RN & Zamzok J. *Periodontology* 2000. Vol. 11, 1996, 85-94

[20] Chen ST and Buser d. Esthetic complications due to implant malpositions: etiology, prevention, and treatment. Stuart J. Froum. *Dental Implant Complications: Etiology, Prevention, and Treatment.* Wiley-Blackwell, UK, 2010, page 134-155.

[21] Stephen T. Chen and Daniel Buser. Esthetic complications due to implant malpositions: etiology, prevention, and treatment. Stuart J. Froum. Dental Implant Complications: *Etiology, Prevention, and Treatment.* Wiley-Blackwell, UK, 2010, page 134-155.

[22] Su-Gwan Kim, Chapter 20 Clinical Complications of Dental Implants 467-490. *Implant Dentistry- A Rapidly Evolving Practice*, Edited by Ilser Turkyilmaz, Published by InTech, Croatia, 2011,

[23] Park SH, Wang HL. Implant Dent. 2005 Sep;14(3):211-20. *Implant reversible complications: classification and treatments.*

[24] Misch, K.; Wang, HL. (2008). Implant surgery complications: etiology and treatment. *Implant Dent*, Vol. 17, No. 2, (Jun 2008), pp. 159-68,

[25] Annibali, S.; Ripari, M., La Monaca, G., Tonoli, F. & Cristalli MP. (2009). Local accidents in dental implant surgery: prevention and treatment. *Int J Periodontics Restorative Dent.* Vol. 29, No. 3, (June 2009), pp. 325-31.

[26] Su-Gwan Kim, Chapter 20 Clinical Complications of Dental Implants 467-490. *Implant Dentistry- A Rapidly Evolving Practice,* Edited by Ilser Turkyilmaz, Published by InTech, Croatia, 2011

In: Current Trends in Periodontics and Implant Dentistry ISBN: 978-1-62618-819-8
Editors: Vishal Anand and Minkle Gulati

Chapter X

Lipoproteins of Human Cariogenic Bacteria are Responsible for Inflammation-Inducing Activity Mediated by Toll-Like Receptor 2

Hideo Kataoka*
Department of Oral Microbiology, Showa University School of Dentistry, Japan

Abstract

Streptococcus mutans and *S. sobrinus* have been implicated as the most important etiologic agents of human dental caries. The mechanism of caries induction by these bacteria has been well characterized; however, little is known about the relationship between periodontal inflammation and these bacteria, although it has been shown that bacterial lipoproteins trigger an innate immune response mediated via the Toll-like receptor 2 (TLR2) displayed on the host cell. In this chapter,the induction of inflammation triggered by *S. mutans* and *S. sobrinus* is characteraized. Lipoproteins were extracted from cells of *S. mutans* 109c and *S. sobrinus* NIDR6715 by treatment with Triton X-114. Interleukin 8 (IL-8) production by THP-1 cells stimulated with either bacterial cells or extracted lipoproteins was measured by ELISA (Enzyme-linked immunosorbent assay). Nuclear factor-kappa B (NF-κB) activation in Human embryonic kidney (HEK) 293 cells transiently producing TLR2 was determined by relative luciferase reporter assay. Results of these experiments revealed that cells of both streptococcal species induced IL-8 production and NF-κB activation via TLR2. Lipoproteins extracted from *S. mutans* and *S. sobrinus* also induced IL-8 production and NF-κB activation via TLR2. This TLR2-mediated activation was abolished by pre-treatment of the lipoprotein fraction with a lipoprotein lipase. These results strongly suggest that lipoproteins of human cariogenic bacteria *S. mutans* and *S. sobrinus* induce inflammatory responses through TLR2.

* Corresponding author.

Keywords: *Streptococcus mutans, Streptococcus sobrinus,* inflammation, lipoprotein, Toll-like receptor 2

Introduction

Periodontal inflammatory diseases, including gingivitis and periodontitis, are induced and developed by accumulation of dental plaque. Thus, prevention and treatment of periodontal diseases requires characterization of the inflammation-inducing mechanism(s) associated with dental plaque bacteria. The bacterial composition of dental plaque varies with time. Initially, dental plaque is predominated by species of streptococci. As plaque matures, increasing proportions of *Actinomyces* and gram-negative anaerobic bacteria, such as *Fusobacterium nucleatum*, are observed. [1] As several gram-negative anaerobic bacteria are considered to be causative agents of periodontal inflammatory diseases, the inflammation-inducing activities of these bacteria have been well-studied. However, the role of oral streptococci is poorly understood, even though they play an important role in the initial stages of plaque formation. It was recently reported that *Streptococcus gordonii*, widely known as one of the commensal oral gram-positive bacterium existing in dental plaque, harbor immunostimulatory components that activate murine dendritic cells. [2]

This chapter describes work showing that oral streptococci harbor inflammation-inducing activity, consistent with the potential role of oral streptococci as causative agents of periodontal inflammatory diseases. The *mutans* streptococci, including *Streptococcus mutans* and *S. sobrinus,* are also oral streptococci and well-known as cariogenic bacteria. [3, 4] However, it remains unclear whether these bacteria induce inflammation in human tissues. In human organs, Toll-like receptors (TLRs) have been demonstrated to play a key role in initiating inflammatory responses. TLRs are host type-1 transmembrane proteins that detect microbes by recognition of various microbial components, collectively defined as pathogen-associated molecular patterns (PAMPs). [5] Upon recognition of microbes through TLRs, these host cells release inflammatory cytokines, which are involved in initiation and amplification of the inflammatory responses in the host organism. To date, more than 10 classes of TLRs have been identified. Among them, TLR2 has been reported to recognize the broadest range of PAMPs, including lipoprotein/lipopeptide, lipoteichoic acid, lipoarabinomannan, and yeast zymosan. [6-10] Interestingly, TLR2 also has been implicated in the inflammatory response triggered by several periodontopathic gram-negative bacteria, [11-15] suggesting that TLR2 plays a key role in initiating periodontal inflammation. However, the relationship between TLR2 and specific oral gram-positive bacteria is poorly understood.

Recently it has been demonstrated that *Actinomyces viscosus*, an oral gram-positive bacterium frequently isolated from dental plaque, activates human macrophages and oral epithelial cells, and that TLR2 plays a key role in this response. [16] Additionally, it has been shown that bacterial lipoproteins from *A. viscosus* act as ligands of TLR2 to induce this response. Based on those results, it can be hypothesized that *mutans* streptococci induce inflammation by a mechanism similar to that of *A. viscosus*. In the work described in this chapter, it was examined whether *mutans* streptococci induce inflammation in human macrophages, and what roles host TLR2 and bacterial lipoproteins play in this process. This work characterizes the pathogenicity of *mutans* streptococci not as cariogenic bacteria, but as periodontopathic organisms.

Materials and Methods

Bacterial Strain and Culturing

S. mutans 109c [17] *and S. sobrinus* NIDR6715 [18] were cultured at 37°C under anaerobic conditions in Todd-Hewitt (Bacto^{TM}, NJ) agar or broth (Todd–Hewitt agar (THA) or Todd–Hewitt broth (THB), respectively). Specifically, strains were grown on plates for 3 days, then inoculated into broth and incubated overnight. The bacterial cells were then harvested by centrifugation (15,000 × *g*, 5 min, 4°C), washed in phosphate-buffered saline (PBS), and resuspended at an optical density of 0.5 at 600 nm, corresponding to a cell density of approximately 1.0 × 10 [7] colony-forming units (CFU)/ml.

Cell Culture

Human embryonic kidney (HEK) 293 cells were obtained from the American Type Culture Collection (Manassas, VA, USA) as strain CRL-1573. The cells were cultured in Dulbecco's modified Eagle medium (DMEM; Sigma-Aldrich, St. Louis, MO) supplemented with 10% heat-inactivated fetal bovine serum (FBS), penicillin G (100 U/ml), and streptomycin (100 μg/ml). A human acute monocytic leukemia cell line, THP-1 (RCB1189) was purchased from the Cell Engineering Division of RIKEN BioResource Center (Tsukuba, Ibaraki, Japan). The cells were cultured in Roswell Park Memorial Institute (RPMI) 1640 medium (Wako, Tokyo, Japan) supplemented with 10% heat-inactivated FBS. All cell cultures were performed at 37°C in a humidified 5% CO_2 atmosphere.

Extraction of Lipophilic Fraction of *S. mutans* and *S. sobrinus*

S. mutans and S. sobrinus cells were treated with Triton X-114 (TX-114; Sigma-Aldrich) to extract the lipophilic fraction. Specifically, bacteria were cultured in THB and harvested as described above. The cell pellet was resuspended in buffer solution (150 mM NaCl and 10 mM Tris-HCl, pH 8.0). The cell suspensions were mixed with 1/10 volume of 20% (vol/vol) aqueous TX-114 working stock solution. The mixture was rotated at 4°C for 2 h and cell debris was removed by centrifugation (15,000 × *g*, 5 min, 4°C). The supernatant was incubated for 5 min at 37°C and re-centrifuged to separate the lower (lipophilic) phase from the upper (aqueous) phase. Excess methanol was added to the lower phase to precipitate the lipophilic fraction; the mixture was incubated overnight at -80°C prior to centrifugation (15,000 × *g*, 30 min, 4°C) and discarding of the supernatant. The precipitated lipophilic fraction was then resuspended in PBS. The protein concentration of the lipophilic fraction was measured by BCA (Bicinchoninic Acid) assay using Bio-Rad Protein Assay (Bio-Rad Laboratories, Hercules, CA). To determine the stimulatory activity of lipoproteins contained in the lipophilic fraction, aliquots of this fraction were incubated (37°C, 6 h) in the presence or absence of lipoprotein lipase from *Pseudomonas* sp.(98,100 U/ml; Sigma-Aldrich) prior to use in stimulation.

ELISA

THP-1 cells were plated at 4.0×10^5 cells per well in 24-well plates in the presence of 10 nM phorbol 12-myristate 13-acetate (Sigma-Aldrich) and cultured for 24 h (to induce differentiation into macrophages). These cells were washed three times with serum-free RPMI 1640 and then stimulated for 6 h with cells of *S. mutans* and *S. sobrinus* (at 1.0×10^4, 1.0×10^5, and 1.0×10^6 CFU/ml) in serum-free medium. After stimulation, the culture supernatants were collected by centrifugation (7,000 × *g*, 10 min, 4°C). The amounts of interleukin 8 (IL-8) in the culture supernatants were determined by ELISA (ELISA Development Kit Human IL-8; PeproTech, Rocky Hill, NJ).

Luciferase Reporter Assay

HEK293 cells were plated at 1.0×10^5 cells/well in 24-well plates. One day later, the cells were transfected transiently with 30 ng of an Nuclear factor-kappa B(NF-κB)-dependent firefly luciferase-encoding reporter plasmid (pNF-κB-Luc; Stratagene, San-Diego, CA), 3.5 ng of a *Renilla* luciferase-encoding reporter plasmid (pRL-TK; Promega, Madison, WI), and 150 ng of pEF6-TLR2 (TLR2 cloned into the pEF6 vector); [16] transfection was performed for 24 h using METAFECTENE Transfection Reagent (Biontex Laboratories, GmbH, München, Germany). On the following day, the cells were washed with serum-free medium and stimulated for 6 h with *S. mutans* and *S. sobrinus* (at 1.0×10^4, 1.0×10^5, and 1.0×10^6 CFU/ml) in serum-free medium. Luciferase activity was determined using a Dual-Luciferase reporter assay system (Promega) according to the manufacturer's instructions. The activity of firefly luciferase was normalized to that of *Renilla* luciferase.

Statistical Analysis

Statistical analysis was performed using Ekuseru-tokei® (2012 software, Social Survey Research Information Co., Ltd., Tokyo, Japan). ELISAs were performed in triplicate (N=3); individual figures provide data as mean ± standard deviation (SD) from a single experiment. The statistical differences were assessed by Student's *t*-test. For Figure 1 and 2, multiple groups were compared using a two-tailed one-way analysis of variance (ANOVA) with Dunnett's test where significance was indicated. P values of ≤ 0.05 were considered statistically significant.

Results and Discussion

Both *S. mutans* and *S. sobrinus* Induce IL-8 Production in Human Macrophages

To determine whether cells of *mutans* streptococci induce the production of inflammatory cytokines in host cells, a human macrophage cell line (THP-1) was stimulated with cells of *S. mutans* and *S. sobrinus.* Exposure to bacterial cells induced the production of the inflammatory cytokine IL-8 by THP-1 cells in a dose-dependent manner (Fig. 1). Thus, bacterial cells of *S. mutans* and *S. sobrinus* are capable of inducing inflammation in human macrophages. IL-8 is one of the initial mediators that induce neutrophil infiltration into inflamed tissues; previous work has shown that IL-8 mRNA levels are elevated in the infiltrated macrophages of inflamed gingiva, compared to those in healthy gingiva. [19] These results suggest that the ability to induce IL-8 production may be an important property of *S. mutans* and *S. sobrinus, so as* to characterize them as periodontophathic bacteria.

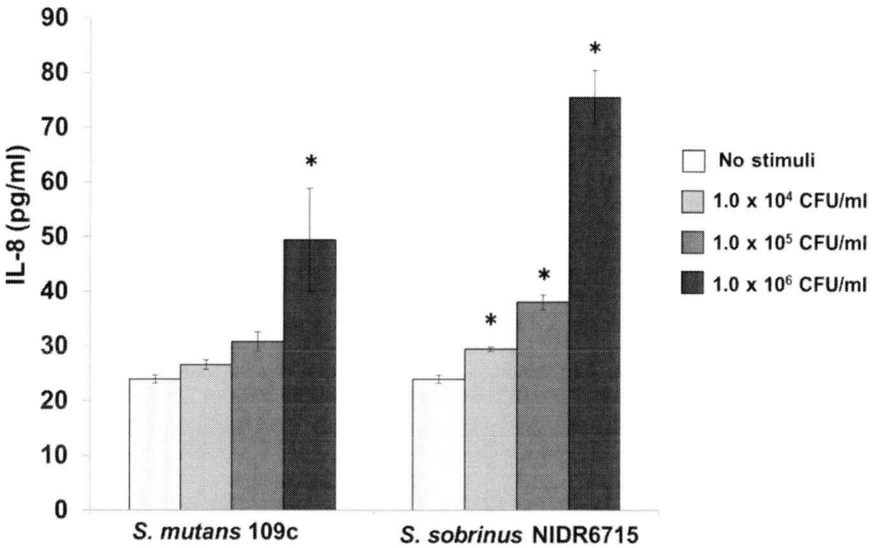

Figure 1. *S. mutans* and *S. sobrinus* cells induce IL-8 production. The production of IL-8 in the culture supernatants of THP-1 stimulated with S. mutans and S. sobrinus cells was measured by ELISA. Asterisks indicate statistically significant differences ($P < 0.05$).

Both *S. mutans* and *S. sobrinus* Induce Inflammatory Responses in a TLR2-Dependent Manner

It was examined whether the *S. mutans* and *S. sobrinus*-induced inflammatory responses were mediated by TLR2. For this purpose, HEK293, a human embryonic kidney cell line that does not produce TLR2 under standard culture conditions was used. [18] For this experiment, HEK293 cells were transiently transfected with the human *TLR2* gene together with an NF-κB-dependent (i.e., TLR2-activated) luciferase-encoding reporter gene; the transfected cells then were exposed to *S. mutans* and *S. sobrinus.* These bacterial cells induced NF-κB activation in HEK293 transfected with the *TLR2* gene in a dose-dependent manner (Fig. 2). In contrast, these bacterial cells failed to induce NF-κB activation in cells transfected with pEF6 control vector. These results showed that TLR2 recognizes *S. mutans* and *S. sobrinus* cells and induces inflammatory responses in host cells. Notably, bacterial activation of NF-κB-dependent expression in *TLR2*-transfected cells was dose-dependent (i.e., higher reporter expression was seen at higher bacterial cell density). This observation suggests that TLR2 is a key mediator for transducing signals from *S. mutans* and *S. sobrinus*, although it remains formally possible that another receptor (one that is not expressed in HEK293) may also mediates the recognition of *S. mutans* and *S. sobrinus*. In addition, this result suggests that *S. mutans* and *S. sobrinus* display TLR2 ligands on the bacterial cell surfaces.

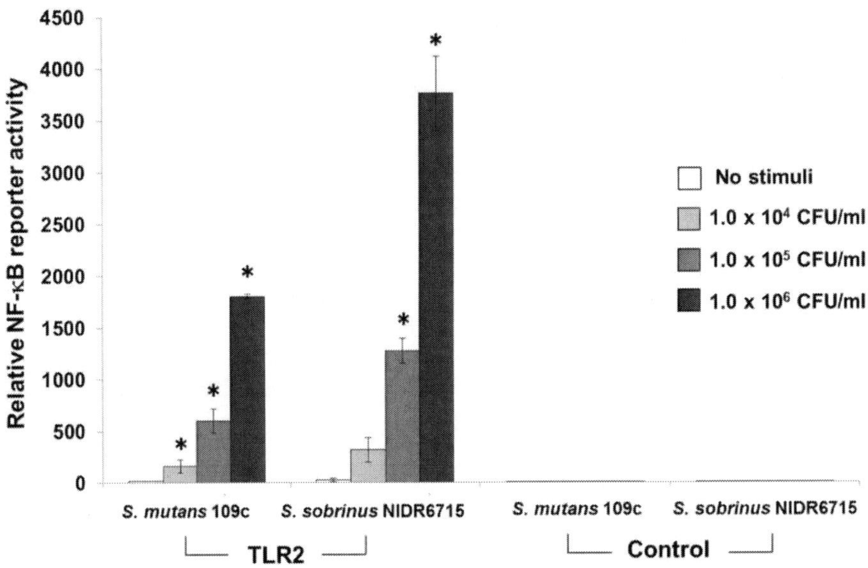

Figure 2. *S. mutans* and *S. sobrinus* cells activate NF-κB in a TLR2-dependent manner. HEK293 was transfected with TLR2-encoding plasmid or control plasmid, along with a NF-κB reporter plasmid and a control reporter plasmid. Transfected cells were then stimulated with S. mutans and S. sobrinus cells, and NF-κB-regulated gene expression was measured as relative luciferase activity. Asterisks indicate statistically significant differences ($P < 0.05$).

Lipoproteins of *S. mutans* and *S. sobrinus* are Responsible for Inducing IL-8 Production

It was also investigated whether lipoproteins of *S. mutans* and *S. sobrinus* were responsible for inducing inflammatory cytokine production in host cells. THP-1 cells were stimulated by lipophilic fractions of *S. mutans* and *S. sobrinus*, and IL-8 production in the culture supernatant was measured by ELISA. The lipophilic fractions induced production of these cytokines in a dose-dependent manner, and pre-treatment of the fraction with lipoprotein lipase eliminated the stimulatory activity of the fractions in this assay (Fig. 3). These results show that lipoproteins of *S. mutans* and *S. sobrinus* have the ability to induce inflammatory responses in host cells, although this experiment does not rule out a possible role for other components of these bacteria.

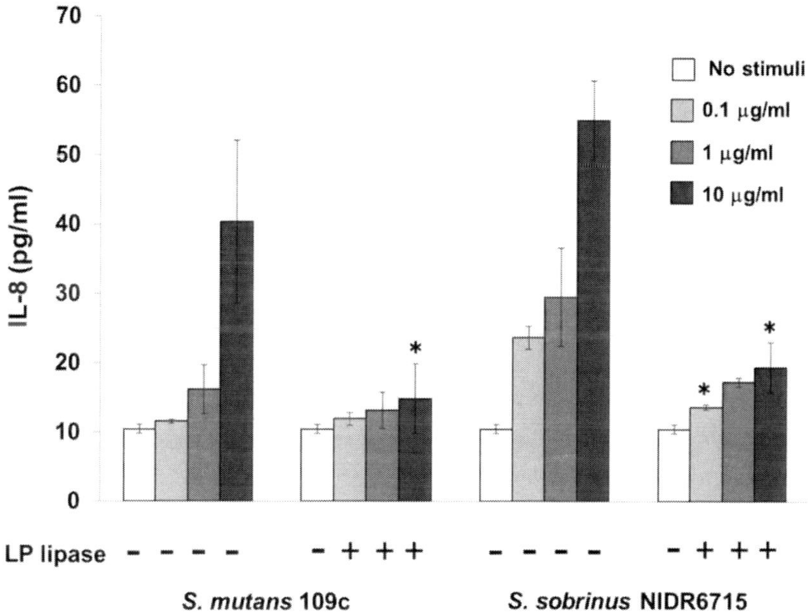

Figure 3. Lipoproteins extracted from *S. mutans* and *S. sobrinus* induce IL-8 production. The production of IL-8 in the culture supernatants of THP-1 stimulated by the lipophilic fraction (or by the fraction treated with lipoprotein lipase) was measured by ELISA. Asterisks indicate statistically significant differences ($P < 0.05$).

Lipoproteins of *S. mutans* and *S. sobrinus* Induce Inflammatory Responses in a TLR2-Dependent Manner

Next, It was examined whether lipoproteins of *S. mutans* and *S. sobrinus* are recognized as ligands by TLR2. To confirm TLR2 dependency, TLR2-dependent NF-κB activation by lipoproteins of *S. mutans* and *S. sobrinus* as described above was assessed. As shown in Fig. 4, lipophilic fractions activated NF-κB in *TLR2*-transfected cells in a dose-dependent manner, and this activity was diminished by lipoprotein lipase pretreatment of the fractions. These results strongly suggest that the inflammatory response induced by lipoproteins of *S. mutans* and *S. sobrinus* is mediated via TLR2. The crude nature of the fractions used in this experiment precluded characterization of the specific lipoprotein that provided the inflammation-inducing activity. However, it has been shown that TX-114 extraction is an efficacious method for extracting bacterial lipoproteins, and that lipoprotein lipase treatment of this fraction impedes the induction of inflammation, [21,22] providing an independent confirmation that lipoproteins included in the TX-114 fraction are responsible for inducing inflammation. This finding cannot rule out the possibility that unfractionated components also may be capable of inducing inflammatory responses. However, both whole cells and lipoproteins of *S. mutans* and *S. sobrinus* exhibited TLR2 dependency. Kim *et al.* have recently demonstrated that cells of *S. mutans* Ingbritt stimulate Tumor necrosis factor-alpha (TNF-α) and interleukin-1beta (IL-1β) production in the mouse macrophage cell line, RAW264.7 cells, by activating p38/c- Jun N-terminal kinase (JNK) and Extracellular signal–Regulated Kinase (ERK)/p38/JNK, and NF-κB through TLR2 and TLR4, respectively. [23]

However, the bacterial components that are capable of stimulating macrophages has not been shown in this chapter. The results of this work suggest that lipoproteins of *S. mutans* and *S. sobrinus* may be an inflammation-inducing factor.

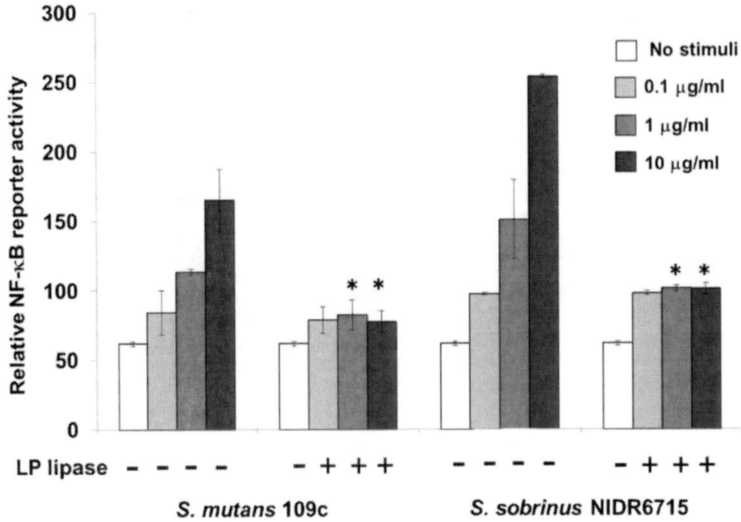

Figure 4. Lipoproteins extracted from *S. mutans* and *S. sobrinus* activate NF-κB in a TLR2-dependent manner. HEK293 was transfected with TLR2-encoding plasmid or control plasmid, along with a NF-κB reporter plasmid and a control reporter plasmid. Transfected cells were then stimulated by the lipophilic fraction of S. mutans and S. sobrinus, and NF-κB-regulated gene expression was measured as relative luciferase activity. Asterisks indicate statistically significant differences ($P < 0.05$).

Acknowledgments

This work was supported in part by a Grant-in-Aid for Young Scientists (B) (No. 21791796), by a Grant-in-Aid for Scientific Research (C) (No. 22592048), and by the Private University High Technology Research Center Project (No. S1001010).

Conclusion

This chapter demonstrates a novel periodontopathy of *S. mutans* and *S. sobrinus*, that is, lipoproteins of these bacteria may be TLR2 ligands, consistent with a possible role for these bacteria as causative agents of periodontal inflammatory diseases.

References

[1] Ritz HL. Microbial population shifts in developing human dental plaque. *Arch Oral Biol.* 1967;12:1561-1568.

[2] Mayer ML, Phillips CM, Townsend RA, Halperin SA, Lee SF. Differential activation of dendritic cells by Toll-like receptor agonists isolated from the gram-positive vaccine vector *Streptococcus gordonii*. *Scand J Immunol.* 2000;69:351-356.

[3] Hamada S, Slade HD. Biology, immunology and cariogenicity of *Streptococcus mutans*. *Microbiol Rev.* 1980;44:331-384.

[4] Loesche WJ. Role of *Streptococcus mutans* in human dental decay. *Microbiol Rev.* 1986;50:353-380.

[5] Takeda K, Kaisho T, Akira S. Toll-Like Receptors. *Annu Rev Immunol.* 2003;21:335-376.

[6] Alliprantis AO, Yang RB, Mark MR, Suggett S, Devaux B, Radolf JD et al. Cell activation and apoptosis by bacterial lipoproteins through toll-like receptor-2. *Science.* 1999;285:736-739.

[7] Takeuchi O, Kaufmann A, Grote K, Kawai T, Hoshino K, Morr M. Cutting edge: preferentially the R-stereoisomer of the mycoplasmal lipopeptide macrophage-activating lipopeptide-2 activates immune cells through a toll-like receptor 2- and MyD88-dependent signaling pathway. *J Immunol.* 2000;164:554-557.

[8] Schroder NW, Morath S, Alexander C, Hamann L, Hartung T, Zähringer Uet al. Lipoteicoic acid (LTA) of *Streptococcus pneumoniae* and *Staphylococcus aureus* activates immune cells via Toll-like receptor (TLR)-2, lipopolysaccharide-binding protein (LBP), and CD14, whereas TLR-4 and MD-2 are not involved. *J Biol Chem.* 2003;278:15587-15594.

[9] Levitz SM. Interaction of Toll-like receptors with fungi. *Microbes Infect.* 2004;6:1351-1355.

[10] Wang T, Lafuse WP, Zwilling BS. Regulation of Toll-like receptor 2 expression by macrophages following *Mycobacterium avium* infection. *J Immunol.* 2000;165:6308-6313.

[11] Sun Y, Shu R, Li CL, Zhang MZ. Gram-negative periodontal bacteria induce the activation of Toll-like receptor 2, 4 and cytokine production in human periodontal ligament cells. *J Periodontol.* 2010;81:1488-1496.

[12] Kikkert R, Laine ML, Aarden LA, van Winkelhoff AJ. Activation of toll-like receptors 2 and 4 by gram-negative periodontal bacteria. *Oral Microbiol Immunol.* 2007;22:145-151.

[13] Wang M, Shakhatreh MA, James D, Liang S, Nishiyama S, Yoshimura F et al. Fimbrial proteins of *Porphyromonas gingivalis* mediate in vivo virulence and exploit TLR2 and complement receptor 3 to persist in macrophages. *J Immunol.* 2007;179:2349–2358.

[14] Myneni SR, Settem RP, Connell TD, Keegan AD, Gaffen SL, Sharma A. TLR2 signaling and Th2 responses drive *Tannerella forsythia*-induced periodontal bone loss. *J Immunol.* 2011;187:501-509.

[15] Burns E, Eliyahu T, Uematsu S, Akira S, Nussbaum G. TLR2-dependent inflammatory response to *Porphyromonas gingivalis* is MyD88 independent, whereas MyD88 is required to clear infection, *J Immunol.* 2010;184:1455-1462.

[16] Shimada E, Kataoka H, Miyazawa Y, Yamamoto M, Igarashi T. Lipoproteins of Actinomyces viscosus induce inflammatory responses through TLR2 in human gingival epithelial cells and macrophages. *Microb Infect.* 2012;14:916-921.

[17] Sato Y, Yamamoto Y, Kizaki H. cloning and sequence analysis of the gbpC gene encoding a novel glucan-binding protein of *Streprtococcus mutans. Infect Immun.* 1997;65:668-675.

[18] Igarashi T, Yamamoto A, Goto N. PCR for detection and identification of *Streptococcus sobrinus. J Med Microbiol.* 2000;49:1069-1074.

[19] Matsuki Y, Yamamoto T, Hara K. Detection of inflammatory cytokine messenger RNA (mRNA)-expressing cells in human inflamed gingiva by combined in situ hybridization and immunohistochemistry. *Immunol.* 1992;76:42-47.

[20] Kirschning CJ, Wesche H, Ayres TM, Rothe M. Human Toll-like receptor 2 confers responsiveness to bacterial lipopolysaccharide. *J Exp Med.* 1998;188:2091-2097.

[21] Hashimoto M, Tawaratsumida K, Kariya H, Aoyama K, Tamura T, Suda Y. Lipoprotein is a predominant Toll-like receptor 2 ligand in *Staphylococcus aureus* cell wall component. *Int Immunol.* 2006;18:355-362.

[22] Li Q, Kumar A, Gui JF, Yu FSX. *Staphylococcus aureus* lipoproteins trigger human corneal epithelial innate response through toll-like receptor-2. *Microb Pathog.* 2008;44:426-434.

[23] Kim JS, Kim KD, Na HS, Jeong SY, Park HR, Kim S et al. Tumor necrosis factor-α and interleukin-1β expression pathway induced by Streptococcus mutans in macrophage cell line RAW 264.7. *Mol Oral Microbiol.* 2012;27:149-159.

In: Current Trends in Periodontics and Implant Dentistry
Editors: Vishal Anand and Minkle Gulati
ISBN: 978-1-62618-819-8

Chapter XI

Diversity of Oral Spirochetes and Their Role as Periodontopathogens

***Meng You*[*], *Rory M. Watt and W. Keung Leung*[†]**
Faculty of Dentistry, The University of Hong Kong, Hong Kong SAR, China

Abstract

Periodontal disease, as typified by periodontitis, has a varied and highly complex polymicrobial etiology. Oral spirochete bacteria, all of whose members belong to the genus *Treponema*, constitute one bacterial group that has been consistently associated with the occurrence and severity of periodontal infections. However, disease associations may be complex, as diverse communities of oral spirochete bacteria have been shown to be present within the human oral cavity. This chapter primarily discusses the positive association of oral spirochetes with periodontal diseases; their diversity within periodontal environments; as well as putative virulence factors that may play important roles contributing to the initiation and progression of periodontal diseases.

Keywords: Etiology, periodontitis, *Treponema,* virulence

Oral Spirochetes and Their Association with Periodontal Diseases

Spirochetes were first observed and described by van Leeuwenhoek in human "spittle" nearly 300 years ago, and these helical-shaped and motile bacteria have been considered to

[*] Current address: Department of Oral Radiology and State Key Laboratory of Oral Diseases, West China College of Stomatology, Sichuan University, Chengdu 610041, China. Tel: +86-13518206937, E-mail: fionayoum@gmail.com.
[†] Correspondence: Faculty of Dentistry, The University of Hong Kong, room 1B25, Prince Philip Dental Hospital Hospital, 34 Hospital Road, Hong Kong SAR, China. Tel: +852-2859-0417, Fax: +852-2858-2532, E-mail: ewkleung@hkucc.hku.hk.

constitute a unique taxonomic grouping for more than a century. Members of this morphologically-distinct class of microbes are found within various animal and human niches; forming pathogenic, opportunistic pathogenic or non-pathogenic relationships with their respective host organisms. All spirochete bacteria that reside in the human oral cavity belong to the genus *Treponema*. Consequently, they are frequently (and often interchangeably) also referred to as oral treponemes. Previous studies have generally reported low detection frequencies for oral spirochetes, noting that low numbers of spirochete cells are typically present within healthy periodontal sites. In contrast, oral spirochetes in general; as well as specific treponeme species such as *Treponema denticola*, have been frequently reported to be associated with the manifestation, extent and severity of periodontal diseases. Evidence supporting these disease correlations has come from a variety of detection methods, including direct microscopic observation of spirochete cells, culture-based approaches, as well as culture-independent molecular approaches including immunological assays, DNA hybridization probes, polymerase chain reaction (PCR) technologies; and most recently DNA sequencing studies.

Early Studies: Direct Microscopic Observation of Spiriochetes

Studies involving the direct microscopic observation and enumeration of microbial cells with a 'spirochete-like' helical or flat wave morphology, have noted that they can often be highly abundant in periodontally-diseased sites. Spirochetes have been reported to account for 20–50% of the total bacterial cell count in subgingival plaque sampled from inflamed periodontal pockets, compared to less than ca. 1% in subgingival plaque sampled from healthy sites. [1-4] Armitage and coworkers reported a positive co-relationship between the proportions of spirochete cells detected in subgingival plaque with clinical measures or indeces, such as gingival exudate levels; periodontal pocket depth; loss of periodontal attachment, and bleeding on probing scores.[3] Moreover, periodontal therapies which successfully reduced periodontal inflammation; such as the administration of antimicrobial agents, and/or scaling and root planing; have frequently resulted in a significant reduction in the proportions of subgingival spirochete cells observable microscopically.[5-9] The positive correlations observed using microscopy-based approaches have extended across a spectrum of periodontal inflammations, such as: gingivitis, chronic periodontitis, aggressive periodontitis and acute necrotizing ulcerative gingivitis (ANUG).[3,10,11]

Investigations via Isolation and Cultivation

Oral spirochetes are generally highly fastidious, and are recalcitrant to laboratory isolation and cultivation. With the continued development and refinement of cell cultivation media; in particular the development of the defined (OMIZ-Pat) medium by Wyss and co-workers in 1996; ten oral treponeme species have been successfully isolated from the oral cavity; predominantly from disease-associated dental plaque (see below). Although the use of culture-based approaches presumably leads to a significant underestimation of the actual population of oral spirochetes present, differences in isolation frequencies from periodontal sites during various stages of disease initiation or progression may reveal positive associations. This was illustrated in landmark studies conducted by Moore and colleagues, who reported that *T. denticola* and *Treponema vincentii* were isolated in higher frequencies from dental plaque sampled from diseased pockets versus plaque obtained from healthy sulci.[12,13]

Studies Using Immunological and DNA-Based Approaches

The development of various molecular identification techniques, which circumvent the requirement for laboratory cultivation, have further facilitated the exploration of oral spirochetes functioning as putative periodontopathogens; at the genus, species and even subspecies levels. Several studies have reported the use of immunological approaches to demonstrate positive associations between certain treponeme species (or taxa) with the occurence and severity of periodontal inflammation. [14-16] Monoclonal antibodies (MAbs) initially raised-against the syphilis spirochete *Treponema pallidum* (MAb H9-2) were found to cross-react with reasonable specificity with antigens present on the surface of oral spirochete cells; which were subsequently termed pathogen related oral spirochetes (PROS). These immunological probes revealed that *T. denticola* and certain other PROS spirochetes (including *T. vincentii* taxa) were more numerous and were detected more frequently within periodontitis versus healthy subgingival plaque samples. [14-16]

Genetic approaches such as DNA hybridization and PCR have also been used to investigate associations between oral treponeme taxa and disease. DNA-based hybridization approaches; e.g. the 'checkerboard assay' pioneered by Socransky and colleagues; may be based on the levels of 'whole-genome' similarity with a defined treponeme species, or may focus upon a single highly-conserved microbial gene, which encodes a small-subunit (SSU) molecule of ribosomal RNA (rRNA). These almost exclusively target a specific SSU rRNA molecule known as 16S rRNA. Species or genus-specific PCR-based approaches, as well as fluorescence *in situ* hybridization (FISH) techniques also generally target the 16S rRNA gene. Using these methodologies, particular treponeme species, such as *T. denticola, T. vincentii* and *Treponema socranskii*, have been associated with the extent and severity of periodontal diseases. [17-21] More recently, these have been largely superceded by DNA-sequencing approaches, whereby the 16S rRNA genes present within dental plaque samples are determined, leading to the fairly unambiguous identification of the species present. Such techniques have reveled that there is a large diversity of oral treponeme taxa present in the human oral cavity, which comprise roughly 10% of the total diversity of bacteria detected within subgingival niches. These genetic studies have revealed that the majority of oral spirochetes correspond to as-yet uncultivated species-level phylotypes (see below). Oral spirochete diversity appears to be greatest within subgingval plaques collected from diseased periodontal pockets compared with those obtained from healthy sites. [22-25]

Diversity of Oral Spirochetes

More than 500 bacterial species have been previously estimated to have the capability of colonizing subgingival niches. [24, 26] Similar to other chronic infectious diseases, periodontitis is generally considered to result from microbial dysbiosis, i.e. a 'pathogenic shift' in the composition of the subgingival microbiota that promotes and potentiates disease-related processes. [27, 28] This implies that periodontal infections are not simply caused by increased amounts of dental plaque in the subgingival niches; the composition of the microbial community is of paramount etiologic significance. The generally accepted paradigm for the microbial during the progression of periodontitis is that there is an increase in the proportions of gram-negative, proteolytic anaerobes such as oral spirochetes. [29]

Oral treponeme populations are diverse and highly varied in composition. Under the microscope, oral spirochetes may be classified as being large, medium or small, according to their cell morphology. Although the isolation and cultivation of these fastidious bacterial organisms can be extremely challenging, various media and methods have been developed, and ten treponeme species have been successfully cultivated, characterized and named. With ongoing advancements in molecular identification techniques based on 16S rRNA gene sequencing, over 50 treponeme phylotypes have been identified within subgingival niches. According to the phylogenetic relationships (i.e. implied patterns of shared genetic ancestry) revealed by the bioinformatic analysis of 16S rRNA sequences, oral treponemes have been clustered into 10 groups termed phylogroups, which share at least 90% 16S rRNA gene sequence identity. [22]

Cultivated Oral Spirochetes

To date, the following oral treponeme species have been isolated, cultured and systematically characterized: "*T. vincentii*" and *Treponema medium* [30] in phylogroup 1, *T. denticola* [31] and *Treponema putidum* [32] in phylogroup 2, *Treponema maltophilum* [33] and *Treponema lecithinolyticum* [34] in phylogroup 4, *Treponema amylovorum* [35] in phylogroup 5, *Treponema socranskii* [36] in phylogroup 6, *Treponema parvum* [37] in phylogroup 7, and *Treponema pectinovorum* [38] in phylogroup 8. However, oral spirochete species/strains belonging to phylogroups 3, 9 and 10 have yet to be isolated, cultivated and characterized.

Despite its long-term study and common utilization in laboratory investigations, '*T. vincentii'* is not yet an officially-recognized species, and has no valid standing in current bacterial taxonomy. *T. vincentii* (originally referred to as *Spirochaete vincenti*) was first described as a microorganism associated with ANUG and Vincent's angina (trench mouth) more than a century ago. [39] Since then, *T. vincentii* has been frequently detected in various periodontally-disease sites, as well as within periodontally-healthy sites, and is therefore regarded as a member of the normal periodontal microflora. [40] The other well-charaterized species in phylogroup 1 is *T. medium* which was firstly formally described in 1997. [30] It was isolated from subgingival plaque sampled from a patient with chronic periodontitis. Similar to *T. vincentii*, it is a medium-size treponeme with around five to seven periplasmic flagella. Unlike *T. vincentii*, *T. medium* was shown to be a saccharolytic species, which ferments carbohydrates. The identification frequency and proportions of *T. vincentii* and *T. medium* were reported to be positively associated with the presence and severity of periodontal inflammation, indicating that they may be of etiological relevance to periodontal disease. [18,19,4] Moreover, strains (taxa) belonging to both *T. vincentii* and *T. medium* were identified as PROS (see above).[42, 43]

Belonging to phylogroup 2, *T. denticola* is the most-highly studied oral treponeme species. As it is comparatively easy to cultivate, is widely used as a model spirochete organism. It was first described by Brumpt in 1925, and its taxonomic standing was established in 1993. [31] It is a small-sized, proteolytic but asaccharolytic treponeme with two to three periplasmic flagella. It is most frequently isolated from inflamed periodontal pockets. Although *T. denticola* may not directly cause periodontal disease by itself, it may still be termed a periodontopathogen, as it has been consistently associated with periodontal disease. [21, 41, 44-47] A variety of virulence mechanisms and disease-associated factors have been reported for this treponeme species, which have been reviewed elsewhere. [48] The isolation and systematic characterization of the only other phylogroup 2 species, *T. putidum* was reported in 2004. [32] It is a medium-sized proteolytic treponeme, and has been isolated from periodontitis and ANUG lesions. This species shares ca. 98.5% 16S rRNA gene sequence similarity with *T. denticola*, making them close relatives, from a phylogenetic perspective. However, the flagellin (a cell surface protein) patterns of *T. putidum* strains are notably different to those of *T. denticola* strains, and they also lack sialidase or dentilisin activities, which are presented in most *T. denticola* strains. This species has also been identified in endodontic infections. [49]

The small saccharolytic spirochetes from phylogroup 4: *T. maltophilum* and *T. lecithinolyticum,* were both originally isolated from human periodontal lesions, and were respectively reported in 1996 and 1999. [35, 50] The medium-size saccharolytic *T. amylovorum* representing phylogroup 5, was formally reported in 1997 by Wyss and co-workers. [35] All three of these species have previously been demonstrated to be associated with periodontitis, particularly aggressive periodontitis, as well as endodontic infections. [18 , 51 ,52]

T. socranskii is small saccharolytic spirochete belonging to phylogroup 6, which requires rumen fluid or short-chain volatile fatty acids for growth. Four subspecies have been identified for this species: *T. socranskii* subsp. *socranskii*, *T. socranskii* subsp. *buccale, T. socranskii* subsp. *paredis,* and *T. socranskii* subsp. *04.* [36,53] Previous studies have indentified *T. socranskii* in periodontal niches of both diseased as well as healthy subjects. [36] However, association studies have indicated that this species is detected more frequently within deep pockets, particularly in aggressive periodontitis. [18, 54-57]

The only validly-named species in phylogroup 7, *T. parvum* is small, glucuronic or galacturonic acid-dependent spirochete, which was originally isolated from lesions of human periodontitis and ANUG in 2001. [58] This species has also been detected in endodontic infections and may be involved in the disease etiology. [59] As the closest characterized relative to *T. parvum*, *T. pectinovorum* (placed within phylogroup 8) was originally isolated from humans periodontitis lesions in 1983. [60] This species requires a fermentable carbohydrate energy source such as pectin. The association of this species with periodontal disease and endodontic infections has been previously established, and its putative virulence determinants have been explored. [51, 61-64]

Phylogenetic Diversity of Oral Spirochetes

DNA sequencing-based investigations have demonstrated that oral spirochete populations are highly diverse, with the as-yet cultivated species representing just a small proportion of the total diversity. Choi and colleagues published the first focused report concerning the composition of oral spirochete communities. They used a PCR-based approach to construct a plasmid clone library of 16S rRNA gene sequences, to identify the spirochetes present in the plaque obtained from a lesion of a patient with destructive periodontitis. Subsequent bioinformatic (computational biology) analysis revealed 23 clusters of spirochetes were present (using a 98% 16S rRNA gene sequence similarity cut-off). [65] In 2000, Dewhirst and coworkers greatly extended our understanding of oral spirochete diversity, through the genetic analysis of 'species' present across a range of periodontal health/disease conditions. [22] By defining a phylotype as a set of closely related 16S rRNA gene sequences sharing >99% similarity, they identified 10 cultivated and 47 as-yet-uncultivated phylotypes, which all belonged to the genus *Treponema*. Shortly-thereafter, Paster and coworkers detected 76 oral 'species' of treponeme in human subgingival plaque; with 10 known species, 9 cultivable but not-yet named (sub)-species, and 57 uncultivated 'species'. [24] Recently, Dewhirst *et al.* reported the analysis of the 34,753 oral clones contained within their Human Oral Microbiome Database (HOMD). They subsequently identified 73 treponeme phylotypes; which they referred to as Operational Taxonomic Units (OTUs, see below).[66] Using a high-throughput pyrosequencing ('next-generation' DNA sequencing) technique, Keijser *et al.* performed a large-scale analysis to survey the bacterial diversity in oral ecosystems. They found that 118 treponeme phylotypes were present in their pooled sample obtained from individuals with reportedly good oral health.[67] In a recent study using a 16S rRNA clone-based approach, 110 species-level treponeme phylotypes in plaque sample collected from twenty subjects were detected. [25] Taken collectively, these studies clearly reveal the complexity and variablility of oral *Treponema* in the human oral cavity.

Results from a variety of studies performed over the years have suggested or implied that there is a positive correlation between the diversity of treponeme species and the severity of periodontal disease. In one study, cell enumeration using dark-field microscopy indicated that there was an increase in the variety of spirochete morphotypes (small, medium, large) present in subgingival plaque from periodontitis subjects compared with controls. [1] In other studies, a greater number of treponeme species were detected in patients with periodontal disease than in those without disease; and the detection frequency was also higher in periodontal lesions compared with healthy sulci.[18, 19 ,41 ,57 ,68] However, many of the DNA hybridization probes or PCR-based methods employed in these studies have had a limited target range, or have focused on specific species previously shown to be associated with periodontal disease (e.g *T. denticola*); thus introducing a bias, or limiting their scope. In comparison, 16S rRNA gene sequencing methods are relatively un-biased, and broad-range in scope.

In 2000, Dewhirst and coworkers found treponeme diversity was much higher in ANUG (32 OTUs) and periodontitis subjects (28 OTUs) than in periodontally healthy (10 OTUs) and HIV-periodontitis subjects (5 OTUs), using a 16S rRNA clone-based approach. In a recent 16S rRNA gene sequence-based study using 'spirochete-selective' primers, treponeme populations present within pooled subgingival plaque samples from ten periodontitis subjects and ten periodontitis-free controls (2 healthy, 8 mild gingivitis, no periodontal attachment loss) were comprehensively analayzed and compared. [25] It was found that both subject groups had diverse treponeme communities present in their subgingival plaque, which comprised many different phylotypes. In agreement with previous studies, the results showed the subgingival plaques sampled from periodontitis subjects contained a significantly higher diversity of oral spirochetes, and the periodontitis and control subjects contained quite distinct populations of spirochetes.

Pathogenic Activities and Virulence Determinants of Oral Spirochetes

Virulence may be defined as the capability of a microorganism to cause or contribute towards disease-related processes. For a periodontal microorganisms, this may be indicated by its capacity to cause damage to host cells or tissues, through direct or indirect means. The pathogenicity of a microorganism may be mediated through specific virulence factors, which are often molecules synthesized and/or secreted by the microorganism. For opportunistic pathogens such as oral *Treponema*, virulence factors may be molecules that enable its adhesion, colonization and proliferation in the local (biofilm) microbiota, its invasion of host tissues; its ability to evade and interfere with the host immune response, and its ability to acquire essential nutrients from the host tissues or local microenvironment. A variety of virulence factors or disease-associated activities (phenotypes) have been identified for oral treponeme, that contribute towards their 'periodontopathogenic' behaviour. [48, 69] Motility, proteolysis and adhesion-related activities play central roles in its ability to colonize, survive, and invade niches within the periodontal environment.

Pathogenic Activities of Oral Spirochetes

Oral spirochetes are highly motile bacteria with chemotactic activities. They make use of motility to enhancc thcir ability to colonize various host and biofilm niches within the subgingival environment; such as to penetrate and invade the periodontal epithelial barrier; to move to more nutrient-rich environments (in a chemotactic manner), as well as to avoid noxious stimuli and components of the host immune and inflammatory reponses.

Adhesion is a common characteristic shared by many pathogens, which is used to facilitate the colonization and invasion of host tissues. Oral treponemes can bind to several extracelluar matrix (ECM) components including fibronectin, fibrinogen, laminin and heparin. [70-72] They can also adhere to host cells such as periodontal epithelium cells and fibroblasts, which facilitate their penetration of host tissue barriers. [73, 74] Furthermore, oral treponemes can coaggregate with other periodontal microorganisms such as *Porphyromonas gingivalis*, *Parviomas micra* and *Fusobacterium nucleatum*. [75-77] The ability to coaggregate with other bacterial species enhances their ability to survive within the subgingival biofilm environment; may facilitate their ability to adhere and invade gingival tissues; enables inter-generic nutritional syntrophies (cross feeding); as well as aiding resistance against mechanical/chemical removal. The interaction of *T. denticola* with other bacteria, especially *P. gingivalis*, during the biofilm formation is considered to be an important step in the formation of 'pathogenic' biofilms involved in the development of periodontal disease.

Moreover, oral treponemes have been well-demonstrated to possess a broad spectrum of pathogenic activities that directly affect host cells and tissues, including: proteolysis; [78-80]

cytotoxicity, [81] perturbation of cytoskeletal and calcium regulation; [82-84] modulation of host proinflammatory and innate immunity responses; [85-87] activation of matrix metalloproteinase (MMP) levels; stimulation of alveolar bone resoption, [88] as well as hemagglutinating and hemolytic activities. [89, 90]

Putative Virulence Determinants of Oral Treponemes

A number of *in vitro* studies have revealed that oral treponemes, particularly the representive species *T. denticola*, produce a variety of proteins and metabolic end products which are detrimental to host cells and tissues during its colonization and invasion. These virulence factors include components involved in cellular motility and chemotaxis such as the endoflagellae and chemotaxis protein A (CheA); adhesins such as the major surface protein (Msp); proteases such as the chymotrpsin-like protease complex (CTLP); hemolysins such as Cystalysin (Hly), as well as other molecules that trigger host inflammatory responses.

Proteins responsible for motility and chemotaxis may be considered as virulence determinants as they are generally essential for host invasion. Similar to other motile (spirochete) bacteria such as *Borrelia burgdorferi*, genes dedicated to motility and chemotaxis account for a significant proportion (ca. 5%) of the entire *T. denticola* genome. [48] These genes encode an assortment of proteins which are responsible for the biosynthesis and export of flagellar components, e.g. rod, sheath, flagellins, basal body. Within the *Treponema* genus, various pairs of periplasmic flagellae (endoflagellae) are present across the different species and strains. These are entirely enclosed within the periplasm; the space between the inner cytoplasmic membrane and outer cell sheath. They are sub-terminally inserted near the cell pole and run towards the mid-cell, winding around the cell body, with their ends sometimes overlapping. This structural arrangement enables oral spirochetes to move within highly viscous media; predominantly via a 'corkscrew-like' motion. [48, 69]

Proteins associated with chemotaxis comprise a system for singal sensing, transduction and adaptation; which is responsible of guiding and promoting positive or negative directional motiliy in response to enviromental simuli. This system includes DmcA and DmcB, which are methyl-accepting chemotaxis proteins (MCPs); as well as the phosphokinase chemotaxis protein A (CheA), which is is resposible for 'energizing' chemotactic motility. [91, 92] Although the mechanism has not been fully established, the Che and Dmc pathways interact to modulate chemotactic motility, with the MCPs most likely regulating the ativities of the CheA phosphoknase.

Dentilisin, which is the functional proteolytic unit of the CTLP complex, has been proposed to function as one of the major virulence factors of *T. denticola*. [93] This surface protease cleaves proteins at phenylalany/alanyl and prolyl/alanyl bonds, thereby contributing to the progression of periodontal disease by degrading host (glyco)-proteins. [93, 94] The active protease properties of dentilisin have been shown to facilitate the ability of *T. denticola* to penetrate the host epithelial barrier. This protein (complex) also modulates the host immune response by degrading inflammatory factors such as interleukin-1 beta (IL-1 β), IL-6, and tumor necrosis factor alpha (TNF-α). [95] The CTLP complex comtains three accessory proteins : PrcA1, PrcA2 and PrcB which are required for full PrtP activities. [96] By testing chymotrypsin-like activities using chromogenic substrates (e.g. SAAPFNA), dentilisin homologues have also been detected in other treponeme species such as *T. socranskii* and *T. lecithinolyticum*.

Msp is the most abundant protein in the outer sheath of various oral treponeme species including strains of *T. denticola* and *T. vincentii*. It is considered to be a key virulence factor, and it has been reported to directly participate in a wide variety of pathogenic processes. Msp is a well-known immunogenic adhesin with pore forming and cytotoxic activities. [81, 97-99] It modulates host immune response through perturbing actin assembly within host cells, subsequently impairing neutrophil chemotaxis and phagocytic activities. [82, 84, 100-103] Msp also directly or indirectly mediates coaggregation with other disease-associated periodontal organisms such as *F. nucleatum* and *P. gingivalis*. [77] The biological functions of proteins mainly depend on their physical (multimeric) structures and amino acid composition. Msp, with the assistance of the CTLP complex, assembles into regular hexagonal arrays on the cell surface, with around 20 nm center-to-center distances. [97,104] This structure resembles the typical multimeric arrangement of transmembrane porins, and it has indeed been shown to functions as a porins *in vitro*. [97,105] It has been proposed that some of the predicted secondary structural units within the Msp protein form a β-barrel structure that forms a hydrophilic membrane-spanning pore. [98] Genes homologous to those encoding the Msp protein have been identified in several oral treponeme species and strains. Although these Msp homologs appear to possess similar functional activities, such as attachment, nutrient intake and cytotoxicity; there is considerable sequence variability in their molecular mass, amino acid compositions and antigenic properties. [99,106] It appears likely that Msp proteins have evolved in a strain- or species-specific manner. The composition of Msp protein forms and functions has been investigated in several different *T. denticola* strains. Msp homologues were classified into three distinct groups according to their molecular mass and antigenic reactivities. Three identified serotypes were respectively represented by the 53 kDa Msp of *T. denticola* ATCC 35405, the 55 kDa Msp of *T. denticola* ATCC 33520, and the 62 kDa Msp of *T. denticola* OTK. [99] It has been proposed that the Msp proteins of the first two serotypes contain 3 distinct domains, based on their sequence conservation and biophysical properties; namely the conserved N-terminal and C-terminal domains, and a central variable domain. [107] The *T. denticola* ATCC 35405 and ATCC 33520 Msp serotypes share high levels of sequence identity in the N-terminal and C-terminal domains, but contain highly distinct central variable regions (only 41% amino acid identity). The Msp sequence of *T. denticola* OTK is quite distinct from the former two serotypes, and appears to have a notably different domain structure.

In ongoing studies, we have determined full and partial-length *msp* gene sequences for a diverse selection of phylogroup 1 and 2 treponeme strains, including *T. vincentii*, *T. medium* and *T. putidum*. To achive this, we designed and utilized pairs of consensus PCR-primers that were capable of amplifying ca. 600-900 bp framgments of the *msp* genes present in several species. These primers were also used to analyze the dominant *msp* genotypes present within the subgingival plaque sampled from a clinical cohort of periodontitis and control subjects. Data indicated that there was a large diversity of *msp* genotypes present, especially within the periodontitis subjects, which comprised a large number of previously-undescribed 'species'.

Conclusion and Prospects

Oral spirochetes have long been indicated to be positively associated with various forms of periodontal desease. However, subgingival spirochete populations are diverse and highly variable within both periodontally-diseased and disease-free individuals. Their isolation, cultivation and characterization are often highly challenging; and hence their clinical distributions may be best analyzed using molecular approaches. Spirochetes emerge in the periodontal microflora as late colonizers and are primarily localized proximal to the host's gingival tissues. By utilizing various virulence-related mechanisms, they are often found at the invasive frontiers of 'pathogenic' biofilms. The strategies employed by spirochetes, in concert with other late colonizing microbes, to overcome mechanical/chemical removal and local environmental stresses remain to be clarified. Further dedicated research is required in order to better-define changes in treponeme community structure associated with periodontal disease prevalence, initiation, and progression.

References

[1] Listgarten MA, Hellden L. Relative distribution of bacteria at clinically healthy and periodontally diseased sites in humans. *J Clin Periodontol.* 1978;5(2):115-32.

[2] Listgarten MA, Levin S. Positive correlation between the proportions of subgingival spirochetes and motile bacteria and susceptibility of human subjects to periodontal deterioration. *J Clin Periodontol.* 1981;8(2):122-38.

[3] Armitage GC, Dickinson WR, Jenderseck RS, Levine SM, Chambers DW. Relationship between the percentage of subgingival spirochetes and the severity of periodontal disease. *J Periodontol.* 1982;53(9):550-6.

[4] Lembariti BS, Mikx FH, van Palenstein Helderman WH. Microscopic spirochete counts in untreated subjects with and without periodontal tissue destruction. *J Clin Periodontol.* 1995;22(3):235-9.

[5] Slots J, Mashimo P, Levine MJ, Genco RJ. Periodontal therapy in humans. I. Microbiological and clinical effects of a single course of periodontal scaling and root planing, and of adjunctive tetracycline therapy. *J Periodontol.* 1979;50(10):495-509.

[6] Mousques T, Listgarten MA, Phillips RW. Effect of scaling and root planing on the composition of the human subgingival microbial flora. *J Periodontal Res.* 1980;15(2):144-51.

[7] Rams TE, Keyes PH. A rationale for the management of periodontal diseases: effects of tetracycline on subgingival bacteria. *J Am Dent Assoc.* 1983;107(1):37-41.

[8] Loesche WJ, Giordano JR, Hujoel P, Schwarcz J, Smith BA. Metronidazole in periodontitis: reduced need for surgery. *J Clin Periodontol.* 1992;19(2):103-12.

[9] Loesche WJ, Grossman N, Giordano J. Metronidazole in periodontitis (IV). The effect of patient compliance on treatment parameters. *J Clin Periodontol.* 1993;20(2):96-104.

[10] Carranza FA, Jr., Saglie R, Newman MG, Valentin PL. Scanning and transmission electron microscopic study of tissue-invading microorganisms in localized juvenile periodontitis. *J Periodontol.* 1983;54(10):598-617.

[11] Courtois GJ, 3rd, Cobb CM, Killoy WJ. Acute necrotizing ulcerative gingivitis. A transmission electron microscope study. *J Periodontol.* 1983;54(11):671-9.

[12] Moore WE, Holdeman LV, Cato EP, Smibert RM, Burmeister JA, Ranney RR. Bacteriology of moderate (chronic) periodontitis in mature adult humans. *Infect Immun.* 1983;42(2):510-5.

[13] Moore WE, Holdeman LV, Cato EP, Smibert RM, Burmeister JA, Palcanis KG, et al. Comparative bacteriology of juvenile periodontitis. *Infect Immun.* 1985;48(2):507-19..

[14] Simonson LG, Goodman CH, Bial JJ, Morton HE. Quantitative relationship of *Treponema denticola* to severity of periodontal disease. *Infect Immun.* 1988;56(4):726-8.

[15] Riviere GR, Wagoner MA, Baker-Zander SA, Weisz KS, Adams DF, Simonson L, et al. Identification of spirochetes related to *Treponema pallidum* in necrotizing ulcerative gingivitis and chronic periodontitis. *N Engl J Med.* 1991;325(8):539-43.

[16] Riviere GR, Weisz KS, Simonson LG, Lukehart SA. Pathogen-related spirochetes identified within gingival tissue from patients with acute necrotizing ulcerative gingivitis. *Infect Immun.* 1991;59(8):2653-7.

[17] Socransky SS, Haffajee AD, Smith C, Dibart S. Relation of counts of microbial species to clinical status at the sampled site. *J Clin Periodontol.* 1991;18(10):766-75.

[18] Moter A, Hoenig C, Choi BK, Riep B, Gobel UB. Molecular epidemiology of oral treponemes associated with periodontal disease. *J Clin Microbiol.* 1998;36(5):1399-403.

[19] Willis SG, Smith KS, Dunn VL, Gapter LA, Riviere KH, Riviere GR. Identification of seven *Treponema* species in health- and disease-associated dental plaque by nested PCR. *J Clin Microbiol.* 1999;37(3):867-9.

[20] Socransky SS, Smith C, Haffajee AD. Subgingival microbial profiles in refractory periodontal disease. *J Clin Periodontol.* 2002;29(3):260-8.

[21] Yoshida A, Kawada M, Suzuki N, Nakano Y, Oho T, Saito T, et al. TaqMan real-time polymerase chain reaction assay for the correlation of *Treponema denticola* numbers with the severity of periodontal disease. *Oral Microbiol Immunol.* 2004;19(3):196-200.

[22] Dewhirst FE, Tamer MA, Ericson RE, Lau CN, Levanos VA, Boches SK, et al. The diversity of periodontal spirochetes by 16S rRNA analysis. *Oral Microbiol Immunol.* 2000;15(3):196-202.

[23] Paster BJ, Dewhirst FE. Phylogenetic foundation of spirochetes. *J Mol Microbiol Biotechnol.* 2000;2(4):341-4.

[24] Paster BJ, Boches SK, Galvin JL, Ericson RE, Lau CN, Levanos VA, et al. Bacterial diversity in human subgingival plaque. *J Bacteriol.* 2001;183(12):3770-83.

[25] You M. *Diversity of oral spirochetes in subgingival niches.* PhD Thesis. Hong Kong: The University of Hong Kong; 2012.

[26] Moore WE, Moore LV. The bacteria of periodontal diseases. *Periodontol* 2000. 1994;5:66-77.

[27] Schaudinn C, Gorur A, Keller D, Sedghizadeh PP, Costerton JW. Periodontitis: an archetypical biofilm disease. *J Am Dent Assoc.* 2009;140(8):978-86.

[28] Zarco MF, Vess TJ, Ginsburg GS. The oral microbiome in health and disease and the potential impact on personalized dental medicine. *Oral Dis.* 2012;18(2):109-20.

[29] Marsh PD. Microbial ecology of dental plaque and its significance in health and disease. *Adv Dent Res.* 1994;8(2):263-71.

[30] Umemoto T, Nakazawa F, Hoshino E, Okada K, Fukunaga M, Namikawa I. *Treponema medium* sp. nov., isolated from human subgingival dental plaque. *Int J Syst Bacteriol.* 1997;47(1):67-72.

[31] Chan EC, Siboo R, Keng T, Psarra N, Hurley R, Cheng SL, et al. Treponema denticola (ex Brumpt 1925) sp. nov., nom. rev., and identification of new spirochete isolates from periodontal pockets. *Int J Syst Bacteriol.* 1993;43(2):196-203.

[32] Wyss C, Moter A, Choi BK, Dewhirst FE, Xue Y, Schupbach P, et al. *Treponema putidum* sp. nov., a medium-sized proteolytic spirochaete isolated from lesions of human periodontitis and acute necrotizing ulcerative gingivitis. *Int J Syst Evol Microbiol.* 2004;54(Pt 4):1117-22.

[33] Siqueira JF, Jr., Rocas IN, Cunha CD, Rosado AS. Novel bacterial phylotypes in endodontic infections. *J Dent Res.* 2005;84(6):565-9.

[34] Wyss C, Choi BK, Schupbach P, Moter A, Guggenheim B, Gobel UB. *Treponema lecithinolyticum* sp. nov., a small saccharolytic spirochaete with phospholipase A and C activities associated with periodontal diseases. *Int J Syst Bacteriol.* 1999;49:1329-39.

[35] Wyss C, Choi BK, Schupbach P, Guggenheim B, Gobel UB. *Treponema amylovorum* sp. nov., a saccharolytic spirochete of medium size isolated from an advanced human periodontal lesion. *Int J Syst Bacteriol.* 1997;47(3):842-5.

[36] Smibert RM, Johnson JL, Ranney RR. Treponema socranskii sp. nov., *Treponema socranskii* subsp. *socranskii* subsp. nov., *Treponema socranskii* subsp. *buccale* subsp. nov., and *Treponema socranskii* subsp. *paredis* subsp. nov. isolated from the human periodontia. *Int J Syst Bacteriol.* 1984;34(4):457-62.

[37] Wyss C, Dewhirst FE, Gmur R, Thurnheer T, Xue Y, Schupbach P, et al. *Treponema parvum* sp. nov., a small, glucoronic or galacturonic acid-dependent oral spirochaete from lesions of human periodontitis and acute necrotizing ulcerative gingivitis. *Int J Syst Evol Microbiol.* 2001;51(Pt 3):955-62.

[38] Smibert RM, Burmeister JA. *Treponema pectinovorum* sp. nov. isolated from humans with periodontitis. *Int J Syst Bacteriol.* 1983;33:852-6.

[39] Blanchard R. Spirilles, Spirochètes et autres microorganismes à corps spiralé. *Semaine Médicale.* 1996;xxvi:1-5.

[40] Klein HS. What role do *Treponema vincenti* play in certain diseases of the gingiva? *Acta Odontol Scand.* 1946;7:92-6.

[41] Asai Y, Jinno T, Igarashi H, Ohyama Y, Ogawa T. Detection and quantification of oral treponemes in subgingival plaque by real-time PCR. *J Clin Microbiol.* 2002;40(9):3334-40.

[42] Choi BK, Wyss C, Gobel UB. Phylogenetic analysis of pathogen-related oral spirochetes. *J Clin Microbiol.* 1996;34(8):1922-5.

[43] Wyss C. Flagellins, but not endoflagellar sheath proteins, of *Treponema pallidum* and of pathogen-related oral spirochetes are glycosylated. *Infect Immun.* 1998;66(12):5751-4.

[44] Sela MN. Role of *Treponema denticola* in periodontal diseases. Crit *Rev Oral Biol Med.* 2001;12(5):399-413.

[45] Sakamoto M, Umeda M, Benno Y. Molecular analysis of human oral microbiota. *J Periodontal Res.* 2005;40(3):277-85.

[46] Haffajee AD, Teles RP, Socransky SS. Association of *Eubacterium nodatum* and *Treponema denticola* with human periodontitis lesions. *Oral Microbiol Immunol.* 2006;21(5):269-82.

[47] Mineoka T, Awano S, Rikimaru T, Kurata H, Yoshida A, Ansai T, et al. Site-specific development of periodontal disease is associated with increased levels of *Porphyromonas gingivalis*, *Treponema denticola*, and *Tannerella forsythia* in subgingival plaque. *J Periodontol.* 2008;79(4):670-6.

[48] Dashper SG, Seers CA, Tan KH, Reynolds EC. Virulence factors of the oral spirochete *Treponema denticola*. *J Dent Res.* 2011;90(6):691-703.

[49] Sakamoto M, Siqueira JF, Jr., Rocas IN, Benno Y. Diversity of spirochetes in endodontic infections. *J Clin Microbiol.* 2009;47(5):1352-7.

[50] Wyss C, Choi BK, Schupbach P, Guggenheim B, Gobel UB. *Treponema maltophilum* sp. nov., a small oral spirochete isolated from human periodontal lesions. *Int J Syst Bacteriol.* 1996;46(3):745-52.

[51] Willis SG, Smith KS, Dunn VL, Gapter LA, Riviere KH, Riviere GR. Identification of seven *Treponema* species in health- and disease-associated dental plaque by nested PCR. *J Clin Microbiol.* 1999;37(3):867-9.

[52] Siqueira JF, Jr., Rocas IN. PCR-based identification of *Treponema maltophilum*, *T. amylovorum*, *T. medium*, and *T. lecithinolyticum* in primary root canal infections. *Arch Oral Biol.* 2003;48(7):495-502.

[53] Paster BJ, Dewhirst FE, Coleman BC, Lau CN, Ericson RL. Phylogenetic analysis of cultivable oral treponemes from the Smibert collection. *Int J Syst Bacteriol.* 1998;48(Pt 3):713-22.

[54] Riviere GR, Smith KS, Carranza N, Jr., Tzagaroulaki E, Kay SL, Dock M. Subgingival distribution of *Treponema denticola*, *Treponema socranskii*, and pathogen-related oral spirochetes: prevalence and relationship to periodontal status of sampled sites. *J Periodontol.* 1995;66(10):829-37.

[55] Sakamoto M, Takeuchi Y, Umeda M, Ishikawa I, Benno Y, Nakase T. Detection of *Treponema socranskii* associated with human periodontitis by PCR. *Microbiol Immunol.* 1999;43(5):485-90.

[56] Takeuchi Y, Umeda M, Sakamoto M, Benno Y, Huang Y, Ishikawa I. *Treponema socranskii*, *Treponema denticola*, and *Porphyromonas gingivalis* are associated with severity of periodontal tissue destruction. *J Periodontol.* 2001;72(10):1354-63.

[57] Moter A, Riep B, Haban V, Heuner K, Siebert G, Berning M, et al. Molecular epidemiology of oral treponemes in patients with periodontitis and in periodontitis-resistant subjects. *J Clin Microbiol.* 2006;44(9):3078-85.

[58] Wyss C, Dewhirst FE, Gmur R, Thurnheer T, Xue Y, Schupbach P, et al. *Treponema parvum* sp. nov., a small, glucuronic or galacturonic acid-dependent oral spirochaete from lesions of human periodontitis and acute necrotizing ulcerative gingivitis. *Int J Syst Evol Microbiol.* 2001;51(Pt 3):955-62.

[59] Rocas IN, Siqueira JF, Jr. Occurrence of two newly named oral treponemes - *Treponema parvum* and *Treponema putidum* - in primary endodontic infections. *Oral Microbiol Immunol.* 2005;20(6):372-5.

[60] Smibert RM, Burmeister JA. *Treponema pectinovorum* sp. nov. isolated from humans with periodontitis. *Int J Syst Bacteriol.* 1983;33(4):852-6.

[61] Walker SG, Ebersole JL, Holt SC. Identification, isolation, and characterization of the 42-kilodalton major outer membrane protein (MompA) from *Treponema pectinovorum* ATCC 33768. *J Bacteriol.* 1997;179(20):6441-7.

[62] Walker SG, Ebersole JL, Holt SC. Studies on the binding of *Treponema pectinovorum* to HEp-2 epithelial cells. *Oral Microbiol Immunol.* 1999;14(3):165-71.

[63] Kesavalu L, Falk CW, Davis KJ, Steffen MJ, Xu X, Holt SC, et al. Biological characterization of lipopolysaccharide from *Treponema pectinovorum. Infect Immun.* 2002;70(1):211-7.

[64] Siqueira JF, Jr., Rocas IN. *Treponema* species associated with abscesses of endodontic origin. *Oral Microbiol Immunol.* 2004;19(5):336-9.

[65] Choi BK, Paster BJ, Dewhirst FE, Gobel UB. Diversity of cultivable and uncultivable oral spirochetes from a patient with severe destructive periodontitis. *Infect Immun.* 1994;62(5):1889-95.

[66] Dewhirst FE, Chen T, Izard J, Paster BJ, Tanner AC, Yu WH, et al. The human oral microbiome. *J Bacteriol.* 2010;192(19):5002-17.

[67] Keijser BJ, Zaura E, Huse SM, van der Vossen JM, Schuren FH, Montijn RC, et al. Pyrosequencing analysis of the oral microflora of healthy adults. *J Dent Res.* 2008;87(11):1016-20.

[68] Colombo APV, Boches SK, Cotton SL, Goodson JM, Kent R, Haffajee AD, et al. Comparisons of subgingival microbial profiles of refractory periodontitis, severe periodontitis, and periodontal health using the human oral microbe identification microarray. *J Periodontol.* 2009;80(9):1421-32.

[69] Fenno JC, McBride BC. Virulence factors of oral treponemes. *Anaerobe.* 1998;4(1):1-17.

[70] Dawson JR, Ellen RP. Tip-oriented adherence of *Treponema denticola* to fibronectin. *Infect Immun.* 1990;58(12):3924-8.

[71] Haapasalo M, Singh U, McBride BC, Uitto VJ. Sulfhydryl-dependent attachment of *Treponema denticola* to laminin and other proteins. *Infect Immun.* 1991;59(11):4230-7.

[72] Haapasalo M, Hannam P, McBride BC, Uitto VJ. Hyaluronan, a possible ligand mediating *Treponema denticola* binding to periodontal tissue. *Oral Microbiol Immunol.* 1996;11(3):156-60.

[73] Keulers RA, Maltha JC, Mikx FH, Wolters-Lutgerhorst JM. Attachment of *Treponema denticola* strains to monolayers of epithelial cells of different origin. *Oral Microbiol Immunol.* 1993;8(2):84-8.

[74] Leung WK, Haapasalo M, Uitto VJ, Hannam P, McBride BC. The surface proteinase of *Treponema denticola* may mediate attachment of the bacteria to epithelial cells. *Anaerobe.* 1996;2(1):39-46.

[75] Grenier D. Demonstration of a bimodal coaggregation reaction between *Porphyromonas gingivalis* and *Treponema denticola. Oral Microbiol Immunol.* 1992;7(5):280-4.

[76] Kolenbrander PE, Parrish KD, Andersen RN, Greenberg EP. Intergeneric coaggregation of oral *Treponema* spp. with *Fusobacterium* spp. and intrageneric coaggregation among *Fusobacterium* spp. *Infect Immun.* 1995;63(12):4584-8.

[77] Rosen G, Genzler T, Sela MN. Coaggregation of *Treponema denticola* with *Porphyromonas gingivalis* and *Fusobacterium nucleatum* is mediated by the major outer sheath protein of Treponema denticola. *FEMS Microbiol Lett.* 2008;289(1):59-66.

[78] Uitto VJ, Grenier D, Chan EC, McBride BC. Isolation of a chymotrypsinlike enzyme from Treponema denticola. *Infect Immun.* 1988;56(10):2717-22.

[79] Ellen RP, Song M, McCulloch CA. Degradation of endogenous plasma membrane fibronectin concomitant with *Treponema denticola* 35405 adhesion to gingival fibroblasts. *Infect Immun.* 1994;62(7):3033-7.

[80] Cogoni V, Morgan-Smith A, Fenno JC, Jenkinson HF, Dymock D. *Treponema denticola* chymotrypsin-like proteinase (CTLP) integrates spirochaetes within oral microbial communities. *Microbiol.* 2012;158(Pt 3):759-70.

[81] Fenno JC, Hannam PM, Leung WK, Tamura M, Uitto VJ, McBride BC. Cytopathic effects of the major surface protein and the chymotrypsinlike protease of *Treponema denticola. Infect Immun.* 1998;66(5):1869-77.

[82] Wang Q, Ko KS, Kapus A, McCulloch CA, Ellen RP. A spirochete surface protein uncouples store-operated calcium channels in fibroblasts: a novel cytotoxic mechanism. *J Biol Chem.* 2001;276(25):23056-64.

[83] Amin M, Ho AC, Lin JY, Batista da Silva AP, Glogauer M, Ellen RP. Induction of de novo subcortical actin filament assembly by *Treponema denticola* major outer sheath protein. *Infect Immun.* 2004;72(6):3650-4.

[84] Amin M, Grove DA, Kapus A, Glogauer M, Ellen RP. An actin-stabilizing peptide conjugate deduced from the major outer sheath protein of the bacterium *Treponema denticola. Cell Motil Cytoskeleton.* 2007;64(9):662-74.

[85] Deng QD, Han Y, Xia X, Kuramitsu HK. Effects of the oral spirochete *Treponema denticola* on interleukin-8 expression from epithelial cells. *Oral Microbiol Immunol.* 2001;16(3):185-7.

[86] Asai Y, Jinno T, Ogawa T. Oral treponemes and their outer membrane extracts activate human gingival epithelial cells through toll-like receptor 2. *Infect Immun.* 2003;71(2):717-25.

[87] Asai Y, Hashimoto M, Ogawa T. *Treponemal glycoconjugate* inhibits Toll-like receptor ligand-induced cell activation by blocking LPS-binding protein and CD14 functions. *Euro J Immunol.* 2003;33(11):3196-204.

[88] Choi BK, Lee HJ, Kang JH, Jeong GJ, Min CK, Yoo YJ. Induction of osteoclastogenesis and matrix metalloproteinase expression by the lipooligosaccharide of *Treponema denticola. Infect Immun.* 2003;71(1):226-33.

[89] Chu L, Song M, Holt SC. Effect of iron regulation on expression and hemin-binding function of outer-sheath proteins from *Treponema denticola. Microb Pathog.* 1994;16(5):321-35.

[90] Chu L, Ebersole JL, Kurzban GP, Holt SC. Cystalysin, a 46-kilodalton cysteine desulfhydrase from *Treponema denticola*, with hemolytic and hemoxidative activities. *Infect and Immun.* 1997;65(8):3231-8.

[91] Li H, Arakawa S, Deng QD, Kuramitsu H. Characterization of a novel methyl-accepting chemotaxis gene, dmcB, from the oral spirochete *Treponema denticola. Infect Immun.* 1999;67(2):694-9.

[92] Lux R, Sim JH, Tsai JP, Shi W. Construction and characterization of a cheA mutant of *Treponema denticola. J Bacteriol.* 2002;184(11):3130-4.

[93] Ishihara K, Miura T, Kuramitsu HK, Okuda K. Characterization of the *Treponema denticola* prtP gene encoding a prolyl-phenylalanine-specific protease (dentilisin). *Infect Immun.* 1996;64(12):5178-86.

[94] Fenno JC, Hannam PM, Leung WK, Tamura M, Uitto VJ, McBride BC. Cytopathic effects of the major surface protein and the chymotrypsinlike protease of *Treponema denticola*. *Infect Immun*. 1998;66(5):1869-77.
[95] Miyamoto M, Ishihara K, Okuda K. The *Treponema denticola* surface protease dentilisin degrades interleukin-1 beta (IL-1 beta), IL-6, and tumor necrosis factor alpha. *Infect Immun*. 2006;74(4):2462-7.
[96] Bian XL, Wang HT, Ning Y, Lee SY, Fenno JC. Mutagenesis of a novel gene in the prcA-prtP protease locus affects expression of *Treponema denticola* membrane complexes. *Infect Immun*. 2005;73(2):1252-5.
[97] Egli C, Leung WK, Muller KH, Hancock RE, McBride BC. Pore-forming properties of the major 53-kilodalton surface antigen from the outer sheath of *Treponema denticola*. *Infect Immun*. 1993;61(5):1694-9.
[98] Fenno JC, Muller KH, McBride BC. Sequence analysis, expression, and binding activity of recombinant major outer sheath protein (Msp) of *Treponema denticola*. *J Bacteriol.* 1996;178(9):2489-97.
[99] Fenno JC, Wong GW, Hannam PM, Muller KH, Leung WK, McBride BC. Conservation of msp, the gene encoding the major outer membrane protein of oral *Treponema spp*. *J Bacteriol.* 1997;179(4):1082-9.
[100] Batista da Silva AP, Lee W, Bajenova E, McCulloch CA, Ellen RP. The major outer sheath protein of *Treponema denticola* inhibits the binding step of collagen phagocytosis in fibroblasts. *Cell Microbiol*. 2004;6(5):485-98.
[101] Puthengady Thomas B, Sun CX, Bajenova E, Ellen RP, Glogauer M. Modulation of human neutrophil functions in vitro by *Treponema denticola* major outer sheath protein. *Infect Immun*. 2006;74(3):1954-7.
[102] Jobin MC, Virdee I, McCulloch CA, Ellen RP. Activation of MAPK in fibroblasts by *Treponema denticola* major outer sheath protein. *Biochem Biophys Res Commun.* 2007;356(1):213-8.
[103] Magalhaes MA, Sun CX, Glogauer M, Ellen RP. The major outer sheath protein of *Treponema denticola* selectively inhibits Rac1 activation in murine neutrophils. *Cell Microbiol*. 2008;10(2):344-54.
[104] Masuda K, Kawata T. Isolation, properties, and reassembly of outer sheath carrying a polygonal array from an oral treponeme. *J Bacteriol.* 1982;150(3):1405-13.
[105] Jeanteur D, Lakey JH, Pattus F. The bacterial porin superfamily: sequence alignment and structure prediction. *Mol Microbiol.* 1991;5(9):2153-64.
[106] Weinberg A, Holt SC. Chemical and biological activities of a 64-kilodalton outer sheath protein from *Treponema denticola* strains. *J Bacteriol.* 1991;173(21):6935-47.
[107] Edwards AM, Jenkinson HF, Woodward MJ, Dymock D. Binding properties and adhesion-mediating regions of the major sheath protein of *Treponema denticola* ATCC 35405. *Infect Immun*. 2005;73(5):2891-8.

In: Current Trends in Periodontics and Implant Dentistry
Editors: Vishal Anand and Minkle Gulati
ISBN: 978-1-62618-819-8

Chapter XII

Influence of Herpes Viruses in the Human Periodontitis: The Hypothesis of Bacteria-Virus Synergy

Ronaldo Luis Thomasini**, Fabiana Souza Maximo Pereira and Mauro Martins Teixeira
Department of Biochemistry and Immunology, Institute of Biological Sciences, Universidade Federal de Minas Gerais, Brazil

Abstract

The human chronic periodontitis is a disease that leads to tooth loss in the patients and naturally implicates in a decrease of self esteem and many other healthy problems related to this disease. Some species of bacteria are implicated in the pathogenesis of the periodontitis; however, the presence of these bacteria does not merely explain the inflammatory processes completely. Some authors have suggested that association between bacteria and viruses, especially herpes viruses, could play a role in the pathogenesis of periodontitis affecting the immune response against microbes. In this chapter the association between herpes virus, specifically cytomegalovirus, and human chronic periodontitis has been investigated. Twenty chronic periodontitis affected patients and 12 healthy subjects were biopsied during surgical treatment and tissue fragment analyzed by polymerase chain reaction and imunohistochemistry to detect cytomegalovirus DNA and antigen, respectively. None of the samples collected from healthy subjects presented positive results to cytomegalovirus either by polymerase chain reaction or immunohistochemistry. Yet, samples from 30% of the periodontitis affected patients were positive to cytomegalovirus DNA, though none of them showed a positive result for cytomegalovirus antigen. The results suggested that cytomegalovirus could play a role in the pathogenesis of periodontitis; however, patients probably presented latent

* Correspondence: Groelandia street, 276 – Sion, Post Code: 303120-060, Belo Horizonte, Minas Gerais, Brazil. Email: ronaldothomasini@yahoo.com.br.

infection instead of active infection. Due to this contrast, additional studies are necessary for better investigation of the association between herpersviruses and chronic periodontitis.

Keywords: Herpes viruses, chronic periodontitis, pathogenesis

Introduction

Periodontitis is associated with specific bacterial species along with polymicrobial colonization of the tooth surfaces. Some bacteria such as *Actinobacillus actinomycetemcomitans* and *Porphyromonas gingivalis* are included among the species with higher periodontopathic potential. [1, 2] However, the amount of bacterial plaque itself does not completely explain the clinical and pathological features of periodontitis. Some authors have suggested that the presence of herpes viruses in periodontal sites could play a role in the pathogenesis of human periodontitis. [3-5]

Herpes viruses are ubiquitous and after primary infection can persist in latent states in the host in different types of cells including immune system cells. Herpes virus have been frequently isolated from immunocompromised patients as well as after organ transplantation and some authors have suggested that viruses may act directly or indirectly by immunomodulation and influence the immune response due to viral replication in lympho- cytes and monocytes/macrophages. [6-9]

The cytomegalovirus (CMV) and Epstein - Barr virus (EBV) are the most often studied members of the herpes viruses in periodontal sites but Human herpes simplex virus (HSV) has been occasionally studied. Recently, human herpes virus 6 and 7 (HHV-6 and HHV-7), have also been investigated due to fact that these viruses are frequently detected in saliva. [3-5, 10] It has been suggested that herpes viruses can affect defense mechanisms against other microorganisms in immunocompromised individuals by modulation of immune system or by directly causing inflammation. Similarly, cells harboring herpes viruses in sites of periodontal inflammation can contribute to the development and course of periodontitis. [11-13]

Cytomegalovirus can induce direct cytopathic effects in fibroblasts, keratinocytes, endothelial cells, polymorphonuclear neutrophils, T lymphocytes, macrophages and possibly it can affect bone cells too. In periodontitis-affected patients, T cells are activated and lymphocytic specific responses are driven by the nature of the initial antigenic stimulus. This process is supported by a complex cascade of events, which involves cytokines, chemokines and other inflammatory mediators that can be altered due to cytomegalovirus infection. The balance between pro-inflammatory and anti-inflammatory activities driven by different lymphocyte subpopulations seems to be crucial for the pathogenesis of periodontitis. [14]

The cytophatic effects of HSV are well described in the literature and HSV infection or reactivation at the periodontal sites can lead to similar effects as observed in other tissues. EBV produces several modifications in infected cells, which includes immortalization and polyclonal expansion of B-lymphocytes. A possible EBV infection or reactivation in periodontal sites can lead to either excessive or inefficient response against microbial agents. Regarding other herpes viruses, the expression of different cellular antigens can be drastically altered in HHV-6 infected tissues where the viral infection can up regulate CD4 and down modulate CD3 in the T cells. HHV-6 can also affect the physiology of secondary lymphoid organs by direct infection of T lymphocytes and modulation of membranes receptors and chemokine immunomodulators. [13, 3]

Citotoxicity and other effects caused by HHV-7 infection in T-CD4+ subpopulation *in vitro* and *in vivo* have been described as an adaptative mechanism for evading the host immune system by this virus.

Local immunomodulatory effects caused by herpesviral infection can facilitate the bacterial proliferation, increase its virulence and induce the release of cytokines and chemokines from inflammatory and connective tissue. Moreover, virus and bacteria can act in synergy to produce the pathology. Yet, the presence of herpes viruses in the periodontitis-affected sites could merely reflect latent virus within the cells of periodontal tissue or within the cells of inflammatory infiltrate derived from this pathology. In contrast, immune system cells in the inflammatory infiltrate could be affected by viral infection. [3, 13]

This chapter investigates and describes the association between cyto- megalovirus and chronic periodontitis using polymerase chain reaction and imunohistochemistry in samples collected from periodontitis affected patients and a healthy control group.

Methods

Patients

Twenty chronic periodontitis-affected patients were enrolled for the investigation. Patients who presented with chronic periodontitis based on clinical and radiographic findings [15] were eligible to participate. All patients were systemically healthy and had not received periodontal treatment or antibiotics for at least 6 months prior to the clinical examination and sampling. Each patient contributed one biopsy, collected from a clinically affected site involving epithelium and connective tissue facing the sulcus and periodontal pocket. [16]

In 12 healthy subjects (healthy controls), tissue samples were harvested from periodontally healthy sites. All healthy subjects presented probing depth $\leq$ 3 mm, with no attachment loss nor gingival bleeding on probing; gingival biopsies were obtained from the sulcular region during tooth extraction procedures.

The demographic data of the patients and healthy subjects included are shown in Table 1. The tissue fragments were rinsed several times with sterile saline and divided into two parts: one part was fixed in 10% buffered formalin and the other was stored frozen (-70°C) in sterile flasks for DNA extraction.

Table 1. Demographic data of the patients (affected group and healthy subjects) included in the study

Group	Total	Sex (male/female)		Age (years)	
	n	n	(%)	Interval	Median
Chronic periodontitis affected	20	7/13	(35/65)	39-69	52
Healthy individuals	12	6/6	(50/50)	20-40	34

Cytomegalovirus Polymerase Chain Reaction (Nested-PCR)

DNA Extraction from Periodontal Samples

The non-fixed tissue fragments were finely minced using blade scalpel and incubated over-night at 56ºC with 100μL of lysis buffer (Tris-HCl pH 8.3 10 mM, NaCl 150 mM, EDTA 1 mM, 0.2% sodium dodecyl sulphate and 100 μg of proteinase K). Two hundred microliters of a phenol-chlorofom mixture (1:1) was added to lysis product, mixed, and then centrifuged at 10.000 rpm for 10 minutes.

The aqueous phasis was washed with phenol-chloroform twice and then DNA was precipited with cold isopropanol by centrigugation at 10.000 rpm for 15 minutes at 4ºC. The precipite was dried at room temperature, rehydrated with 50 μL of nuclease free water and the DNA was quantified by espectro- photometry using a Nanodrop® (Thermo Scientific, DE, USA) espectrophometer.

PCR using a primer to beta-globin gene was carried out in all samples to avoid false negative results due to presence of PCR inibithors and failed DNA extraction. Samples that did not present expected positivity to beta-globin gene were excluded from sampling. Finally, DNA samples were stored frozen at -70°C until analysis.

First PCR Round

DNA extracted as described above was submitted to PCR reaction. Briefly, 5 μL of 10x Mg^{++} taq PCR buffer, 1 mM of DNTPs, 1 U *Taq* DNA polymerase (Genscript, NJ, USA), 5 pM of each forward and reverse primers (forward 5'CCA AGC GGC CTC TGA TAA CCA AGC C 3' and reverse 5'CAG CAC CAT CCT CCT CTT CCT CTG G 3') (Invitrogen, Sao Paulo, Brazil) [16] and 5 μL of DNA sample were used to a total volume of 50 μL reaction. The conditions of reaction were initial denaturing step at 94°C for 10 minutes following by 40 cycles of 30 seconds at 94°C, 1 minute at 55°C and 30 seconds at 72°C. A final extension step at 72°C was carried out for 10 minutes.

Second PCR Round

Five microliters of 10x Mg^{++} taq PCR buffer, 1 mM of DNTPs, 1 U *Taq* DNA polymerase (Genscript, NJ, USA), 5 pM of each forward and reverse primers (forward 5'CCA CCC GTG GTG CCA GCT CC3' and reverse 5'CCC GCT CCT CCT GAG CAC CC3') (Invitrogen, Sao Paulo, Brazil) [16] and 1 μL of DNA template from first PCR step were used to a total volume of 50 μL reaction. The conditions of reaction were: initial denaturing step at 94ºC for 10 minutes followed by 40 cycles of 30 seconds at 94°C, 1 minute at 60°C and 30 seconds at 72ºC. A final extension step at 72°C was carried out for 10 minutes.

All PCR reactions were performed in a Peltier Thermal Cycler (MJ Research, Waltham, MA, USA).

Agarosis Gel Electrophoresis

Ten microliters of second PCR reaction was electrophoresed in 2% agarosis gel stained with ethidium bromide (0.5 μg/mL) and then examined under UV light using molecular weight ladder as reference. The referred primers resulted in a DNA fragment of 159 base pairs.

Cytomegalovirus Immunohistochemistry

Tissue Preparation and Antigen Retrieval

The formalin-fixed fragment tissue was dehydrated following standard histotechnical protocol and then paraffin-embedded. The blocks containing fragment tissue were sectioned in microtome (6 μm) and sections transferred to silane pre-treated slides (Sigma-Aldrich, MO, USA). The slides were dewaxed by immersion in xylol, rehydrated and washed with phosphate-buffered-saline (PBS). The antigen retrieval was carried out by incubation of slides in citrate buffer (sodium citrate, pH 6.0) at 95°C for 50 minutes in water-bath.

Immunohistochemistry

To avoid interference by unspecific binding, the slides containing the tissue sections were incubated with 1% bovine serum albumin (BSA) in PBS for 15 minutes. The tissue section was covered with monoclonal antibodies against cytomegalovirus (C-10 and C-11, Biotest, Frankfurt, Germany) and incubated at 37°C for 2 hours in humid chamber. The slides were washed 3 times with PBS and immersed in methanol containing 0.3% of hydrogen peroxide for 15 minutes to block endogenous peroxidase activity.

The slides were washed 3 times with PBS and tissue sections covered with rabbit anti-mouse horseradish conjugate (Z0456, Dako, Copenhagen, Denmark) and incubated at 37°C for 1 hour in humid chamber. The slides were washed 3 times and covered with goat anti-rabbit horseradish conjugate (81-6120, Zymed, CA, USA) and incubated at 37°C for 1 hours in humid chamber. The slides were washed in PBS and reaction revealed by incubation with amino-ethyl-carbazole containing 0.03% of hydrogen peroxide for 30 minutes in dark room. The slides were washed with deionized water, counterstained with Harris´s hematoxylin and examined under light microscope (Leica DM2000, Wetzlar, Germany). The cells stained in brown were considered to be positive for cytomegalovirus antigens. Cytomegalovirus-negative tissue and cytomegalovirus-positive tissue biopsied from a HIV-infected patient with gastrointestinal cytomegalovirus disease was employed to each bath of reaction as negative and positive quality control, respectively.

Morphological Analysis

One slide of each tissue fragment was stained by Giemsa for histopathological examination. The total area of the slides was examined under light microscope (Leica

DM2000, Wetzlar, Germany) and classified by type of infiltrate (chronic or acute) and scores of infiltration intensity.

The scores of infiltration were classified as following: 0 = absence of infiltrate, 1 = discrete infiltratation (few inflammatory cells near to the junction tissue), 2 = moderate infiltration (many inflammatory cells scattered by overall of the tissue) and 3 = intense infiltration (more than 1/3 of tissue cells are inflammatory type). [18]

Statistical Analysis

Data were presented by descriptive analysis and statistical analysis of categorical variables was performed by chi-squired or Fisher's exact test.

Results

DNA quantification, and 260/280 and 260/230 absorbance ratios were considered satisfactory to PCR analysis in all the samples. PCR to beta-globin gene was positive in all the DNA samples extracted from periodontal tissues indicating good quality DNA extraction and absence of PCR inibithors.

All samples collected from periodontitis affected patients presented chronic infiltrate in different scores. The percentages of scores 0, 1, 2 and 3 were 0, 21, 21 and 58%, respectively. Samples collected from healthy subjects as expected presented no significant level of infiltration.

Cytomegalovirus DNA was detected in 30% (6/20) of periodontitis affected patients and was undetected in healthy subjects ($p=0.04$). Differences on the positivity concerning sex, age, probing depth and degree of inflammation were not statistically significant.

None of the samples were positive to cytomegalovirus antigen by immunohistochemical analysis. Negative and positive controls showed results as expected.

Discussion

Some authors have suggested that herpes viruses especially cytomegalo- virus could play a role in the pathogenesis of human periodotitis. [3-5] Immune system cells harboring herpes viruses in the periodontal inflamed sites could contribute to development and evolution of periodontitis. [11-13]

In a Brazilian cohort, Casarin *et al.* (2010) [19] found 37-39.1% of positive cases to cytomegalovirus by PCR in diabetes type 2 and Imbronito et al. (2008), [20] described 50% of CMV positive cases in non-diabetes individuals diagnosed with chronic periodontitis. Chalabi et al. (2008) [21] found cytomegalovirus DNA in 59% of patients but only when the probing depth was lower than 6 mm. However, in this chapter, no correlation was found with probing depth and presence of cytomegalovirus DNA. Bilichodmath et al. (2009) [22] found 26.3% of cytomegalovirus DNA in chronic periodontitis affected patients. Grenier et al.

(2009) [23] and Watanabe et al. (2007) [24] reported lower frequencies, 11% and 6% of cytomegalovirus DNA, respectively.

Obviously, to compare different studies, many factors must be considered such as sample size, sensitivity of primers designed to PCR, systemic disease, immunosenescence, ethnical origin and whether periodontitis type was chronic or aggressive. In addition, apical and marginal periodontitis should be considered distinctly of one another.

Cytomegalovirus has the potential to suppress indirectly the antigen specific cytotoxic T cells. By infecting other types of cells in the periodontal tissue which can release cytokines influencing T-CD8+ cells, it can cause a decrease in the number of T CD8+ cells affecting cells mediated immune functions. The immunosuppressive effect related to direct damage of lymphocytes inducing production of auto-antibodies and inflammatory mediators have also been described. [11]

A model described as 'herpes viral-bacterial pathogen' was proposed in which herpes viral infection could facilitate the bacterial proliferation and its virulence or induce the release of cytokines and chemokynes from inflammatory cells and connective tissue. [13, 25]

Cytopathic effects, immune evasion, immunopathogenicity, latency, reactivation and cellular tropism are the most important aspects related to herpes virus concerning periodontitis. Among several processes, activation of T cells and osteoclasts could be important to inflammation and bone resorption. [26] Cells harboring cytomegalovirus could play a role in the pathogenesis of chronic periodontitis. However, in this chapter, the samples were not positive to expression of cytomegalovirus antigen by immunohistochemistry in epithelial cells, connective tissue and inflammatory cells. Usually, viral antigens are not significantly expressed in latent states. On the other hand, active infection expresses high levels of viral antigen detectable by immunohistochemistry.

Relatively, few studies based on antigen detection, [27, 28] analyses of the RNA and quantitative PCR [29, 30] have been reported. The presence of antigens, viral DNA transcription and high viral load on the samples are more closely related to active infection than qualitative methods.

Sabóia-Dantas et al. (2007) [27] demonstrated that CMV was significantly more frequent in apical periodontitis lesions from HIV-positive patients (67%) than in lesions from HIV-negative patients (8%) Sunde et al. (2008) [29] did not find cytomegalovirus antigen in a cohort of apical periodontitis affected patients. Sabeti et al. (2009) [28] found CMV infection in 67% samples from periapical lesions, in 40% of periapical monocytes/macrophages and in 54% periapical T lymphocytes, but not in periapical B lymphocytes.

Most of the studies are concerned with PCR as first method to cytomegalovirus detection in DNA extracted from tissue and crevicular fluid. Qualitative PCR has received several critics when used for diagnosis of viral antigens, which can cause latent infection in the host. The higher sensitivity of PCR can detect low viral load in cells harboring virus in latent states and it could explain the presence of cytomegalovirus DNA in the samples. The presence of cytomegalovirus DNA could merely indicate the higher amount of inflammatory cells, which are a natural reservoir of this virus. The absence of cytomegalovirus DNA in the healthy samples could also be explained by the lesser amount of inflammatory cells, which are a target to cytomegalovirus latency. The presence of cytomegalovirus in saliva is also an important factor to be considered. Although the samples were washed several times with saline solution to remove contaminants, the contamination of the tissue samples with saliva cannot be completely discarded.

Although the periodontal inflammatory infiltrate harboring latent cytomegalovirus could be the most probable hypothesis, this data should be evaluated carefully. The positive and negative control to the immunohisto- chemistry resulted as expected and it can be an indicative of well-controlled reaction conditions. However, other types of monoclonal antibodies could be used as well as other techniques for detection of antigen-antibody binding such as direct immunofluorescent assay, flow cytometry and western blot. In addition, other molecular methods distinctly of qualitative PCR such as real time PCR and *in situ* hybridization could be carried out to confirm this finding.

Cytomegalovirus can reactivate transiently and intermittently in the host and the evaluation in a single sample of each patient cannot discard completely the reactivation of cytomegalovirus. Other herpes viruses such as HSV, EBV, HHV-6 and HHV-7 in periodontitis are still under investigation using molecular and immunological techniques.

Conclusion

Herpes viruses could play a role on the pathogenesis of human periodontitis. However, the data suggest presence of cytomegalovirus in latent infection instead of active infection. The association of cytomegalovirus as well as another herpes viruses remain to be better investigated.

References

[1] Zambon J. J., Haraszthy V. I., Hariharan G., Lally E. T., Demuth D. R. The microbiology of early-onset periodontitis: association of highly toxic Actinobacillus actinomycetemcomitans strains with localized juvenile periodontitis. *J Periodontol.* 1996;67:282-290.

[2] Haffajee A. D., Socransky S. S. Microbial etiological agents of destruc- tive periodontal diseases. *Periodontol* 2000. 1994;5:78-111.

[3] Contreras A., Nowzari H., Slots J. Herpes virus in periodontal pocket and gingival tissue specimens. *Oral Microbiol Immunol.* 2000;15:15-18.

[4] Cassai E., Galvan M., Trombelli L., Rotola A. HHV-6, HHV-7, HHV-8 in gingival biopsies from chronic adult periodontitis patients. *J Clin Periodontal.* 2003;30:184-191.

[5] Rotola A., Cassai E., Farina R., Caselli V., Lazzarotto T., Trombelli L. Human herpes virus 7, Epstein-Barr virus and human cytomegalovirus in periodontal tissue of periodontally diseased and healthy subjects. *J Clin Periodontal.* 2008;35:831-837.

[6] Ihira M., Yoshikawa T., Suzuki K. et al. Correlation between human herpes virus 6 and 7 infections after living related liver transplantation. *Microbio. Immunol.* 2001;45(3): 225-232.

[7] Mendez J. C., Dockrell D. H., Espy M. J. et al. Human β-Herpes virus interactions in solid organ transplant recipients. *J Infect Dis.* 2001; 183:179-184.

[8] Feldstein A. E., Razonable R. R., Boyce T. G. et al. Prevalence and clinical significance of human herpes virus 6 and 7 active infection in pediatric liver transplant patients. *Pedriatr Transp.* 2003;7:125-129.

[9] Peigo M. F., Thomasini R. L., Puglia A. L. P., Costa S. C. B., Bonon S. H. A., Boin I. F. S. Human herpes virus-7 in Brazilian liver transplant recipients: a follow-up comparison between molecular and immuno- logical assays. *Transpl Infect Dis.* 2009; 11:497-502.

[10] Contreras A., Madirossian A., Slots J. Herpes viruses in HIV-periodontitis. *J Clin Periodontol.* 2001;28:96-102.

[11] Contreras A., Umeda M., Chen C., Bakker I., Morrison J. L., Slots J. Relationship between herpes virus and adult periodontitis and periodontopathic bacteria. *J Perio dontol.* 1999;70:478–484.

[12] Kamma J. J., Slots J. Herpesviral–bacterial interactions in aggressive periodontitis. *J Clin Periodontol.* 2003;30:1–6.

[13] Slots J. Herpesviral – bacterial synergy in the pathogenesis of human periodontitis. *Curr Opin Infect Dis.* 2007;20:278–283.

[14] Slots J. Human viruses in periodontitis. *Periodontol* 2000. 2010;53:89-110.

[15] Armitage G. C. Development of a classification system for periodontal diseases and conditions. *Ann Periodontl.* 1999;4:1-6.

[16] Demmler G. J., Buffone C. J., Schimbor C. M. et al. Detection of cytomegalovirus in urine newbornes by using polymerase chain reaction DNA amplification. *J Infect Dis.* 1988;158:1177-1184.

[17] Cassai E., Galvan M., Trombelli L., Rotola A. HHV-6, HHV-7, HHV-8 in gingival biopsies from chronic adult periodontitis patients. *J Clin Periodontal.* 2003;30:184-191.

[18] Liu R., Bal H. S., Desta T., Krothapalli N., Alyassi M., Luan Q., Graves D. T. Diabetes Enhances Periodontal Bone Loss through Enhanced Resorption and Diminished Bone Formation. *J Dent Res.* 2006;85:510.

[19] Casarin R. C. V., Duarte P. M., Santos V. R., Lima J. A., Gagnon G., Casati M. Z. et al. Influence of glycemic control and Epstein-Bar and Cytomegalovirus infection in periodontal pocket of type 2 diabetic subjects. *Arch Oral Biol.* 2010;55:902-906.

[20] Imbronito A. V., Okuda O. S., Freitas N. M., Lotufo F. M., Nunes F. D. Detection of Herpes viruses and periodontal pathogens in subgingival plaque of patients with chronic periodontitis, generalized aggressive periodontitis, or gingivitis. *J Periodontol.* 2008;79 (2):2313-2321.

[21] Chalabi M., Moghin S., Mogharehabed A., Najafi F., Rezaie F. EBV and CMV chronic periodontitis: a prevalence study. *Arch Virol.* 2008; 153:1917-1919.

[22] Bilichodmath S., Mangalekar S. B., Sharma D. C. G., Prabhakar A. K., Reddy S. B., Kalburgi N. B. Herpes virus in chronic and aggressive periodontitis patientsin an Indian population. *J Oral Sci.* 2009;51:79-86.

[23] Grenier G., Gagnon G., Grenier D. Detection of herpetic viruses in gingival crevicular fluid of patients suffering from periodontal diseases: prevalence and effect of treatment. *Oral Microbiol Immunol.* 2009;24:506-509.

[24] Watanabe S. A., Correia-Silva J. F., Horta M. C. R., Costa J. E., Gomez R. S. EBV-1 and HCMV in aggressive periodontitis in Brazilian patients. *Braz. Oral Res.* 2007;21 (4):336-341.

[25] Slots J., Kamma J. J., Sugar C. The herpes virus-Porphyromonas gingivalis-periodontitis axis. *J Periodontol Res.* 2003;38:318-232.

[26] Slots J. Oral viral infections of adults. *Periodontol* 2000. 2009;49:60-86.

[27] Sabóia-Dantas C. J., Coutrin T. L. F., Sampaio-Filho H. R., Siqueira J. R. J. F. Herpes virus in asymptomatic apical periodontitis lesions: an immnunohistochemical approach. *Oral Microbiol Immunol.* 2007;22: 320-325.

[28] Sabeti M., Daneshmand A., Simon J. H., Slots J. Cytomegalovirus-infected inflammatory cells in dental periapical lesions. *Oral Microbiol Immunol.* 2009;24:434–436.

[29] Botero J. E., Contreras A., Parra B. Effects of cytomegalovirus infection on the mRNA expression of collagens and matrix metalloproteinases in gingival fibroblasts. *J Periodontal Res.* 2008;43(6):649-57.

[30] Sunde P. T., Olsen I., Enersen M., Beiske K., Grinde B. Human cytomegalovirus and Epstein-Barr virus in apical and marginal periodontitis: a role in pathology? *J Med Virol.* 2008;80:1007-1011.

In: Current Trends in Periodontics and Implant Dentistry ISBN: 978-1-62618-819-8
Editors: Vishal Anand and Minkle Gulati

Chapter XIII

Mechanical Periodontal Therapy in Chronic Periodontitis Patients with Postmenopausal Osteoporosis Using Alendronate

Leyla Kuru[1], Ebru Rabia Toprakseven[1], Ülkü Noyan[1], Tanju Kadir[2] and Bahar Eren Kuru[1,*]

[1]Department of Periodontology, Dental Faculty,
Marmara University, Istanbul, Turkey
[2]Department of Basic Science, Division of Microbiology,
Dental Faculty, Marmara University, Istanbul, Turkey

Abstract

The objective of this chapter was to present the effect of mechanical periodontal treatment on clinical, microbiological and radiological parameters in chronic periodontitis patients with postmenopausal osteoporosis using oral alendronate. A total of 20 female patients were included. All of the patients were diagnosed as postmenopausal osteoporosis with a T score ≤ -2.5 and defined to be in need of alendronate treatment by their gynecologists. The test group (n=10) consisted of patients who confirmed to undergo oral alendronate treatment whereas the control group (n=10) was made up with patients refusing any type of medication. Both of the groups received mechanical periodontal therapy. At baseline and 6 months after periodontal treatment, periodontal condition was assessed, subgingival microbial samples were evaluated by culturing, bone mineral density (BMD) of lumbar spine, femur and mandible was analysed by dual energy xray absorptiometry and mandibular cortical width (MCW) was measured by dental panoramic radiographs. Clinical evaluation revealed statistically significant periodontal improvements within both groups ($p<0.01$). Intergroup comparisons revealed

* Marmara Üniversitesi Dişhekimliği Fakültesi Periodontoloji A. D. Büyükçiftlik sok. No 6 Nişantaşı 34365 İstanbul, Türkiye, Phone (business): 00 90 212 231 91 20/514. Fax: 00 90 212 246 52 47. E-mail: bkuru@marmara.edu.tr.

a statistically significant difference for sulcus bleeding index only ($p<0.05$). The proportion of obligate anaerobes decreased significantly in both groups ($p<0.05$), however, no significant difference was found between the groups. While BMDs were decreased in the control group, significant increases were observed in the test group ($p<0.01$). Similarly, the MCW increased in the test group but decreased in the control group. Furthermore, a significant positive relationship was detected between the mandibular BMD and MCW ($p<0.05$). The results presented in this chapter suggest that oral alendronate therapy may have an adjunctive effect to mechanical periodontal treatment in terms of resolution of gingival inflammation in postmenopausal women with chronic periodontitis and osteoporosis. In addition, no side effect of orally administered alendronate was observed during this period.

Keywords: Alendronate, bone density, chronic periodontitis, osteoporosis

Introduction

Periodontitis is a chronic inflammatory disease affecting the periodontal tissues including gingiva, cementum, periodontal ligament and alveolar bone, often accompanied by significant bone loss. While mild to moderate forms of periodontal disease affect a majority of adults, a total of 5 to 20% of the population has severe, generalized periodontitis. [1] The pathogenesis involves predominantly Gram-negative bacteria in a biofilm that initiates a localized inflammatory host reaction, leading to release of inflammatory mediators, destruction of attachment apparatus, periodontal pocket formation and alveolar bone resorption and, ultimately tooth loss. [2] Osteoporosis, a chronic disease characterised by low bone mass and deterioration of the microarchitecture of the skeletal tissue predisposing to increased risk of fracture, [3] has been estimated to develop in 1 out of 4 women over the age of 50 years. [4] It is characterized by low bone mineral density (BMD), measured as 2.5 standard deviations below the mean value of peak bone mass in gender- and race-matched young adults. [5]

In recent years, there has been ever increasing interest in the relationship between periodontitis and systemic osteoporosis both of which are closely associated with advanced age and accompanied by bone loss. [6-9] Smoking and certain diseases and medications that may interfere with healing also appear to be relevant risk factors, [6, 10] while common etiological agents affect their natural history. [11] Additionally, osteoporosis has been considered to be a risk factor for the progression of periodontal disease and loss of teeth. [12-15] Postmenopausal studies also suggest a positive association of osteoporosis with_clinical signs of periodontitis or periodontal disease severity, [7, 8, 16-18] periodontal infection with at least one of the five established periodontal pathogens, [19] lower BMD and tooth loss. [13, 14] In a recent review, it has been suggested that reduced BMD in osteoporosis patients is a shared risk factor for periodontitis rather than a causal factor. [9]

A number of studies of periodontal therapy in experimental models have demonstrated that systemically administrated bisphosphonates, which inhibit the activity of bone-resorbing osteoclast cells *in vitro*, significantly inhibit alveolar bone loss *in vivo*. [20-25] Additionally, in a clinical trial using the bisphosphonate risedronate, postmenopausal women with osteoporosis showed significantly less plaque accumulation, gingival inflammation and alveolar bone loss. [26] However, while the aminobisphosphonate alendronate has also been reported to have anti-inflammatory and antibacterial properties, [21, 27] the effects of this drug along with periodontal treatment on clinical parameters including gingival inflammation and microbial dental plaque are much less certain. [22, 28] In recent clinical studies, the efficacy of alendronate gel as an adjunctive local drug delivery system to mechanical periodontal treatment in patients with chronic periodontitis or aggressive periodontitis have been investigated and revealcd promising clinical outcomes. [29, 30] Thus, futher studies are warranted on the potential role for alendronate as an adjunct to conventional periodontal therapy. [28, 31-33] This chapter was therefore written to present the clinical, microbiological and radiographical effects of alendronate orally administred during mechanical periodontal treatment in patients with chronic periodontitis and postmenopausal osteoporosis.

Materials and Methods

Study Population

Twenty non-smoking women, 50 to 65 years old (mean age 56.2 ±3.8 years) with chronic periodontitis and postmenopausal osteoporosis were included. Inclusion criteria were females between ages 50-65 and within 10 years of menopause, diagnosed as having (1) postmenopausal osteoporosis with a T score $\leq$ -2.5 (5); and (2) chronic periodontitis based on clinical and radiographic evaluations, [34] having a minimum of 15 teeth and at least 3 single rooted teeth with probing depth (PD)$\geq$5 mm. Exclusion criteria included any systemic disease other than osteoporosis, treatment with glucocorticoids, NAIDS, hormone replacement therapy, antibiotics or periodontal treatment within the last 6 months, any drug known to affect periodontal tissues or to alter bone calcium metabolism.

A total of 276 women were screened from new referrals to the Medical Faculty of Marmara University. Twenty-five out of 54 patients eligible according to the inclusion criteria, accepted to attend the investigation. Five were excluded due to the intake of antibiotics for reasons not related to periodontal treatment.

The patients in the test group (n=10) were treated with mechanical periodontal therapy and started to use oral alendronate (Fosamax, 70 mg, once a week, Merck Sharp Dohme S.p.A., Pavia, Italy) on day 0, while the control group patients (n=10) who refused to use oral alendronate were treated with mechanical periodontal therapy only.

The protocol was approved by the Ethics Commitee of the Medical Faculty, Marmara University, and conducted in accordance with the ethical standards of the Helsinki Declaration. All the procedures were described thoroughly to the patients and the informed consent was signed by each of them.

Clinical Periodontal Assessment

At baseline, the age, height and weight of all subjects were recorded, and body mass index (BMI) was calculated as weight divided by the square of height (kg/m^2). Periodontal assesment was performed at baseline and 6 months after mechanical periodontal treatment. The following measurements were taken by an investigator other than those treating the patients: plaque index (PI), sulcus bleeding index (SBI), PD and relative attachment level

(RAL). PI was assessed at four locations for each tooth (mesio-buccal, mid-buccal, distobuccal and mid-lingual/palatal aspects) as described by Silness and Löe. [35] The appearance of gingiva and existence of gingival bleeding upon gentle probing were evaluated according to Mühlemann and Son [36] and assigning a score of 0 to 5 for SBI, with 0 indicating a healthy appearance and no bleeding. PD and RAL were measured with a periodontal probe (PCPUNC15, Hu-Friedy Ins. Co, USA) using an individual occlusal stent as a reference point for probe placement.

Periodontal Therapy

Mechanical periodontal treatment included oral hygiene instructions, scaling and root planing, removal of iatrogenic factors and occlusal adjustment. Patients were advised to brush their teeth using a modified Bass method and use dental floss for interdental cleaning. Scaling and root planing procedures were performed using ultrasonic (Cavitron® EMZ, Nyon, Switzerland) and hand instruments (Gracey curets, SG 3/4, 7/8, 11/12, 13/14, Hu-Friedy Ins. Co., Chicago, IL, USA) on days 0 (baseline) and 7. Oral hygiene instructions were re-inforced when necessary during the 6 months period.

Microbial Sampling and Assessment

Following the gentle removal of supragingival plaque and drying, microbiological samples were obtained at baseline and 6 months using a sterile paper point #40 inserted to the depth of the pocket of periodontal sites which had an initial PD $\geq$5 mm. Sample preparation and culturing were carried out. [37, 38] Briefly, each sample was aseptically transferred to 4.5 ml of PBS (phosphate buffered saline), immediately homogenized using a vortex mixer at maximal setting for 30 s and then serially tenfold diluted. From each dilutions (10^{-1},10^{-2}, … 10^{-5}) two portions of 0.1 ml were taken and plated sperately onto trypticase soy agar (Oxoid) medium supplemented with 5% defibrinated sheep blood, 0.0005% hemin (Sigma) and 0.00005% menadione (Sigma).

The first trypticase soy agar plate was incubated anaerobically at 37°C for 7 to 10 days in Gas Pak Jars (AnaerogenGen kit, Oxoid), while the other was incubated at 37°C in 5% CO_2 for 4 days. The total viable count (TVC) was determined as the total number of bacterial colonies on plates anaerobically incubated. All the microbiologic data were transformed into colony forming units/milliliter (CFU/ml) of transport medium. In addition, obligate anaerobic bacteria was calculated as the TVC minus the total counts of colonies on plates incubated in 5% CO_2 condition and expressed as a percentage of TVC. Samples were taken from 3 periodontal sites of each participant.

Radiological Measurements

BMD (g/cm^2) was measured at the lumbar spine (L2 to L4), proximal femur (neck, Ward's triangle and trochanter) and mandible using DEXA (I'acn Unigamma X-ray Plus, Milano, Italy) at baseline and 6 months. The mandibular BMD was also assessed by DEXA using the method described by Horner et al. [39] Dental panoramic radiographs were taken for all subjects and the mandibular cortical width (MCW) below the mental foramen was measured bilaterally at baseline and 6 months, according to Taguchi et al. [40]

Table 1. Demographic data of patients at baseline

	Test Group	Control Group	p
Number of subjects (n)	10	10	-
Age (years)	56.00 ± 3.68	56.60 ± 4.38	NS
BMI (kg/m^2)	25.26 ± 4.09	25.78 ± 2.49	NS
Number of missing teeth	4.00 ± 2.40	5.90 ± 2.72	NS

Mann-Whitney U test, p 0.05
Numbers are given as mean ± standard deviation
BMI= body mass index
NS= not significant

Statistical Analysis

SPSS for Windows, (Release 10.0, SPSS Inc., USA) was used for all data analyses. *P* values < 0.05 were considered statistically significant. Lack of significance is indicated by not significant (NS). Full-mouth means were the basis for periodontal data analysis. The means for each periodontal parameter was also calculated separately for periodontal sites selected for microbial sampling. Three microbial samples from each patient were examined separately and the mean was calculated on per-patient basis. Comparisons between the groups were carried out using the Mann-Whitney U test, and comparisons between the baseline and 6 months within each group were performed using the Wilcoxon test. Associations between clinical and radiological parameters were evaluated using the Pearson Correlation test.

Results

Patient characteristics and baseline periodontal parameters of the test and control groups were similar and there were no statistically significant differences between the groups ($p>0.05$) (Table 1, 2). All clinical measurements including PI, SBI, PD and RAL improved significantly in both groups ($p<0.01$), however only the change of SBI within the test group was found to be significantly different than that of the control group ($p<0.05$). Moreover, this occurred both in full mouth values as well as in periodontal sites with initial PD ≥5 mm.

The number of total anaerobically grown microorganisms expressed as TVC showed significant reductions in both groups ($p<0.05$) (Table 3). While the proportion of obligate anaerobes in TVC decreased significantly in both groups after 6 months compared with their respective baseline values ($p<0.05$), facultative anaerobes concommitantly increased ($p<0.05$) (Table 3). However, no significant differences were found between the groups ($p>0.05$).

As shown in Table 4, the BMD of the lumbar spine, femur and mandible all increased at 6 months in the test group ($p<0.01$). In contrast, decreases were observed in all BMD levels in the control group, with a statistical significance only in the femur BMD ($p<0.01$). Intergroup comparison revealed significant differences in the BMD changes between the groups at 6 months (p<0.01). Thus, positive correlations were found between the BMD of spine versus BMD of femur and mandible (Table 5). In addition, while the MCW of the test group increased, it decreased in the control group with no significant difference between the groups (Table 4). However, a significant positive relationship was detected between the mandibular BMD and the MCW (p<0.05) (Table 5). No correlations were found between the clinical periodontal parameters and radiographic measures (data not shown).

Table 2. Comparison of clinical periodontal parameters of the all sites and the sites with PD≥5 mm between the groups at baseline and changes after 6 months

		Test Group (mean ± SD)	Control Group (mean ± SD)	p
PI- Full mouth	baseline	1.75 ± 0.28	2.05 ± 0.52	NS
	change	-1.28 ± 0.36	-1.41 ± 0.58	NS
PI- PD≥5 mm	baseline	2.07 ± 0.49	2.43 ± 0.56	NS
	change	-1.14 ± 0.75	-1.52 ± 0.54	NS
SBI- Full mouth	baseline	2.36 ± 0.55	1.85 ± 0.47	NS
	change	-1.63 ± 0.60	-1.16 ± 0.42	<0.05
SBI- PD≥5 mm	baseline	3.43 ± 0.72	2.95 ± 0.69	NS
	change	-1.76 ± 0.76	-1.11 ± 0.52	<0.05
PD- Full mouth	baseline	2.66 ± 0.52	2.95 ± 0.41	NS
	change	-0.83 ± 0.41	-1.04 ± 0.35	NS
PD- PD≥5 mm	baseline	5.23 ± 0.23	5.44 ± 0.19	NS
	change	-2.01 ± 0.73	-2.60 ± 0.91	NS
RAL- Full mouth	baseline	6.61 ± 0.73	7.24 ± 0.74	NS
	change	-0.64 ± 0.66	-0.86 ±0.40	NS
RAL- PD≥5 mm	baseline	8.39 ± 0.85	9.07 ± 0.41	NS
	change	-1.69 ± 0.65	-1.51 ± 0.68	NS

Mann-Whitney U test, p 0.05.

Table 3. Comparison of TVC (x10[4] CFU/ml), proportions of obligate and facultative anaerobes (expressed as % of tvc) of subgingival microbial samples before and 6 months after therapy

	Test Group			Control Group		
	baseline	**6 month**	**p**	**baseline**	**6 month**	**p**
TVC Mean	28.9	0.8	<0.05	21.1	1.3	<0.05
Range	0.2-170.6	0.04-2.5		0.3-90.1	0.7-4.3	
Obligate anaerobe Mean	60.5	5.4	<0.01	81.3	8.9	<0.01
Range	0-99.9	0-21.4		24.2-99.9	0-30.2	
Facultative anaerobe Mean	39.5	94.6	<0.01	18.7	91.0	<0.01
Range	0.1-100	78.6-100		0.1-99.9	69.8-100	

Wilcoxon test, p 0.05.

Table 4. Changes in BMDs of lumbar spine, femur and mandible, and MCW in both groups

	Bone mineral density (gr/cm^2)		
	Alendronate group (mean ± SD)	**Control group (mean ± SD)**	**p$^{\Delta}$**
Lumbar spine baseline	0.83 ± 0.05	0.91 ± 0.10	NS
6 month	0.90 ± 0.07	0.89 ± 0.12	-
change	0.07 ± 0.05	-0.02 ± 0.04	<0.01
p^{+}	<0.01	NS	
Femur baseline	0.51 ± 0.18	0.70 ± 0.20	NS
6 month	0.64 ± 0.20	0.64 ± 0.21	-
change	0.12 ± 0.07	-0.06 ± 0.07	<0.01
p^{+}	<0.01	<0.01	
Mandible baseline	1.38 ± 0.18	1.37 ± 0.26	NS
6 month	1.55 ± 0.16	1.33 ± 0.24	-
change	0.17 ± 0.13	-0.04 ± 0.03	<0.01
p^{+}	<0.01	NS	
Mandibular cortical width (mm)			
baseline	4.10 ± 0.81	3.94 ± 0.67	NS
6 month	4.15 ± 0.81	3.84 ± 0.75	NS
change	0.03 ± 8.10	-0.09 ± 0.24	NS
p^{+}	NS	NS	

NS= not significant.

$^{+}$Comparison within the group (Wilcoxon test).

$^{\Delta}$ Comparison between the groups (Mann-Whitney U test).

P 0.05.

Table 5. Correlations of radiographic measurements

		BMD Spine	BMD Femur	BMD Mandible	MCW
BMD Spine	r		0.554	0.480	0.088
	p		**0.032**	**0.011**	0.714
BMD Femur	r	0.480		0.390	0.051
	p	**0.032**		0.089	0.83
BMD Mandible	r	0.554	0.390		0.488
	p	**0.011**	0.089		**0.029**
MCW	r	0.088	0.051	0.488	
	p	0.714	0.83	**0.029**	

BMD= bone mineral density.

MCW= mandibular cortical width.

Discussion

Both periodontal disease and osteoporosis are major health concerns in older populations. Although osteoporosis is not an etiological factor for periodontitis, it may influence the severity of existing periodontal disease in a host with poor bone resistance. [12, 18] On the other hand, periodontitis has been found to be a strong and independent predictor for incident tooth loss in postmenopausal women. [41] As the population ages, the impact of both periodontitis and osteoporosis will be more profound. Pharmacotherapy for osteoporosis has been focused mainly on interventions that could reverse excessive bone resorption. One alternative is the use of bisphosphonates, non-biodegradable analogs of pyrophosphates that include potent inhibitors of bone resorption and have a high affinity for calcium.

Therefore, they bind to calcified bone matrix and then are taken up by osteoclasts, leading to their inactivation and programmed cell death. [20] Alendronate has been shown to be effective in increasing or maintaining BMD in early postmenopausal women [42] and to reduce significantly vertebral and non-vertebral fractures among women with osteoporosis. [43, 44] In addition to several uses of bisphosphonates, a recent attention has been drawn to their potential use in the management of periodontal disease-associated bone loss. [24-26, 28-31] Reddy et al. [22] suggested a combined approach of conventional periodontal therapy and alendronate administration which may provide a strong adjunctive effect in the management of periodontitis.

Mechanical periodontal treatment including thorough removal of supra- and subgingival bacterial deposits by scaling and root planing is the main step of periodontal therapy and the first recommended approach to the control of periodontal infections. [45] This treatment is still considered to be the gold standard to which other treatment methods are compared. In addition to obtaining a high level of personal oral hygiene, scaling and root planing clinically induces PD reduction, decrease in the number of gingival sites with bleeding on probing, attachment gain, and a shift from a predominantly Gram-negative obligate anaerobe to a Gram-positive subgingival microbiota. [37, 46, 47] In this chapter, alendronate administred as an adjunct to mechanical treatment revealed significant improvements in all clinical parameters with respect to baseline values, as expected. The significantly low SBI values found in the test group is consistent with previous cross-sectional and prospective studies showing improved levels of gingival inflammation. [26, 29, 30, 33] One possible mechanism for significantly less gingival inflammation is that alendronate may reduce the activity of matrix metalloproteinases, [48] particularly by inhibiting matrix metalloproteinase-8 expression [49] and increasing tissue inhibitor of metalloproteinase-1 expression [49] thereby decreasing collagen breakdown. The low SBI level can also be explained by decreased activity of myeloperoxidase, a lysosomal enzyme most abundantly present in neutrophil granulocytes producing cytotoxic agents. [21]

Microbiological findings of this chapter showed that high proportion of obligate anaerobes were present in subgingival flora of deep periodontal pockets in postmenopausal osteoporotic women. Although bacterial species were not identified in this chapter, established periodontal pathogens *Prevotella intermedia*, *Tannerella forsythia*, *Porphyromonas gingivalis* and *Fusobacterium nucleatum* in the red or orange complexes described by Socransky et al [50] are obligate anaerobic microorganism. Thus, it is likely that the proportion of periodontopathogen bacteria decreased significantly 6 months after mechanical treatment in both the groups. On the other hand, periodontal treatment resulted in a subgingival flora with high proportion of facultative anaerobes. A body of evidence indicates that mechanical therapy is relatively effective in suppressing periodontal pathogens and in promoting clinical improvement. [47] However, any additional effect of oral alendronate was not obtained on the number and proportions of microorganisms in subgingival plaque within the limits of patient population and investigation period.

Significant reductions in obligate anaerobes were attributed to the positive antimicrobial effect of mechanical scaling and root planing procedures.

BMD measurements are being used today routinely to diagnose osteoporosis. Although bisphosphonates have been established as effective pharmacologic agents for prevention and treatment of osteoporosis [42, 51] role of antiresorptive drugs including alendronate on BMD and MCW of the mandible has attracted little attention. [52] The present chapter demonstrated that 6-month alendronate use resulted in significant gain of BMD levels of spine, femur as well as mandible. In this chapter, the mandibular BMD was found to correlate with the BMD of lumbar spine in accordance with previous findings. [53-55]

Dental panoramic radiographs have been investigated for their potential use in detecting low BMDs so that on a routine dental examination dentists might be able to identify postmenopausal women with increased risk of osteoporosis. [40, 56] On the other hand, MCW has been found to be associated with lumbar BMD suggesting the possibility that cortical width may not reflect the increased bone turnover after menopause but rather peak bone mass in young age. [40] In addition, the sensitivity and specificity of MCW were reported to increase when its assessment was combined with the mandibular cortical index based on the appearance of the lower border of mandibular inferior cortex. [57]

Dental panoramic radiographs was used for the diagnosis of periodontal disease along with the clinical periodontal examination and for the evaluation of the effect of alendronate on the height of the mandibular inferior cortex. MCW of the test group demonstrated a 0.03 ± 8.10 mm increase, whereas it decreased 0.09 ± 0.24 mm in the control group. However, this finding did not reach statistical significance, probably because of the small sample size. Nevertheless, it was found that MCW was positively correlated with the BMD of mandible but not with that of the spine or femur. This finding was in accordance with the previous study of Horner and Devlin [58] but contradicts with the findings of Taguchi et al [54] and Taguchi et al [40] who has demonstrated a strong association between the MCW and lumbar BMD. However, a recent study suggested that mandibular cortical measures on dental panoramic radiographs were associated with an increased risk of osteoporotic fracture. [59]

Recently, prominence has been given to an uncommon adverse reaction affecting the mandible and maxilla, called osteochemonecrosis of the jaw, especially in those patients with multiple myeloma or metastatic breast cancer receiving high doses of bisphosphonates as palliation for bone metastases. [60, 61] The risk of developing this severely debilitating complication is revealed to be increased in patients who underwent tooth extraction or other oral surgery, however, osteochemonecrosis was also presented in a report of a simple case who received mechanical periodontal treatment. [62] The clinical presentation of osteochemonecrosis was reported to include bone exposure, pain, suppuration and inflammation in women around 70 years of age taking alendronate for 4.5 years. [63] Nevertheless, none of the participants of the test group developed such a complication, most probably due to the relatively low potency and low dose of this drug, and lack of contributing factors, such as poor oral hygiene, older age and smoking. [62, 63] The duration of the follow-up or the administration of alendronate at the same time with the mechanical treatment treatment could be other factors influencing the result.

In conclusion, the findings in this chapter suggest that systemic oral alendronate therapy may support mechanical periodontal treatment in terms of resolution of gingival inflammation in postmenopausal women with chronic periodontitis and osteoporosis. However, the local use of this medication could be of preferable mode of administration. Further studies are warranted to clarify the effects of local administration of alendronate as an adjunct to periodontal therapy.

Acknowledgments

This study was supported by a grant from Marmara University Scientific Research Project Comission with the number SAĞ-DKR-100105-0029.

References

[1] American Academy of Periodontology. Epidemiology of periodontal diseases (position paper). *J Periodontol.* 1996;67:935-945.

[2] Carranza F. A., Camargo P. M. *The periodontal pocket.* In: Newman M. G., Takei H. H., Klokkevold P. R., Carranza F. A., editors. Carranza's clinical periodontology, 10th edn, China: Saunders Elsevier, 2006. p. 434-451.

[3] World Health Organization. Assessment of fracture risk and its application to screening for postmenopausal osteoporosis. *Report of a WHO Study Group (Technical report series).* Geneva, Switzerland: 1994;WHO:1-129.

[4] Melton L. J. 3rd, Chrischilles E. A., Cooper C., Lane A. W., Riggs B. L. Perspective. How many women have osteoporosis? *J Bone Miner Res.* 1992;7:1005-1010.

[5] Anonymous. Consensus Development Conference: diagnosis, prophy- laxis, and treatment of osteoporosis. *Am J Med.* 1993;94:646-650.

[6] Jeffcoat M. K. Osteoporosis: A possible modifying factor in oral bone loss. *Ann Periodontol.* 1998;3:312-321.

[7] Persson R. E., Hollender L. G., Powell L. V., MacEntee M. I., Wyatt C. C. L., Kiyak H. A. et al. Assessment of periodontal conditions and systemic disease in older subjects I. Focus on osteoporosis. *J Clin Perio dontol.* 2002;29:796-802.

[8] Wactawski-Wende J. Periodontal diseases and osteoporosis: Association and mechanisms. *Ann Periodontol.* 2001;6:197-208.

[9] Megson E., Kapellas K., Bartold P. M. Relationship between perio- dontal disease and osteoporosis. *Int J Evid Based Healthc.* 2010;8: 129-39.

[10] Payne J. B., Reinhardt R. A., Nummikoski P. V., Dunning D. G., Patil K. D. The association of cigarette smoking with alveolar bone loss in postmenopausal females. *J Clin Periodontol.* 2000;27:658-664.

[11] Garcia R. I., Henshaw M. M., Krall E. A. Relationship between periodontal disease and systemic health. *Periodontol* 2000. 2001;25:21-36.

[12] Payne J. B., Reinhardt R. A., Nummikoski P. V., Patil K. D. Longitudinal alveolar bone loss in postmenopausal osteoporotic/osteopenic women. *Osteoporos Int.* 1999; 10:34-40.

[13] Tezal M., Wactawski-Wende J., Grossi S. G., Ho A. W., Dunford R., Genco R. J. The relationship between bone mineral density and periodontitis in postmenopausal women. *J Periodontol.* 2000;71:1492-1498.

[14] Wactawski-Wende J., Grossi S. G., Trevisan M., Genco R. J., Tezal M., Dunford R. G. et al. The role of osteopenia in oral bone loss and periodontal disease. *J Periodontol.* 1996;67(10Suppl):1076-1084.
[15] Taguchi A., Tanimoto K., Suei Y., Otani K., Wada T. Oral signs as indicators of possible osteoporosis in elderly women. *Oral Surg Oral Med Oral Pathol Oral Radiol Endod.* 1995;80:612-616.
[16] Mohammad A. R., Brunsvold M., Bauer R. The strength of association between systemic postmenopausal osteoporosis and periodontal disease. *Int J Prosthodont.* 1996;9:479-483.
[17] Brennan R. M., Genco R. J., Hovey K. M., Trevisan M., Wactawski-Wende J. Clinical attachment loss, systemic bone density, and subgingival calculus in postmenopausal women. *J Periodontol.* 2007b; 78:2104-2111.
[18] Gomes-Filho I. S., Passos Jde S., Cruz S. S., Vianna M. I., Cerqueira Ede M., Oliveira D. C. et al. The association between postmenopausal osteoporosis and periodontal disease. *J Periodontol.* 2007;78:1731-1740.
[19] Brennan R. M., Genco R. J., Wilding G. E., Hovey K. M., Trevisan M., Wactawski-Wende J. Bacterial species in subgingival plaque and oral bone loss in postmenopausal women. *J Periodontol.* 2007a;78:1051-1061.
[20] Tennenbaum Akesson K. New approaches to pharmacological treatment of osteoporosis. *Bull World Health Organ.* 2003;8:657-664.
[21] Menezes A. M. A., Rocha F. A. C., Chaves H. V., Carvalho C. B. M., Riberio R. A., Brito G. A. C. Effect of sodium alendronate on alveolar bone resorption in experimental periodontitis in rats. *J Periodontol.* 2005;76:1901-1909.
[22] Reddy M. S., Weatherford T. W. 3rd, Smith CA, West BD, Jeffcoat M. K., Jacks T. M. Alendronate treatment of naturally-occurring periodontitis in beagle dogs. *J Periodontol.* 1995;66:211-217.
[23] Yaffe A., Iztkovich M., Earon Y., Alt I., Lilov R., Binderman I. Local delivery of an amino bisphosphonate prevents the resorptive phase of alveolar bone following mucoperiosteal flap surgery in rats. *J Periodontol.* 1997;68:884-889.
[24] Binderman I., Adut M., Yaffe A. Effectiveness of local delivery of alendronate in reducing alveolar bone loss following periodontal surgery in rats. *J Periodontol.* 2000;71:1236-1240.
[25] Goya J. A., Paez H. A., Mandalunis P. M. Effect of topical adminis- tration of monosodium olpadronate on experimental periodontitis in rats. *J Periodontol.* 2006;77:1-6.
[26] Palomo L., Bissada N. F., Liu J. Periodontal assessment of postmeno- pausal women receiving risedronate. *Menopause.* 2005; 12: 685-690.
[27] Teronen O., Heikkilä P., Konttinen Y. T., Laitinen M., Salo T., Hanemaaijer R. et al. MMP inhibition and downregulation by bisphos- phonates. *Ann N Y Acad Sci.* 1999;878:453-465.
[28] El-shinnawi U. M., El-Tantawy S. I. The effect of alendronate sodium on alveolar bone loss in periodontitis (clinical trial). *J Int Acad Perio- dontol.* 2003;5:5-10.
[29] Sharma A., Pradeep A. R. Clinical efficacy of 1% alendronate gel as a local drug delivery system in the treatment of chronic periodontitis: a randomized, controlled clinical trial. *J Periodontol.* 2012a;83:11-18.

[30] Sharma A., Pradeep A. R. Clinical efficacy of 1% alendronate gel in adjunct to mechanotherapy in the treatment of aggressive periodontitis: a randomized, controlled clinical trial. *J Periodontol.* 2012b;83:19-26.
[31] Lane N., Armitage G. C., Loomer P., Hsieh S., Majumdar S., Wang H. Y. et al. Bisphosphonate therapy improves the outcome of conventional periodontal treatment: Results of a 12-month, randomized, placebo-controlled study. *J Periodontol.* 2005;76:1113-1122.
[32] Rocha M., Nava L. E., Torre C. V., Sanchez-Marin F., Garay-Sevilla M. E., Malacara J. M. Clinical and radiographical improvement of perio- dontal disease in patients with type 2 Diabetes Mellitus treated with alendronate: A randomized, placebo-controlled trial. *J Periodontol.* 2001;72:204-209.
[33] Rocha M. L., Malacara J. M., Sánchez-Marin F. J., Vazquez de la Torre C. J., Fajardo M. E. Effect of alendronate on periodontal disease in postmenopausal women: a randomized placebo-controlled trial. *J Perio- dontol.* 2004;75:1579-1585.
[34] Armitage G. C. Development of a classification system for periodontal diseases and conditions. *Ann Periodontol.* 1999;4:1-6.
[35] Silness J., Löe H. Periodontal disease in pregnancy. II. Correlation between oral hygiene and periodontal conditioning. *Acta Odontol Scand.* 1964;22:121-135.
[36] Mühlemann H. R., Son S. Gingival sulcus bleeding: A leading symptom in initial gingivitis. *Helv Odont Acta.* 1971;15:107-112.
[37] Noyan Ü., Yilmaz S., Kuru B., Kadir T., Acar O., Büget E. A clinical and microbiological evaluation of systemic and local metronidazole delivery in adult periodontitis patients. *J Clin Periodontol.* 1997;24:158-165.
[38] Kuru B., Yilmaz S., Noyan U., Acar O., Kadir T. Microbiological features and crevicular fluid aspartate aminotransferase enzyme activity in early onset periodontitis patients. *J Clin Periodontol.* 1999;26:19-25.
[39] Horner K., Devlin H., Alsop C. W., Hodgkinson M., Adams J. E. Mandibular bone mineral density as a predictor of skeletal osteoporosis. *Br J Radiol.* 1996; 69:1019-1025.
[40] Taguchi A., Sanada M., Krall E., Nakamoto T., Ohtsuka M., Suei Y. et al. Relationship between dental panoramic radiographic findings and biochemical markers of bone turnover. *J Bone Miner Res.* 2003;18: 1689-1694.
[41] Tezal M., Wactawski-Wende J., Grossi S. G., Dmochowski J., Genco R. J. Periodontal disease and the incidence of tooth loss in postmenopausal women. *J Periodontol.* 2005;76:1123-1128.
[42] Hosking D., Chilvers C. E., Christiansen C., Ravn P., Wasnich R., Ross P. et al. Prevention of bone loss with alendronate in postmenopausal women under 60 years of age. Early Postmenopausal Intervention Cohort Study Group. *N Engl J Med.* 1998;338:485-492.
[43] Cummings S. R., Black D. M., Thompson D. E., Applegate W. B., Barrett-Connor E., Musliner T. A. et al. Effect of alendronate on risk of fracture in women with low bone density but without vertebral fractures: results from the Fracture Intervention Trial. *JAMA.* 1998;280:2077-2082.
[44] Black D. M., Cummings S. R., Karpf D. B., Cauley J. A., Thompson D. E., Nevitt M. C. et al. Randomised trial of effect of alendronate on risk of fracture in women with

existing vertebral fractures. Fracture Intervention Trial Research Group. *Lancet.* 1996;348:1535-1541.

[45] Cobb C. M. Non-surgical pocket therapy: mechanical. *Ann Periodontol.* 1996;1:443-490.

[46] Greenstein G. Periodontal response to mechanical non-surgical therapy: a review. *J Periodontol.* 1992;63:118-130.

[47] Umeda M., Takeuchi Y., Noguchi K., Huang Y., Koshy G., Ishikawa I. Effects of non-surgical periodontal therapy on the microbiota. *Perio dontol* 2000. 2004;36:98-120.

[48] Nakaya H., Osawa G., Iwasaki N., Cochran D. L., Kamoi K., Oates T. W. Effects of bisphosphonate on matrix metalloproteinase enzymes in human periodontal ligament cells. *J Periodontol.* 2000;71:1158-1166.

[49] Buduneli E., Vardar-Sengül S., Buduneli N., Atilla G., Wahlgren J., Sorsa T. Matrix metalloproteinases, tissue inhibitor of matrix metalloproteinase-1, and laminin-5 gamma2 chain immunolocalization in gingival tissue of endotoxin-induced periodontitis in rats: effects of low-dose doxycycline and alendronate. *J Periodontol.* 2007; 78:127-134.

[50] Socransky S. S., Haffajee A. D., Cugini M. A., Smith C., Kent R. L. Microbial complexes in subgingival plaque. *J Clin Periodontol.* 1998; 25:134-144.

[51] Anonymous. Management of osteoporosis in postmenopausal women: position statement of The North American Menopause Society. *Menopause.* 2010;17:25-54.

[52] Komerik N., Akkaya A., Yildiz M., Buyukkaplan U. S., Kuru L. Oral health in patients on inhaled corticosteroid treatment. *Oral Dis.* 2005; 11(5):303-8.

[53] Jacobs R., Ghyselen J., Koninckx P., van Steenberghe D. Long-term bone mass evaluation of mandible and lumbar spine in a group of women receiving hormone replacement therapy. *Eur J Oral Sci.* 1996; 104: 10-16.

[54] Taguchi A., Suei Y., Ohtsuka M., Otani K., Tanimoto K., Hollender L. G. Relationship between bone mineral density and tooth loss in elderly Japanese women. *Dentomaxillofac Radiol.* 1999;28:219-223.

[55] Takaishi Y., Okamoto Y., Ikeo T., Morii H., Takeda M., Hide K. et al. Correlations between periodontitis and loss of mandibular bone in relation to systemic bone changes in postmenopausal Japanese women. *Osteoporos Int.* 2005;16:1875-1882.

[56] Nakamoto T., Taguchi A., Ohtsuka M., Suei Y., Fujita M., Tanimoto K. et al. Dental panoramic radiograph as a tool to detect postmenopausal women with low bone mineral density: untrained general dental practitioners' diagnostic performance. *Osteo- poros Int.* 2003;14:659-664.

[57] Klemetti E., Kolmakov S., Heiskanen P., Vainio P., Lassila V. Panoramic mandibular index and bone mineral densities in postmenopausal women. *Oral Surg Oral Med Oral Pathol.* 1993;75: 774-779.

[58] Horner K., Devlin H. The relationship between mandibular bone mineral density and panoramic radiographic measurements. *J Dent.* 1998;26:337-343.

[59] Bollen A. M., Taguchi A., Hujoel P. P., Hollender L. G. Case-control study on self-reported osteoporotic fractures and mandibular cortical bone. *Oral Surg Oral Med Oral Pathol Oral Radiol Endod.* 2000;90: 518-524.

[60] Rizzoli R., Burlet N., Cahall D., Delmas P. D., Eriksen E. F., Felsenberg D. et al. Osteonecrosis of the jaw and bisphosphonate treatment for osteoporosis. *Bone.* 2008; 42:841-847.

[61] Soileau K. M. Oral post-surgical complications following the administration of bisphosphonates given for osteopenia related to malig- nancy. *J Periodontol.* 2006; 77: 738-743.

[62] Braun E., Iacono V. J. Bisphosphonates: Case report of non-surgical periodontal therapy and osteochemonecrosis. *Int J Periodontics Resto- rative Dent.* 2006;26:315-319.

[63] Diniz-Freitas M., López-Cedrún J. L., Fernández-Sanromán J., García-García A., Fernández-Feijoo J., Diz-Dios P. Oral bisphosphonate-related osteonecrosis of the jaws: Clinical characteristics of a series of 20 cases in Spain. *Med Oral Patol Oral Cir Bucal.* 2012;17:751-758.

Index

D

E

F

G

H

I

J

K

L

M

Q

R

S

T

U

V

W

X

Y

Z